MW00628319

The Handbook on Child Welfare Practice

Jennifer M. Geiger • Lisa Schelbe

The Handbook on Child Welfare Practice

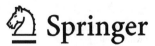 Springer

Jennifer M. Geiger
Jane Addams College of Social Work
University of Illinois Chicago
Chicago, IL, USA

Lisa Schelbe
College of Social Work
Florida State University
Tallahassee, FL, USA

ISBN 978-3-030-73911-9   ISBN 978-3-030-73912-6   (eBook)
https://doi.org/10.1007/978-3-030-73912-6

Cover image: A variety of hand prints together form a seamless tileable pattern. © Robert Kneschke / Alamy Stock Photo

This Springer imprint is published by the registered company Springer Nature Switzerland AG
The registered company address is: Gewerbestrasse 11, 6330 Cham, Switzerland

For Kate Rich, the person who drew me into child welfare practice and taught me everything I know about advocating for and supporting families to keep children safe.

This book is dedicated to all the parents and professionals who do their best every day to improve the lives of children

-JMG

I dedicate this book to Deb Daro for her visionary work and passion for the prevention of child maltreatment and to all of the people involved in the Doris Duke Fellowship for the Promotion of Child Well-Being who seek to continue Deb's legacy.

-LS

Preface

I (Jen) never planned to work in child welfare. When I worked on my Master of Social Work degree, I wanted to be a counselor. When I graduated, there was a job as a child welfare specialist with the Office of the Legal Advocate that housed attorneys who served as Guardians ad Litem. They had a unique model where attorneys and social workers worked together to do what they each did best to represent the best interest of children involved with the child welfare system. I had no idea I would love this work so much. I met countless heroes along the way—parents, foster parents, grandparents, relatives, case managers, therapists, attorneys, judges, and most importantly, the kids. I learned a lot about our broken system that was often left without the resources needed to prevent families from becoming involved with child welfare systems or to help families get back together. I also saw the hard work of many families to reunify, to complete guardianships, and create families through adoption. I was especially inspired by the youth I worked with, which ultimately led me back to school to work on a PhD. It was hard to leave the job, but I kept one foot in the field to make sure my work was meaningful. I have been fortunate to be able to continue doing work that helps us to understand how to better serve vulnerable youth and families. I have also been lucky enough to be able to teach future social workers who want to work with children and families. It takes a special person to do child welfare work. It is not an easy job and families are complex, and having to navigate multiple systems is challenging when the lives of children and families are in our hands. What I've also learned is this work is rewarding, it's emotional, and it matters.

Like Jen, my (Lisa's) journey to child welfare was not planned. When I was a doctoral student, I worked on a research project with youth who were transitioning out of foster care to understand their experiences leaving care. The first interview that I conducted was with a young woman who had recently left foster care after turning 18. Her strength and resilience inspired me; at the same time, I was horrified by how difficult her life was after leaving foster care. The system that had functioned as her parents for years largely abandoned her as she was transitioning to adulthood. It was my first real understanding of the child welfare system as it could impact children and youth, although previously I interacted with the system when I had worked in various agencies serving women who had experienced domestic violence. It was this young woman and the youth I got to know through the research project that motivated me to be part of improving the child welfare system and eliminating—or at least minimizing—the need for the system through child maltreatment prevention.

I have had the privilege of knowing and working with many who share a similar vision to end child maltreatment, many of those who I met through the Doris Duke Fellowship for the Promotion of Child Well-being. It was in the fellowship where Jen and I met and started working together. Part of the vision of ending child maltreatment is ensuring that the child welfare system functions optimally such that the children and families who are involved will be helped and both the likelihood of children's reentry into care and their children's entry into care is minimized. Educating the next generation of the child welfare workforce is central to this vision.

Over the years, we have been teaching courses in social work related to child abuse and neglect and child welfare practice and have struggled to find a recent text to use that would be comprehensive and that would be useful for undergraduates and graduate students at various levels of experience. We envisioned a textbook that could be used across states and at different institutions for instructors to add content and context around policies and practices where they are. When asked to write this text, we wholeheartedly agreed and took it on.

We are so pleased to be able to offer a textbook that we hope provides a solid foundation for what child welfare practice is, its history, and how child welfare professionals play an important role in supporting families and protecting children through prevention, reunification, and permanency. We hope that this text provides aspiring child welfare professionals with the knowledge, skills, and tools to be able to improve the lives of children and their families by understanding the policies, best practices, and hearing from some of the experts in the field. We balance the text with stories from those who have experienced them as youth, parents, professionals and from researchers and policy-makers across disciplines.

It is our hope that faculty who select this textbook will continue to use state-specific content to increase the relevance for the communities their students will likely serve. It is our desire that this textbook is useful to students and others who want to understand child welfare. We hope that this book helps those who are going to be working with children and families to ultimately help children and families and prevent child maltreatment.

Chicago, IL, USA   Jennifer M. Geiger
Tallahassee, FL, USA   Lisa Schelbe

Acknowledgments

There are so many people to acknowledge for their support, input, and guidance throughout the process of writing this book. Thank you to our editors at Springer— Jennifer Hadley at Springer who first approached us and had the confidence in us to write this much-needed textbook, and Janet Kim, for supporting us throughout this process.

We would like to thank the Doris Duke Charitable Foundation and the Doris Duke Fellowship staff, leadership, and fellows. Thank you to Deb Daro for your vision and tireless work to create this network, keeping us all together, and moving us forward. Thank you to Lee Ann Huang for keeping us going and being such a great support and cheerleader for us. The fellowship is how we met 10 years ago and we've since developed such a strong collaborative relationship with researchers, practitioners, and policy-makers working hard to prevent child maltreatment and improve the lives of children and families.

Thank you to our colleagues across the country who gave feedback and offered contributions based on their research and their own personal and professional experiences. We are so excited to highlight the important work from our friends, students, co-workers, and community partners. Thank you to Allison Kipphut and the students from her child welfare practice course at the University of Illinois Chicago who agreed to pilot the text and give us valuable feedback to improve the text. We also want to thank all of the students we've had the honor to work with through their journey into learningmoreaboutthechildwelfaresystem,childmaltreatment,andchildwelfarepractice.–

Special thanks from Jen: I am so fortunate to have an amazing partner who supports everything I do. Thank you, Mike, for valuing my work and being the amazing father you are to our kids. You keep us balanced, happy, and always know what we need. My kids make this work even more meaningful for me and put it all into context. Thanks, Z, R, and H!

Special thanks from Lisa: I want to thank my sisters and parents who are always encouraging of my work. I could not have written this book without their loving support. The daily support from my husband, Chris, made my writing possible. Thank you for all that you did to support this book, including making coffee, cooking meals, listening, offering suggestions, encouraging, and loving me.

Contents

Contributors

Leah Bartley, PhD University of North Carolina at Chapel Hill, Chapel Hill, NC, USA

Breanna M. Carpenter, LMSW, MPA Arizona State University, Phoenix, AZ, USA

Barbara H. Chaiyachati, MD, PhD Children's Hospital of Philadelphia, Philadelphia, PA, USA

Leah Cheatham, PhD, JD University of Alabama, Tuscaloosa, AL, USA

Carly B. Dierkhising, PhD California State University – Los Angeles, Los Angeles, CA, USA

Elizabet Bonilla Escobar, MSW Illinois Department of Children and Family Services, Springfield, IL, USA

Libby Fakier, MBA Atlanta, GA, USA

Lisa Garcia, MSW Waukegan, IL, USA

Justin S. Harty, MSW, LCSW University of Chicago, Chicago, IL, USA

Kris Jacober Arizona Friends of Foster Children Foundation, Phoenix, AZ, USA

Colleen Cary Katz, PhD, LCSW Hunter College, New York, NY, USA

Nicole Kim, MSSW Dallas, TX, USA

Cynthia A. Lietz, PhD, LCSW Arizona State University, Phoenix, AZ, USA

Kizzy Lopez, EdD Fresno Pacific University, Fresno, CA, USA

Brittany Mihalec-Adkins, M.S.Ed Purdue University, West Lafayette, IN, USA

Christina Mondi-Rago, PhD Brazelton Touchpoints Center, Boston, MA, USA
Harvard Medical School, Boston, MA, USA

Terry A. Solomon, PhD University of Illinois Chicago, Chicago, IL, USA

Carol Taylor, MSW, LCSW University of Illinois Chicago, Chicago, IL, USA

Tova B. Walsh, PhD, MSW University of Wisconsin-Madison, Madison, WI, USA

Ashley Wilfong, MSW Fairmont, WV, USA

About the Authors

Jennifer M. Geiger, PhD is an assistant professor at the Jane Addams College of Social Work at the University of Illinois Chicago. Her research focuses on promoting access and success for youth in care and foster care alumni in higher education settings. She also conducts research to support and promote resilience among caregivers (kin and non-relative) for children and youth in care. Dr. Geiger has co-authored 35 peer-reviewed journal articles and 6 book chapters on foster care and child maltreatment. She co-authored *Intergenerational Transmission of Child Maltreatment* and *Assessing Empathy* in 2017.

Dr. Geiger received her Master of Social Work degree in 2004 and PhD in social work in 2014 from Arizona State University (ASU) in Phoenix. Dr. Geiger was a Doris Duke Fellow for the Promotion of Child Well-being and continues to be an active member of the network. Prior to returning to work on her PhD, she worked at the Maricopa County Office of the Legal Advocate as a child welfare specialist. She worked alongside dedicated attorneys appointed to advocate for the best interests of children in foster care and ensure their social-emotional, psychological, educational, and medical needs were met.

Dr. Geiger is the principal investigator (PI) for the Cook County *Permanency Enhancement Project* (PEP), a statewide partnership with the Illinois Department of Child and Family Services, which provides technical assistance to action teams in Cook County to address issues related to racial disproportionality and disparity in the child welfare system and communities. She is the co-founder for the National Research Collaborative for Foster Alumni in Higher Education (NRC-FCA), a national research collaborative to promote access and success for youth in care and alumni in higher education. She helped develop and implement Bridging Success at Arizona State University and the Sparking Success Scholars Program, recruitment and retention programs for foster care alumni, and was Co-PI for Bridging Success Early-Start, a pre-college program for foster care alumni designed to orient new students to college life and expectations at a higher education institution.

Lisa Schelbe, PhD is an associate professor at the Florida State University College of Social Work in Tallahassee. Additionally, she is a faculty affiliate at the Florida Institute for Child Welfare. Dr. Schelbe is co-editor of the *Child Adolescent Social Work Journal* and editor of the American Professional Society on the Abuse of Children (APSAC) *Advisor* and *Alert*. Dr. Schelbe's research focuses on youth aging out of the child welfare system with a special interest in their experiences with post-secondary education and early parenting. She is a qualitative methodologist with experience working on interdisciplinary teams. Dr. Schelbe has written over 35 journal articles and co-authored *Intergenerational Transmission of Child Maltreatment*.

Dr. Schelbe earned her doctorate in social work from University of Pittsburgh in Pennsylvania where she was a Doris Duke Fellow for the Promotion of Child Well-Being. She obtained her Master of Social Work degree from the Brown School at Washington University in St. Louis, Missouri. Dr. Schelbe is a co-director of the Child Well-Being Research Network and served as co-chair of the Leadership Committee for the Doris Duke Fellowship for the Promotion of Child Well-Being. She is a member of ReSHAPING (Research on Sexual Health and Adolescent Parenting IN out-of-home environments Group), an interdisciplinary network of scholars dedicated to research on understanding needs and improving outcomes related to sexual health and parenting for youth who are homeless, trafficked, or in out-of-home environments, whether in child welfare, juvenile justice, or other systems. Dr. Schelbe is co-chair of the National Research Collaborative for Foster Alumni in Higher Education (NRC-FCA).

Chapter 1
Introduction to Child Welfare Practice

Introduction

Child maltreatment is an epidemic. Recent estimates are that approximately one-eighth of children in the United States will experience child abuse or neglect by the age of 18 (Wildeman et al., 2014); however, it is difficult to discern the true numbers and impact of child maltreatment as many incidents are not reported or investigated, and therefore not counted. According to the U.S. Department of Health and Human Services (2020), in 2018 in the United States, approximately 4.3 million reports were made to child protective services annually which involved 7.8 million children. Approximately 678,000 children were identified as experiencing child maltreatment. Three-fifth (60.8%) of the children experienced only neglect. Approximately 1.3 million children received post-response services from a child protective services agency. States reported that a total of 1770 children died in 2018 due to abuse or neglect, which translates to almost 5 children dying each day as a result of child maltreatment. Over 70% of these deaths are children under the age 3. Child fatality rates for African American children are 2.8 times greater than White children and 3.4 greater than Hispanic children. Racial disparities exist in most other statistics pertaining to child maltreatment and the child welfare system, although as will be discussed later does not necessarily mean that there are higher rates of child maltreatment.

Of the cases where maltreatment was substantiated in 2018, approximately 250,000 children were removed from their homes and placed into out-of-home placements (USDHHS, 2020). According to the Adoption and Foster Care Analysis and Reporting System annually in the United States, over 400,000 children are in foster care were in care on September 30, 2019, and over 670,000 children are served in foster care annually (USDHHS, 2020). Of children who left care in 2019, the median time in care was 15.5 months, with 22% of children spending less than 6 months in care, and 30% of children spending more than 2 years in care.

© Springer Nature Switzerland AG 2021
J. M. Geiger, L. Schelbe, *The Handbook on Child Welfare Practice*,
https://doi.org/10.1007/978-3-030-73912-6_1

Child maltreatment is costly to society. In an assessment of the economic burden of child maltreatment in the United States, researchers estimated that each child victim would incur over their lifetime $210,012 in health care, child welfare, criminal justice, special education, and productivity losses (in 2008 dollars; Fang et al., 2012). Child fatalities due to maltreatment were estimated to cost $1,272,900 per child. Considering all of these costs, it was estimated that for the child maltreatment that occurred in 2008, the lifetime costs would be almost $124 billion. A more recent study included the additional costs of disease and disability, and almost quadrupled the cost each child who is maltreated will incur over the lifetime to $830,928 (in 2015 dollars; Peterson et al., 2018). The study also increased the costs of a child fatality to over $16.6 billion per child. With these updated estimates, the economic burden of the lifetime costs of child maltreatment that occurred in 2015 was $428 billion (Peterson et al., 2018). When these recent costs of maltreatment were applied to the number of child maltreatment cases substantiated in 2018 as well as the child fatalities that occurred in the same year, the costs were approximately $592 billion (Klika et al., 2020).

Child maltreatment is a problem worldwide, with the World Health Organization (WHO, 2020) reporting that a quarter of all adults report experiencing physical abuse as a child. UNICEF, also known as the United Nations Children's Fund, works in over 190 countries to ensure child can grow up in safe environments through their advocacy for policies and children's access to services (UNICEF, 2020). Worldwide there are efforts to address child abuse and neglect. The focus of this book is in the United States and how the child welfare system seeks to help children and families before and after abuse and neglect occur.

Child Welfare Systems

The child welfare system includes an array of services seeking to keep children safe and ensure families can successfully care for their children. The services focus on promoting the goals of safety, permanency, and well-being of children. There is not a single child welfare system in the United States, rather each state and tribe has their own organization and set of policies that operate on a state level or other jurisdiction (e.g., county, district, regional). The federal government provides oversight through legislation and monitoring and supports states through funding.

Child welfare agencies are responsible for preventing child maltreatment through the provision of services, education, and support to families. Agencies receive reports of child maltreatment, often through a "hotline" mechanism, and determine if abuse or neglect is occurring. Through an assessment process, agencies determine if a family can safely care for a child. When it is not safe for a child to remain in the home, the agency oversees the child being removed from the home and placed in an out-of-home placement such as foster care or relative care. The agency's responsibilities continue after a child is removed in that the agency ensures the safety, permanency, and well-being of the child while the child is in care. Child welfare agencies continue to work with the child and family with the goal of reunification, adoption, or other permanency option with and without court oversight. Child welfare professionals are responsible for the safety, permanency, and well-being of children.

Systems' Historical Response to Child Maltreatment

Child maltreatment has occurred throughout history across multiple cultures. In ancient history, there were sometimes societal acknowledgment of children's vulnerability, although there were not consistently interventions to ensure that children were cared for. In some ancient societies, child sacrifices were sanctioned. However, across multiple cultures, children who were orphaned were adopted or cared for by other families. The Hammurabi Code, one of the oldest deciphered code of law which was in the ancient society of Mesopotamia (c.1754 BC), included information on adoption of children and the protection of orphans. There are stories of families adopting children like Moses in the book of Exodus (Exodus 2, New International Version). Historically looking at how children have been treated, it is evident that throughout history children have had limited rights and were vulnerable to abuse. In Roman Law (c. 450 BCE), children were considered property of the male head of the household.

Elizabethan Poor Laws (1601), which greatly influenced the policies in the United States, addressed the issues of poverty in England and Wales and developed a formal process by which relief was provided to the poor. While not all specifically related to child maltreatment, the Elizabethan Poor Laws are relevant in that there were guidelines that affected how children were cared for. Perhaps most notable is that the Poor Laws identified those who were considered "deserving poor" as compared to those who were the "non-deserving poor." The non-deserving poor were broadly able-bodied men perceived as capable of work and providing for themselves, including those who were perceived as "lazy" or "drunks." The deserving poor included children, the elderly, those with health problems not caused by themselves (i.e., drinking), and women. The communities would only assist those who were the deserving poor, although assistance was not guaranteed and there were certain requirements. For example, one requirement was that those needing assistance needed to meet a residency requirement, meaning they needed to be from the community. Those who came into the community who were poor and needing assistance were pushed out of the community and not assisted. Some support was available to children and families living in their home, yet some of it was only provided in residential facilities of work houses or almshouses. During this time, evidence exists that some free Black children received assistance, yet they were treated more harshly than White children.

Colonial times in the United States (c. 1600) included many of the practices of Elizabethan Poor Laws to both provide for and control those living in poverty, including children. During this time, there were no formal child protection efforts, and any interventions were sporadic. The Body of Liberties 1641 is the first child abuse law in the United States. It was only for cases of extreme abuse: "If a parent were to 'exercise an unaturall severitie towards them, such children shall have free libertie to complaine to Authoritie for redress'" (sec. 83, as cited in Myers, 2011, p. 272). Within the law, children were permitted to defend themselves against abuse. It is worthy to note that girls had fewer rights than boys and "bastard" children had no rights. Children were viewed as the property of their families (father), were seen as "little adults," and children were expected to work and help support their families.

Two centuries later in the 1800s, concerned citizens developed charitable organizations to address the needs of orphans and poor children in urban centers in the United States. To ensure children did not live in deplorable conditions and were engaged in prosocial behaviors, these organizations attempted to care for children. The focus was not entirely on children who were maltreated yet included those who were. Black children were often excluded from services that were developed for White children. Separate institutions were developed for Black children, such as the Association for the Care of Colored Children which the Society of Friends established in 1822, which cared for Black orphans (Hogan & Siu, 1988). Additionally, African American churches, extended kin networks, and African American families helping other families through aid and support assist with providing for poor and orphaned Black children, sometimes through informal adoptions (Jimenez, 2006).

Orphan trains, established in 1854 under the leadership of Charles Loring Brace, a minister from New York City, were a program to relocate orphans and poor children to the Midwest. Coinciding with the period of Western Expansion, children were placed on trains and sent to families in the Midwest who would assume the responsibility for raising the children. Loring Brace saw many orphaned and homeless children in the city and believed that poverty could be avoided by getting children off the streets and into a rural environment with families. While not without critics, this program continued until 1929 with over 250,000 children placed, despite reports that these children were being treated poorly with little oversight, were separated from their siblings, and that some children with families were taken inadvertently. Further, these Children's Aid Societies were not making efforts toward family reunification or alleviating poverty and harsh living conditions in the city.

It was not until the late nineteenth century that there were formal services in place to address child maltreatment in the United States. In 1875, the New York Society for the Prevention of Cruelty to Children (NYSPCC) was formed as the first child protection agency in the world. The story of Mary Ellen, a 10-year-old child who was severely abused by her foster parents, is credited for impetus to create NYSPCC. She is the first recorded case of child maltreatment within the United States. Within a couple of decades, there were hundreds of child protection organizations in the United States. Once again, it must be stressed that Black children were often excluded from these private charitable organizations, and specific organizations developed in response to serve the needs of Black children. Additionally, there was the practice to send Black children to institutions for delinquent children or to adult prisons, rather than receiving child protection services (Jimenez, 2006). In 1935, the federal government established the Child Welfare Service Program, Title IV-B of the Social Security Act which made grants available to states to address child maltreatment and offered payments for foster care.

Child maltreatment largely came to the attention of professionals and citizens in 1962 with the paper "The Battered-Child Syndrome" written by Dr. Henry Kempe and his colleagues. This seminal work identified child maltreatment as a serious problem. Prior to this, there was not widespread recognition of the problem of child maltreatment. Nor was there any systematic government involvement. Child protection agencies run as non-government child protection entities had previously addressed the needs of children abused and neglected; however, they lacked authority to intervene in cases of child maltreatment.

The early 1960s heralded a new era of child protection. The Social Security Act of 1962 required states to make child welfare services available statewide by 1975. This is a substantial shift to a government involving child welfare system with accountability to the federal government. The Child Abuse Prevention and Treatment Act of 1974 (CAPTA) was passed. This landmark piece of federal legislation became the cornerstone of the modern child welfare system. In it, along with a definition of maltreatment, there was a mandate for states to develop a response to the child maltreatment. In effect, it was the birth of the modern child welfare system. After the passage of CAPTA, each state had developed a child welfare system to respond to child maltreatment and ensure the safety and permanency of children. Since the formation of child welfare systems and this initial legislation, there have been efforts to improve the responses and better protect children.

Key Federal Child Welfare Policies in the United States

Starting with CAPTA, congress has passed significant federal child welfare policies which have shaped the current child welfare system. It should be noted that legislation prior to CAPTA did have implications for child well-being yet is not typically classified as child welfare legislation (e.g., Bezark, 2021). This chapter presents the most important federal legislation to child welfare practice. See Fig. 1.1 for a timeline of key child welfare policies in the United States. It is important to note that what is covered here is not exhaustive. Additionally, it is necessary to remember that child welfare agencies are state-based; thus, state-specific legislation plays a central role in child welfare.

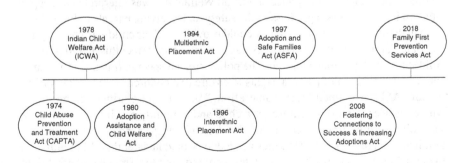

Fig. 1.1 Key child welfare policies in the United States

Adoption Assistance and Child Welfare Act of 1980

States followed CAPTA after its passage. As child welfare systems were removing children from families, it became evident that some children were languishing in care and may not have needed an out-of-home placement. The Adoption Assistance and Child Welfare Act of 1980 prioritized family preservation and permanency. It was an attempt to make sure that children were not unnecessarily removed from their families and when they were removed, there were guidelines to facilitate permanency. The Adoptions Assistance and Child Welfare Act requires child welfare agencies to make "reasonable efforts" to work with families to try to avoid unnecessarily removing children from the home through providing caregivers with resources that will ensure the child's safety and well-being in the home. When children were removed, the legislation required reviews of the status of a child in an out-of-home placement every 6 months. The courts had to determine if a child would be reunified with caregivers, adopted, or remain in foster care within 18 months of the child's placement in foster care. The legislation also required states to make adoption assistance payments for children with special needs, which is defined as children who (1) cannot be reunified with parents, (2) have a special condition that requires assistance, or (3) have not been placed without assistance.

The Adoption Assistance and Child Welfare Act created the Title IV-E program of the Social Security Act which established reimbursements from the federal government to states for foster care and adoption. Under Title IV-E, states could be reimbursed by the federal government for some of the expenditures on children who were in foster care as well as adoption assistance. Adoption assistance reimbursement was reserved for children with "special needs" as defined by individual states, which often was defined as children who may be difficult to be adopted due to their health or mental health needs, or being in a sibling group, of a certain race/ethnicity, or of a certain age. Title IV-E also developed a state-university partnership training component to professionalize the child welfare workforce.

Adoption and Safe Families Act of 1997 (ASFA)

At times, the Adoption Assistance and Child Welfare Act was interpreted as keeping children in their homes regardless of the safety and as giving parents unlimited time to change their behaviors so that they could provide for their children. The Adoption and Safe Family Act of 1997 (ASFA) was an attempt to correct this and to prioritize child safety and promote adoption. The policy created specific timelines for reunification or termination of parental rights to ensure that children were not languishing in care. ASFA redefined "reasonable efforts" and further clarified circumstances where services to prevent removal of a child and to reunify a child were not necessary. Shorter time limits were added for determining permanent placements and terminating parental rights. Hearings needed to be held no later than 12 months after the initial placement. Additionally, states were required to terminate parental rights after a child had been in foster care for 15 of the 22 months, except in cases where it was not in the best interest of the child or if the child was being cared for by a relative. Along with these timelines was the concept of concurrent planning, that in addition to working toward reunification, there could be an additional permanency goal. For example, an additional goal of adoption or guardianship that was also being planned for if the reunification failed. One of the goals of ASFA was to promote the adoption of children in foster care, and states were given incentive funds for increasing adoptions. States efforts to promote adoptions and document the process were required. In addition to focusing on safety and permanency, ASFA stresses the importance of well-being. As a policy, it sought to increase innovation and accountability within child welfare. ASFA amended Title IV-E funding.

With the passage of ASFA, there was an increase in permanency in the number of children exiting foster care. In addition to more timely reunifications, there was an increase in children who were adopted and children placed in guardianships. In the years following ASFA, the number of children adopted out of foster care doubled. There was some concern with the increased number of terminations of parental rights (TPR) due to ASFA's timelines, more children to be "legal orphans" within the system without connections to their parents, and no prospects for adoption.

Family First Prevention Services Act

The Family First Prevention Services Act (Family First) was signed into law in 2018 and is seen as a major shift in child welfare legislation. This legislation is significant as it provides states, territories, and tribes an option to use Title IV-E funding for providing evidence-based prevention services. Previously the funds could only reimburse expenses for "foster care maintenance for eligible children; administrative expenses to manage the program; and training for staff, foster parents, and certain private agency staff; adoption assistance; and kinship guardianship assistance" (NCSL, 2020). Now states, territories, and tribes can be reimbursed for prevention services after an evidence-based, trauma-informed prevention plan is developed and approved. Many states, territories, and tribes are in the process of creating such plans and identifying appropriate evidence-based programs for their jurisdictions.

The prevention services can serve children who are "candidates" for foster care, meaning they are identified in a prevention plan for being at risk of entering foster care but can safely be at home or a kinship placement as well as their families. Additionally, prevention services can be provided to foster youth who are pregnant or parenting. There are no income eligibility requirements. Services may include mental health and substance abuse treatment programs as well as in-home parenting programs. All services must be trauma-informed and be evidence based. Prevention services can be offered for no longer than 12 months, starting when a child is recognized in a prevention plan.

Family First legislation also seeks to reduce the use of congregate care and group care for children and emphasizes family foster homes. With limited exceptions, the federal government will not reimburse states for children in congregate care facilities for more than 2 weeks. The only approved setting is "qualified residential treatment programs" which provide trauma-informed care with registered or licensed professional staff. There are additional limitations on the setting including that the number of children in the placement should be no more than six and there must be formal assessments of a child within 30 days of placement to determine whether a child's needs can be met by family, a family foster home, or another setting.

Federal Child Welfare Policies Addressing Racial and Ethnic Disparities

In addition to the federal legislation broadly addressing child maltreatment, there is legislation designed to address racial and ethnic disparities and populations where system involvement is overrepresented. Before presenting the legislation, a review of racial disparities is necessary to provide context.

Racial Disparities and Disproportionalities in Child Welfare

Historically, there have been differences in how children of different races/ethnicities have been treated by child protective services, and unfortunately differences in the child welfare systems persist. Race continues to play a role in decisions and outcomes in the child welfare system (e.g., Cleveland & Quas, 2020). It must be stressed that there is no evidence that maltreatment occurs at the higher levels in different racial groups. Multiple factors have been identified including poverty, discrimination, biases, and lack of resources. Racial disparities and disproportionalities in child welfare are well documented at every decision point and part of the case (e.g., reporting, screening, investigating, assessing, removing from parents, selecting placement type, reunifying/adopting). Racial disparities mean there are unequal outcomes for different racial groups. Disproportionality is defined as unequal representation of a group compared to its percentage in the total population.

African American children and American Indian children are overrepresented in the child welfare system and consistently have found to have poorer outcomes than children of other races in the system. Approximately a quarter of children in foster care are African American, although they are only 15% of the population of children in the United States (USDHHS, 2020; Child Trends, 2018). American Indian children are in foster care at rates 2.7 greater than the general population; they are 0.9% of the child population, yet 2% of children in foster care (USDHHS, 2020; Child Trends, 2018). It must be emphasized that there is great variation within different states and communities; some systems have higher rates of disparities than others. Nevertheless, national estimates indicate that there is a problem with race and child welfare. It is documented that there are multiple decision points where individual and systematic racism impact children and families involved in the child welfare system (Miller et al., 2013).

Note from the Field

Addressing Racial Disproportionality: Child Welfare Professionals Becoming Part of the Solution

Terry A. Solomon, PhD.

The social unrest we are experiencing requires child welfare workers to reflect on their role in maintaining systems of oppression or creating systems of racial equity. The unjustified police killing of African-American men and women, the denial of medical care for COVID-19 residents of urban communities, and the history of discrimination and persistent low wages, minimum wages, and non-living wages created the perfect storm that capitulated the Black Lives Matter Protest to the world stage. As an African American, I know firsthand of the results of failed public policies resulting in under-resourced schools, substandard housing, poor health care, and economic inequality. These failed public policies have resulted in racial disparities in economic and social well-being. The consequences of the public policies have created generational wealth for the majority of the dominate society and generational poverty for many African Americans. Child welfare workers are members of both groups. Child welfare workers who are privileged want to protect their privileges, and child welfare workers who lived experiences of racial inequities continue to challenge the status quo abuse of institutional and systemic power. Are child welfare workers part of the problem or part of the solution for achieving racial equity for all families?

The social work profession "promotes social change and development, social cohesion, and the empowerment and liberation of people" (International Federation of Social Workers, 2014). It is critical for social work programs to examine how the above principles are integrated in preparing professionals, particularly child welfare workers to work in diverse communities. The racial disparities and disproportionality in child welfare outcomes for families of color require one to examine how the above-stated principles are infused in the education and training of child welfare workers. Recognizing that many of the child welfare workers do not reflect their clientele or the community where they practice, several questions come to mind. Are social work schools preparing child welfare workers to uphold the profession's value of social justice and racial equity, or are we teaching child welfare workers to maintain the status quo training on color blindness? Can child welfare workers confront their individual fears and understand how such fears negatively impact the successful reunification of African American children and all children of color? How can we overlay antiracism tenets with the profession's core values? Child welfare professionals must decide if they answer the call for justice or promote structural racism. Do we want to be part of the problem or part of the solution?

(continued)

The Black Lives Matter Protest is grounded in social work practice and social work action. Institutional and systemic racial equity offers social workers an opportunity to expand its body of work founded on the principles of protest, resistance and reform. It is a call to action for child welfare workers to examine their implicit biases about families of color and to be intentional of improving permanency outcomes for all families. For times such as this, child welfare workers cannot be part of the problem. The greater mandate is for child welfare workers to be part of the solution.

While African American children and American Indian children are overrepresented in child welfare systems, some groups are underrepresented. White children make up 50% of the population yet are only 44% of the children in foster care (USDHHS, 2020; Child Trends, 2018). Nationally, the proportion of Asian-American and Hispanic children involved in child welfare is lower than their proportion in the population. There is not a general consensus about why there is such underrepresentation; and in some geographic areas, the national trends do not match what is occurring at the state and community levels. In some states and in some communities, Hispanic children are overrepresented. As such, it is recommended that without knowing the local context, one should not assume that there are no disparities for Hispanic children.

Attempts through legislation to address the racial disparities are presented below; however, child welfare practices and protocols at the agency, team, and individual level can also play a role in reducing racial disparities and racism in child welfare. Throughout the textbook, information will be included about factors that contribute to disparities as well as child welfare professionals' responsibilities for reducing racial disparities and promoting racial equity.

Indian Children Welfare Act of 1978 (ICWA)

Soon after the enactment of CAPTA, it became readily apparent that American Indian and Alaskan Native children were disproportionally removed from their families and placed with non-American Indian families. There were grave concerns that this not only was detrimental to the individual children but also had the potential to damage the passing of culture down to the younger generations. The Indian Child Welfare Act of 1978 (ICWA) was designed "...to protect the best interest of Indian Children and to promote the stability and security of Indian tribes and families by the establishment of minimum Federal standards for the removal of Indian children and placement of such children in homes which will reflect the unique values of Indian culture, and by providing for assistance to Indian tribes in the operation of child and family service programs"(25 U.S. C. 1902; Pub. L. 95–608, § 3, Nov. 8, 1978, 92 Stat. 3069). ICWA outlined guidelines and minimum standards for states in how to handle cases of child maltreatment and adoption of native children.

Specifically, Indian children were required to be placed in foster or adoptive homes that reflected Indian culture. ICWA created tribal jurisdiction over all child custody proceedings involving an Indian child when requested by a Tribe, parent, or Indian "custodian." State and federal courts were required to honor the Tribal court decrees. The legislation provided assistance to Tribes for child and family programs and resources for the development of organizations or centers designed to improve child welfare services for Indian children and families.

ICWA is credited for progress in the handling of cases involving American Indian children; however, more work needs to be done as large disparities remain. American Indian children are two to three times more likely than White children to be removed from home and placed in foster care. American Indian children are in foster care at a rate 14 times higher than their rate in the general population. There are ongoing concerns with how ICWA is implemented. In 2016, the Bureau of Indian Affairs provided more federal guidelines about how to implement ICWA.

Note from the Field

Balancing Permanency and Honoring Tribal Sovereignty

Richard[1] was 18 months old when he was placed with a foster family when his biological mother was unable to care for him. When interviewed, his mother indicated that his biological father was a member of the Navajo Nation. The Child Welfare Agency was required to notify the Tribe and include them in all legal proceedings and to determine the child's eligibility for membership of the Navajo Nation. Richard was cared for by a White family during his time in foster care. As the case proceeded, his biological mother had been unable to meet the requirements for him to be reunited with her permanently, and the case was moving toward severance and adoption. Due to Richard's membership with the Tribe, the case was under the purview of ICWA, and the Tribe was involved in decisions made about permanency. By this time, Richard had been in the same home with the same caregivers for 3 years, and the foster parents were interested in adopting him. The Navajo Nation legal representatives were opposed to adoption as this would cease Richard's connection to the Navajo Nation and likely impact his cultural relationship to traditions and practices. As a child, Richard was entitled to permanency and stability with his family. Several attempts were made to identify a family who were Native American to adopt Richard; however, the agency was unable to find another permanent placement. After hearings and mediation, the Tribe and the Child Welfare Agency agreed that it would be in his best interest to be adopted by his current caregivers; however, they also implored his caregivers to make every effort to preserve his heritage.

---

[1] All names and other personal identifiers in cases and examples throughout this book have been changed to protect privacy and confidentiality.

Multiethnic Placement Act of 1994 (MEPA) and Interethnic Placement Act of 1996 (IEPA)

The goal of the Multiethnic Placement Act was to reduce delays in permanent placement of children, specifically with children of color. The legislation was created to address (1) the practice of children being placed in foster or adoptive parents of the same race ("race matching") and (2) the practices that created a shortage of foster and adoptive parents who were minorities. With these practices, minority children frequently languished in care. Additionally, with "race matching" children in placement with a foster parent whose race was different could be bonded with the family, and an agency would move them to a different placement that was with foster parents of the same race as the child without consideration of the attachment to the family and the best interest of the child.

The provisions of MEPA prohibit agencies from delaying or denying a foster care or adoption placement due to the parent's or child's race, color, or national origin. However, the legislation allows agencies to consider a child's culture, ethnicity, and race when determining a placement. Thus, race, color, and national origin could be one factor in a decision to place a child in a foster or adoptive home, but it could not be the only factor. As a part of MEPA, states were required to recruit diverse foster and adoptive families that reflected the demographics of children in the state. The requirements of MEPA were necessary for states receiving federal funding. The Interethnic Placement Act (IEPA) amended MEPA, clarifying language about cultural considerations. It specified that race, color, or national origin could not be used in any placement decisions. It added an exception in individual cases where it could be demonstrated that considering race, color, or national origin was in a certain child's best interest. Additionally, the legislation added fines for states which do not follow IEPA guidelines with regard to making placement decisions. It is important to note that Native American children are not covered by MEPA/IEPA, rather they are covered by the Indian Child Welfare Act.

MEPA/IEPA has not been as successful as hoped. In part, this because of there was a misconception that "race matching" was the cause of children of color remaining in care, and by removing the practice, White families would adopt the children of color who needed home. The legislation did not impact the length of time that children of color were in out-of-home placement. Some critics of MEPA/IEPA have stressed that there has been inadequate emphasis on the provisions about recruiting diverse foster and adoptive families. There is also the recognition that people of color face additional barriers when seeking to adopt a child; thus, there may be more people interested in adopting children who have been unable to do.

Goals of Child Welfare

Through legislation, the federal government has identified three goals for child welfare: safety, permanency, and well-being. Together, these goals provide a foundation for child welfare practice. The Children's Bureau, a part of the Administration for Children and Families, conducts Child and Family Services Reviews (CFSR) to review states' compliance with federal child welfare requirements, to determine how children and families engaged in child welfare services are faring, and to assist states in promoting positive outcomes for children and families. The CFSRs focus on the goals of safety, permanency, and well-being.

> The Children's Bureau conducts Child and Family Services Review (CFSR) using the following definitions:
>
> **Safety:** All children have the right to live in an environment free from abuse and neglect.
> **Permanency:** Children need a family and a permanent place to call home.
> **Child and Family Well-Being:** Children deserve nurturing environments in which their physical, emotional, educational, and social needs are met.

Safety

The goal of safety is to have children not abused or neglected and, as possible, to keep them safe in their home. A child is safe when there is no threat of danger, or if there is a threat of danger, there are sufficient safeguards in place to mitigate the threat and protect the child. When considering if the goal of safety is met, child welfare practice considers the response of the child protection services agency in responding to the report, assessing the family, and providing services.

Permanency

The goal of permanency is for every child in an out-of-home placement to have a legally permanent family through reunification, adoption, guardianship, or another planned permanent living arrangement (APPLA). Child welfare agencies ensure permanency through a case plan that prioritizes the child returning home or to another permanent placement and not reentering the system. Placement instability, or the frequent changes among placements, challenges the permanency goal. Thus, efforts are made to ensure a child is not moved among different placements.

Well-Being

In 2012, The Children's Bureau as part of the US Department of Health and Human Services Administration on Children, Youth and Families added well-being as a goal of child welfare. The memo explained: "The Administration on Children, Youth and Families (ACYF) is focused on promoting the social and emotional well-being of children and youth who have experienced maltreatment and are receiving child welfare services. To focus on social and emotional well-being is to attend to children's behavioral, emotional and social functioning – those skills, capacities, and characteristics that enable young people to understand and navigate their world in healthy, positive ways. While it is important to consider the overall well-being of children who have experienced abuse and neglect, a focus on the social and emotional aspects of well-being can significantly improve outcomes for these children while they are receiving child welfare services and after their cases have closed." (p. 1) Well-being includes physical health and development as well as cognitive, behavioral/emotional, and social functioning. Consistently, there are concerns about assessing well-being as it is not as straightforward as safety and permanency.

Note from the Field

A First Look at Poverty

Over 20 years ago, I was an intern shadowing my supervisor during a home visit. I don't remember the family or any details about the case. However, I vividly recall a heavily stained mattress on the floor near the front door of the sparsely furnished apartment. No sheets were on the mattress, but crumpled clothes were on it piled on it. I realized that multiple people slept on this bed and used the clothes for pillows and blankets. I don't remember much else about the home, but I remember feeling sick thinking about the living conditions. It was hard to focus on the conversation my supervisor and the client were having because I was distracted thinking about the living conditions. It was my first exposure to poverty and poor living conditions within someone's home. I had a wide range of intense feelings: anger, disbelief, frustration, guilt, curiosity. Afterward, I processed the visit with my supervisor who helped me acknowledge my privileged background and sort through my feelings. I encountered other homes where the living conditions were similar, and I witnessed worse. Some of the homes were in squalor, unfit for people to live. I remember one apartment where the odors assaulted me when the front door open and I resorted to breathing through my mouth to minimize the smells that made me nauseous. I grew to understand that poverty was not always linked with poor living conditions. I also learned how some of the conditions – including the filth – were based in larger problems. After shadowing a case manager on a home visit to a youth aging out who was living in a subsidized apartment, the case manager reflected that he understood why the young man did not clean the apartment. The cost of a vacuum was great, and the apartment, including the carpet, was in poor condition before the youth moved into it. It was logical for the youth not to clean the floor considering that the apartment was completely rundown. Many of the homes that I visited had problems. I frequently heard clients complain about their "slumlords" and a litany of problems with where they lived. Landlords would not repair the properties. In some cases, health and safety were issues. Numerous homes had problems with mold which caused breathing problems for those living there. In one apartment with a broken window lock that repeatedly had been reported to a landlord, someone had been able to break into and burglarize the apartment. I learned to empathize with people living in poverty and not quickly judge the conditions. Nothing prepared me for the first time I saw poverty in a person's home. While it no longer shocks me, I continue to have the range of feelings when I see people living in poverty where their basic needs are not met. I am upset that people live in homes where conditions threaten their safety and health. I am angry that landlords do not maintain their properties. I am frustrated that families struggle and there is not enough support. I am grateful that I did not know such conditions as a child. I am hopeful that my work can help families escape poverty and children live in an environment where they can thrive.

Child Maltreatment Prevention

If all child maltreatment were prevented, child welfare professionals would be out of work. While we remain a long way from preventing all child maltreatment, the importance of prevention is increasingly recognized. This is the case in the federal legislation Family First that priorities prevention for states. Child welfare systems do not have to wait for abuse and neglect to occur to assist children and families. There is ample evidence that it is cost effective to prevent child maltreatment rather than dealing with its aftermath. A full argument and details about prevention are discussed in depth in Chap. 7; however, throughout the entire textbook, it is important to carry a prevention lens. Child welfare professionals have the obligation to work to prevent child maltreatment.

Child maltreatment is multi-faceted and consists of more than just stopping abuse and neglect occurring in the first place. While preventing maltreatment from occurring definitely is part of prevention efforts, it is also important to prevent it from re-occurring and to mitigate its harmful effects. Making sure that children who have been abused and/or neglected are safe from future maltreatment is part of child maltreatment prevention. Additionally, child maltreatment prevention efforts attempt to reduce the likelihood of poor outcomes due to maltreatment. Often this is done through various interventions. Prevention efforts, as will be discussed in Chap. 7, take place at multiple levels and may be universal, selective, or targeted.

Protective Factors

Protective factors are characteristics of individuals, families, and communities that reduce the likelihood of negative outcomes. Through a rigorous review of child maltreatment research, the Strengthening Families framework identified the following five key protective factors to reduce child maltreatment: parental resistance, social connections, knowledge of parenting and child development, concrete support in times of need, and social and emotional competence of children. Many states have adopted this framework and seek to prioritize helping all families increase these protective factors. More details about protective factors will be provided in Chap. 4.

Child Welfare Practice as a Profession

Working in child welfare provides the opportunity to help children and families. Professionals in the field have the ability to literally save lives and change the life trajectory of some of the most vulnerable people in society: children. However, the high rates of turnover suggest that not everyone who enters the child welfare field was prepared for the work. Attempts to reduce this turnover often target improved training. This book is designed to educate people about what is necessary to understand in child welfare so that they can be successful and help children and families.

Characteristics of a Child Welfare Professional

Not everyone would make a good child welfare professional. Skills can be taught as can protocols and procedures; however, some people are better suited than others to work in child welfare. The Vermont Department for Children and Families (n.d.) identifies the following characteristics of a successful child welfare work: a positive attitude and sense of humor, the ability to maintain a healthy balance between personal and professional life, the ability to work with clients and achieve positive outcomes, good communication, organization, critical thinking, problem solving, and time management skills, professional commitment to clients, resilience, flexibility, and high energy, realistic expectations about the challenges of the work, and the willingness to reflect on own work and learn from others. Many of these characteristics are consistent with social work skills, which is why some child welfare systems require degrees in social work.

Professional Responsibilities

While there may be different titles and responsibilities, child welfare professionals work with children and families to ensure children's safety, permanency, and well-being. Frontline child welfare workers are largely divided into two categories: child protection investigators (CPIs) and case managers. CPIs have the responsibility of conducting assessments in cases referred to the system to determine if a child is safe or at risk for maltreatment. Case managers work with children and families in the system in an ongoing manner. There are additional positions such as hotline personnel and supervisors that are intimately connected to cases as well as a wide range of professionals who work with families to provide services. See Chap. 2 for more information about the different types of positions and their roles within child welfare.

Mandates

There are multiple levels of mandates, policies, and procedures that child welfare professionals must follow. Federal legislation is the overarching policy under which states have specific legislation. There are also agencies policies and guidelines and protocols at the individual unit level. These mandates are all designed to protect children. Mandates outline timelines and requirements for working with children and families. Child welfare professionals must know and follow the mandates in the jurisdictions in which they work. Some states and child welfare agencies have very specific and extensive policies, forms, and procedures to follow to ensure

Note from the Field

Becoming a Child Welfare Professional

Breanna M. Carpenter, LMSW, MPA

I have become passionate about child welfare and keeping families safe and healthy. I am particularly interested in making sure that youth who transition out of foster care have positive outcomes in adulthood. This passion initially grew out of my own experience in foster care. Later, my work as a youth advocate and now professional social worker has expanded my knowledge and understanding of the challenges and the importance of the child welfare system. Decisions made in child welfare are life-defining moments for each individual child, young person, and parent. In my life, I have seen the system from many perspectives, as a youth, a volunteer advocate, and now a professional. What drives me most is a desire to better prepare professionals working in this system. I see it from all perspectives now. Too often the roles are at odds with one another. Parents are at odds with the investigators; courts are at odds with the caseworkers; and foster parents are at odds with the court. Too often people see only one perspective but miss the bigger picture. Through my transition from youth, to advocate to social worker, I have gained a great understanding of all sides of these issues. This understanding drives my passion to do more.

I exited the foster care system at 17 years old when I entered a guardianship with my grandparents. One year later, I went off to college and started my social work degree. January of my freshman year in college, Children's Action Alliance invited me to join their Youth Advisory Board, allowing me to influence state policy and practice. Through this work, I had the opportunity to testify in front of the state legislature over ten times to influence three significant bills related to a college tuition waiver, car insurance, and housing and mental health services for foster youth. My history in foster care was influential in these efforts, as it allowed me to directly use my voice informed by personal experience to influence the system. It is a privilege to use my voice on behalf of others, giving a seat to all youth involved in the child welfare system who will follow.

Although my advocacy work directly leverages my own personal history, my role as a social worker is informed not just by experience but also by theory, research, and professional knowledge and standards. My education and professional experience have created a third transition, one where I moved from a youth advocate to a child welfare professional. It is important to mention that I have been mentored by many experienced social workers, and I would not have developed into a competent professional without their guidance and wisdom. I am looking forward to growing in the field through ongoing professional experience. I look forward to my next transition – one where I can use my experience and knowledge to prepare the next generation of social workers who too are passionate about creating positive change.

consistency in reporting, documentation, and protocol for staff in accordance with the laws and practices in place. These polices are often described and reviewed during child welfare professional training and used as a reference in daily practice.

Ethics

There is no single code of ethics for child welfare professionals; however different states and child welfare systems have ethical guidelines and may have a code of ethics. The National Association of Social Workers (2013) has outlined standards for social work practice in child welfare and provides guidance for handling ethics in child welfare. The standards present expectations on topics including professional development, advocacy, collaboration, confidentiality, cultural competence, assessment, engagement, supervision, and administration. More information on ethics is provided in Chap. 12 on professional development.

Reflection
Is the child welfare profession a good fit?
To determine if someone is a good fit for a career in child welfare, they may want to ask themselves:
- Can I work in a stressful, unpredictable environment?
- Can I meet rigid deadlines?
- Do I function well in ambiguous situations?
- Do I like working with people in crisis?
- Can I handle learning about children who are hurt?
- Do I have strategies to take care of myself?

If the person finds themselves answering yes to these questions, they may be well suited for work in child welfare. Do not worry if they answered no; they still may thrive as a child welfare professional! These questions which were answered no can guide their selection of positions within child welfare as well as their professional development.

Skills in Child Welfare

The work child welfare professionals do demands a wide range of skills. This is in part due to the breadth of the positions and the high variability among cases. There are many concrete skills that child welfare professionals must possess to be success- ful in securing the safety, permanency, and well-being of children. Child welfare workers must possess oral and written communication skills so that they work with children, families, and colleagues. Listening without judgment is central to all of this. Child welfare professionals need to be able to interview, document interac- tions, and create reports. They also need to be able to talk with people, often in set- tings where there are great emotions. Child welfare professionals need to be able to work well with people and be part of a team. They need to be able to deescalate potentially volatile situations. Child welfare professionals need to be able to think quickly and be creative in their problem solving. Fortunately, the skills required in child welfare work can be taught and refined.

Empathy in Child Welfare

Child welfare professionals should use empathy within their work. Empathy is the ability to understand others' experiences while effectively regulating one's emo- tions and maintaining health boundaries and self-other awareness (Gerdes et al., 2010). Empathy is a physiological, emotional, and cognitive process that involves understanding of others' experiences, thoughts, and feelings.

Empathy is a critical skill for child welfare professionals working with children and families who may have very different beliefs and experiences than they do. These differences can lead to misunderstanding and mistreatment and potentially impact case outcomes. This trait and skill is discussed in more depth in Chap. 6 as it relates to developing rapport and relationships with children and families. It is important to understand empathy and its components to better understand the pro- cess of empathy. Empathy is part of our human biology and social interactions. It is a complex process that involves physiological responses, cognitive processes, and behaviors (Segal et al., 2017). Researchers have identified five components that together contribute to the full scope of empathy: affective response, self-other awareness, perspective-taking, affective mentalizing, and emotion regulation.

The brain includes neurological pathways that are capable of physiologically simulating the experiences of others. Often referred to as "mirroring," this ability is unconscious, automatic, and involuntary. For example, if a person starts crying in front of us, even if we do not understand why, we too may feel like crying – not because we are sad, but because we are mirroring what the other person is doing behaviorally. *Affective sharing* can run through all types of emptions (e.g., happy, sad) as well as physical sensations (e.g., feeling pain when watching another person being physically hurt).

Once the affective response occurs, individuals need to recognize the difference between the experiences of another person from our own or have a *self-other aware- ness*. We may feel like crying (as in the example above), but it is the other person's experience and not our own, and it is important to recognize this difference in experience. By acknowledging that the emotions are different moves the empathic response into a cognitive, conscious place.

Assuming that one successfully mirrors and then processes the affective response to understand that it belongs to the other person, it becomes possible to cognitively process what it might be like to personally experience the experiences of another or perspective-take. This is what we commonly refer to as "stepping into the shoes of another." Further, affective mentalizing is the process of cognitively weighing someone else's emotional response or state. We assess others' emotional states through their facial expressions, body language, and/or words. Finally, emotion regulation helps us to move through these affective and cognitive processes without becoming overwhelmed or swept up into someone else's emotions. This is the ability to sense another's feelings without becoming overwhelmed by the intensity of their experience. Understanding empathy and how it is manifested, particularly in a client-professional relationship, is critical to relationship development and maintenance and ensuring the client has adequate support and services. Without empathy, workers may become frustrated with the children and parents they work with when they don't fully understand where a family is coming from, what has led them to their current situation, or what feelings and thoughts surrounding their circumstances (Mullins, 2011). Further, burnout is common given the everyday professional stressors child welfare professionals are exposed to. However, empathy has been shown to be a buffer in some cases for burnout among social workers, possibly because of one's ability to regulate emotions, see the self apart from another, and perspective-taking (Wagaman et al., 2015).

Understanding Trauma

Child welfare professionals serve children (and families) who have experienced trauma. A traumatic event is one that is dangerous and frightening and that poses a threat to a person's life or body. Traumas frequently experienced by children who come to the attention of child protection services include maltreatment, neglect, sudden loss of a loved one, removal from their families, family violence, community violence, illnesses, serious accidents, poverty, homelessness, or exposure to someone with a substance use disorder.

Someone who experiences trauma can have a wide range of responses as they process the trauma. A person's response can depend on various factors including

Practice Highlight
Using Empathy in Child Welfare Work with Biological Parents
Empathy is a critical skill in child welfare practice; however, many overlook the importance of using empathy when working with biological parents.

Child welfare professionals may have negative perceptions of parents involved in the child welfare system, which may be reflected in value judgments in their practice. The parents' perception of the child welfare professional's lack of understanding and ability to empathize with their circumstances can impact service implementation and the success of family interventions.

severity, exposure, chronicity, reactions of others, developmental stage, incidence of multiple traumatic events, and previous experiences. Children's physical, emotional, social, and cognitive development can be impacted by trauma. Their reactions may include depression, anxiousness, behavior changes (e.g., sleeping, eating), physical complaints, issues related to school performance, social relationships, withdrawal or isolation, and/or risky behaviors (e.g., substance use or sexual).

A trauma-informed approach in child welfare is based on the premise that to be able to work with children and families, there is an acknowledgment of trauma(s) and an understanding of how the trauma(s) influence behaviors and thinking. For example, a child who has been removed from her parents because of being sexually abused by her mother's paramour may scream and curse at the group home staff the first day when told it is time to go to school. Without a trauma-informed approach, she could be labeled "noncompliant" and as "acting out." Taking trauma into account, her behaviors can be reframed as reactions to the trauma of the abuse and removal from her home. Rather than describing her as a "bad child," it is possible to see that things were done to her outside of her control and she is reacting to the traumas. It is central that child welfare professionals understand trauma and a trauma-informed approach. Chapter 5 explores trauma and using a trauma-informed approach in depth as it relates to child maltreatment and child welfare.

> Through empathy, child welfare professionals can enhance their relationship while encouraging parent participation in services and ultimately promoting family reunification. There are several ways child welfare professionals can use empathy as a key skill in supporting biological parents. Child welfare professionals should make an effort to acknowledge the parent's emotional response, their feelings about having to be separated from their child, and show understanding of the associated challenges of being involved with the child welfare system. Child welfare professionals can try to better understand the various experiences the parent has had that have led them to their current system involvement and recognize the trauma they may have experienced. Finally, the child welfare professional should ensure they are able to separate their own emotions from those of the parent, acknowledging that they understand those feelings but that they are separate from their own. This will help protect them from overidentification of emotions that may lead to burnout.

Managing Bias and Navigating Professional Identity

Racial and ethnic disparities are well documented within child welfare. Professionals working in child welfare settings must be cognizant of their potential role in perpetuating the inequalities and disparities through biased decision making. Broadly, child welfare professionals must be aware of their biases and how they impact their work with children and families. Biases extend beyond race and ethnicity; other biases may include beliefs about a wide range of other characteristics such as age, family structure, marital status, nationality, gender, sexual orientation, and religion. Personal beliefs and biases can impact practice if they are unchecked. A starting place in ensuring biases do not negatively impact child welfare practice is for workers to understand their personal beliefs and identify where they could be biased. Ensuring that workers continue to check their biases at every interaction and reflect on their thoughts and behaviors also helps improve practices. As one develops into a child welfare professional and gains more experience, one will also learn more about the self, beliefs, and how they might play a role in interactions with children and families. Being honest, reflective, and acknowledging bias, along with a genuine effort to make changes, is a good starting point.

Note from the Field

Changing the System to Improve Outcomes
Nicole Kim, MSSW

After graduating from college, I took a gap year and became licensed as a foster mother. The sound of children crying while they were removed from their families and placed into my arms will stay with me forever. Every removal, no matter the circumstance, was a traumatic experience of loss for the child. In one instance, a mother had attempted to take formula from a grocery store when her WIC balance was depleted. As a result, her child was placed with me. Poverty led to this child's entrance into the child welfare system – and he was not the only one. I cared for children who would save chicken nuggets in their pockets in case we ran out of food. I bathed babies who arrived covered in dried up milk and grime because their families did not have access to clean water and toiletries. I picked sleeping toddlers up from floors because they never had a bed before and were unused to sleeping in one. After fostering 28 children, I knew that I wanted to do whatever I could to strengthen families and address the systemic and structural inequalities that bring too many families into care.

After my time as a foster mother, I became a caseworker. I was often in the field visiting homes, prisons, and hospitals and advocating for children and parents at court hearings. I worked with a young mother who had aged out of foster care, had been abused in care, and did not receive attention from caseworkers until she burned down her foster home. By then, she was pregnant with her child. Soon after giving birth, her child was removed from her care due to her unmet mental health needs and homelessness, which were out of her control. Her story was one that I would see repeated too many times in the lives of the parents I served.

As both a foster parent and caseworker, I wondered – what policies, programs, and financing innovations are needed to prevent system involvement in the first place and to improve the system for those currently involved? What could be done to better train staff and to better support families? My experience inspired me to dedicate my career to the reform of the child welfare system and to find solutions to improve the well-being of the children and families it serves.

Outline of the Book

This text is divided into 12 chapters that are described below. Within each chapter, there is information based on the latest research available. Additionally, there are sidebars that include case studies and experiences from the field. These are included to provide real-life examples of what child welfare professionals experience. Additionally, key information and definitions are highlighted in sidebars. At the conclusion of each chapter is a section to assess understanding and a list of additional resources. Through answering these questions, readers can apply what they learned in the chapters and demonstrate understanding of the material.

Chapter 2 describes how the child welfare system works and the various steps throughout the life of a case in child welfare, including intake, investigations, placement, and adoption. It includes information about various roles within child protection, how to navigate the system, and who some of the key players are in the child welfare system. The chapter explores the importance of working in teams both within child welfare and across systems. It also provides an overview of preparing for and testifying in court.

Chapter 3 focuses on introducing information about normative physical, social-emotional, and cognitive development as well as how this development is interrupted and altered as a result of trauma associated with child maltreatment. The chapter outlines several domains of normative development and behavior as it relates to a child's physical and social environment and key caregiver responsibilities and nurturing. The chapter describes the family life cycle, attachment and bonding, and relationships and describes the research regarding promoting child and adolescent well-being. The chapter also presents parenting styles, discipline, and what the research concludes about healthy and unhealthy parenting and its short-term and long-term implications.

Chapter 4 provides in-depth descriptions of the different types of child abuse and neglect: physical abuse, sexual abuse, psychological and emotional abuse, and neglect (physical, educational, emotional, and medical). In addition, it describes what is known about the short-term and long-term consequences of each type of maltreatment. The chapter discusses how these various types of abuse and neglect can be assessed in various contexts using specific tools and knowledge. Information about important cultural considerations in the identification and assessment of various types of child maltreatment is also included.

Chapter 5 describes trauma-informed practice broadly and applies this framework to child welfare practice. It will present how trauma is defined, how it impacts one's development, and how we can use a trauma-informed approach to reducing the impact of trauma on development and child and adult functioning. The chapter provides information about what is known in the research about adverse childhood experiences (ACEs) and how pervasive and diverse trauma experiences can be. The chapter also presents information about what is known about trauma-informed approaches to prevention and treatment of experiences of child maltreatment.

Chapter 6 discusses the importance of child and family engagement in child welfare practice as well as describes key skills in engaging and interviewing the various parties involved at various stages of a case. Effective strategies for developing and maintaining appropriate and culturally grounded relationships with children and their families are discussed, as well as ways to work with parents/guardians to provide, monitor, and support services. The chapter also discusses various models for engaging families such as Family Group Decision Making (FGDM), Parent Cafes, and Child and Family Teams (CFTs) and how to work closely with various professionals, family, and caregivers involved with the case (e.g., school personnel, medical and behavioral health professionals, and law enforcement). The chapter highlights strategies for working with families who experience mental health challenges and substance abuse and other issues as they relate to child welfare system involvement.

Chapter 7 discusses the importance of child maltreatment prevention in child welfare practice. The chapter outlines several prevention strategies, including evidence-based individual, family, and community-level approaches to preventing maltreatment, the reoccurrence of child maltreatment, and the preservation of families through treatment and provision of services and support. This chapter discusses family preservation models and approaches used by child welfare systems across the United States as well as their goals and what is known about outcomes. Information about the role of the child welfare professional in prevention and family preservation service delivery is also included.

Chapter 8 provides concrete skills needed for assessment and intake in child welfare practice. The chapter explores the various ways safety and risk are assessed by the type of abuse and in different contexts. The chapter documents the assessment tools used by practitioners, such as actuarial- and clinical-based approaches as well as the advantages and disadvantages of each and how they inform decision-making. The chapter also discusses new ways states and child welfare agencies are identifying families in need of services (i.e., predictive analytics). The chapter describes how to conduct family and home assessments and assessing for child and family needs and strengths. The chapter outlines documentation procedures and how to write effective case notes.

Chapter 9 provides a description of the various types of placement options (e.g., relative/kinship, nonrelative family placement, in-home, congregate care, etc.) and the frequency and trends related to placement. The chapter discusses policies that inform placement options and decision making. The chapter describes child removal and placement process. This chapter also presents the importance of placement in least restrictive environments, with siblings, with family/kin, culturally appropriate settings, and in homes closest to a child's neighborhood and school. It provides research about placement stability and strategies for finding and promoting the best placements based on the child's needs. It describes the process of recruiting, training, and licensing foster parents.

Chapter 10 outlines policies and procedures related to permanency options for children and families. The chapter outlines the types of permanency outcomes and ways to identify permanency goals alongside family members and professionals to ensure timely permanence. The chapter discusses service planning to meet permanency goals as well as establishing concurrent permanency plans and the importance of family reunification. The chapter discusses meeting service goals, rates of permanency, and foster care reentry.

Chapter 11 describes how to work with special populations involved with the child welfare system (e.g., youth in care; children with disabilities; lesbian, gay, bisexual, transgender, or queer/questioning [LGBTQ] youth; immigrant or refugee children) to ensure professionals work collaboratively alongside them to ensure their voice is heard and that as practitioners, child welfare professionals are providing optimal services to ensure child and family well-being. The chapter also discusses best practices when working with siblings and youth experiencing human and sex trafficking.

Chapter 12 discusses the importance of clinical supervision in child welfare practice and highlights ways that supervisors and child welfare workers and other professionals can best structure and benefit from clinical supervision. It describes effective models of strengths-based supervision and how to enhance supervision interactions and its impact on family-centered practice and other child welfare practice outcomes. The chapter also outlines strategies and planning in professional development for child welfare professionals, including various issues related to promoting self-care, professional development (education and training), legal and ethical issues, licensing, and ensuring child welfare practitioner safety at home and on the job. The chapter discusses issues related to longevity, burnout and secondary traumatic stress, job satisfaction, retention, and professional goals and what the research says about promoting healthy personal and professional practices for child welfare professionals.

Conclusion

Child maltreatment continues to be a major social problem today. Child welfare agencies seek to address all types of child maltreatment. They do so by following the framework provided by federal legislation. The modern child welfare system's goal is to ensure safety, permanency, and well-being for children. Child welfare professionals in various capacities seek to meet these ideals. Regardless of their specific job responsibilities, child welfare professionals need to be able to engage children and families. This can best be done through using empathy in their work and managing their biases. The work of child welfare professionals is important as it directly can save children's lives and offer them a better future.

Acknowledgments The authors thank Breanna M. Carpenter, LMSW, MPA; Nicole Kim, MSSW; and Terry A. Solomon, PhD, for their contributions to Chap. 1.

Discussion Questions

1. Why is child maltreatment considered a major public health concern?
2. What are the economic impacts of child maltreatment?
3. How has society's view of child maltreatment and child welfare changed in the last century?
4. What are the reasons for racial disparities and disproportionality in child welfare?
5. What are the three goals of child welfare? How are they related and how are they different?

Suggested Activities

1. Read the *Miami Herald*'s investigative report "Innocents Lost" about how child welfare policies can impact child maltreatment: https://media.miamiherald.com/static/media/projects/2014/innocents-lost/
2. Visit the University of Minnesota's Center for Advanced Studies in Child Welfare (https://cascw.umn.edu/) and view video: "Child Protection Work in Minnesota: A Realistic Job Preview" and read other resources around professional development as a child welfare worker. Write a reflection about how you see yourself in a child welfare role. Ask yourself about how your experiences, interests, and training have prepared you for this role. Explore what role you would like to serve in child welfare and what you may need to do to get there.
3. Go online to see if your state has a child fatalities dashboard. For example, see South Carolina's: http://reports.dss.sc.gov/SSRSReportServer/Pages/ReportViewer.aspx?%2fChild+Fatalities
   Look at the child deaths in the state and identify trends for the state you live in (i.e., age of children, causes of death, circumstances, etc.)
4. Access the Kempe et al. (1962) article from your institution's library. Consider ways that it is relevant today and ways that it may be outdated. Discuss with a peer, professor, or field instructor.
   Kempe, C. H., Silverman, F. N., Steele, B. F., Droegemueller, W., & Silver, H. K. (1962). The battered-child syndrome. *Journal of American Medical Association*, *181*(1), 17–24. Available: https://www.kempe.org/wp-content/uploads/2015/01/The_Battered_Child_Syndrome.pdf
5. Read Klika, et al. (2020). Identify the amount of money that your state is spending on child maltreatment. Write an essay your thoughts about how much money is being spent.
   Klika, J. B., Rosenzweig, J., & Merrick, M. (2020). Economic Burden of Known Cases of Child Maltreatment from 2018 in Each State. *Child and Adolescent Social Work Journal*, 37(3), 227–234. (Available: https://rdcu.be/cbo5D).

Additional Resources

American Professional Society on the Abuse of Children: https://www.apsac.org/
Child Welfare Information Gateway. (2018). *What is child welfare? A guide for educators*. Washington, DC: U.S. Department of Health and Human Services, Children's Bureau. https://www.childwelfare.gov/pubs/cw-educators/

Child Welfare Information Gateway. (2013). *How the child welfare system works.* Washington, DC: U.S. Department of Health and Human Services, Children's Bureau. https://www.childwelfare.gov/pubs/factsheets/cpswork/

Child Welfare Information Gateway. (2013). *Understanding child welfare and the courts.* Washington, DC: U.S. Department of Health and Human Services, Children's Bureau. https://www.childwelfare.gov/pubPDFs/cwandcourts.pdf

Child Welfare Information Gateway. (2019). *Major Federal legislation concerned with child protection, child welfare, and adoption.* Washington, DC: U.S. Department of Health and Human Services, Children's Bureau. https://www.childwelfare.gov/pubs/otherpubs/majorfedlegis/

National Association of Social Workers, Standards for Social Work Practice in Child Welfare. https://www.socialworkers.org/LinkClick.aspx?fileticket=zV1G_96nWoI%3D&portalid=0

Child Welfare Information Gateway, Multidisciplinary Teams: https://www.childwelfare.gov/topics/responding/iia/investigation/multidisciplinary/

Child Welfare Information Gateway, Child and Family Well-being: https://www.childwelfare.gov/topics/systemwide/well-being/

Child's Bureau (2014). Integrating safety, permanency and well-being series. https://www.acf.hhs.gov/cb/resource/well-being-series

Child and Family Services Review, CFSR Information Portal. https://www.cfsrportal.acf.hhs.gov/

Children's Bureau, Child & Family Services (CFSRs). https://www.acf.hhs.gov/cb/monitoring/child-family-services-reviews

References

Bezark, M. (2021). 'Our arithmetic was unique': The Sheppard-Towner Act and the constraints of federalism on data collection before the new deal. *Journal of Policy History, 33*(2), 183–204.

Child Trends. (2018). *Racial and ethnic composition of the child population.* https://www.childtrends.org/indicators/racial-and-ethnic-composition-of-the-child-population

Cleveland, K. C., & Quas, J. A. (2020). Juvenile dependency court: The role of race in decisions, outcomes, and participant experiences. In M. C. Stevenson, B. L. Bottoms, & K. C. Burke (Eds.), *The legacy of race for children: Psychology, public policy and law* (pp. 71–90). Oxford University Press.

Fang, X., Brown, D. S., Florence, C. S., & Mercy, J. A. (2012). The economic burden of child maltreatment in the United States and implications for prevention. *Child Abuse & Neglect, 36*(2), 156–165. https://doi.org/10.1016/j.chiabu.2011.10.006

Gerdes, K. E., Segal, E. A., & Lietz, C. A. (2010). Conceptualising and measuring empathy. *British Journal of Social Work, 40*(7), 2326–2343. https://doi.org/10.1093/bjsw/bcq048

Hogan, P. T., & Siu, S. F. (1988). Minority children and the child welfare system: An historical perspective. *Social Work, 33*(6), 493–498. https://doi.org/10.1093/sw/33.6.493

International Federation of Social Workers. (2014). *Global definition of social work.* https://www.ifsw.org/what-is-social-work/global-definition-of-social-work/

Jimenez, J. (2006). The history of child protection in the African American community: Implications for current child welfare policies. *Children and Youth Services Review, 28*(8), 888–905. https://doi.org/10.1016/j.childyouth.2005.10.004

Kempe, C. H., Silverman, F. N., Steele, B. F., Droegemueller, W., & Silver, H. K. (1962). The battered-child syndrome. *Journal of American Medical Association, 181*(1), 17–24. https://doi.org/10.1001/jama.1962.03050270019004

Klika, J. B., Rosenzweig, J., & Merrick, M. (2020). Economic burden of known cases of child maltreatment from 2018 in each state. *Child and Adolescent Social Work Journal, 37*(3), 227–234. https://doi.org/10.1007/s10560-020-00665-5

Miller, K. M., Cahn, K., Anderson-Nathe, B., Cause, A. G., & Bender, R. (2013). Individual and systemic/structural bias in child welfare decision making: Implications for children and families of color. *Children and Youth Services Review, 35*(9), 1634–1642. https://doi.org/10.1016/j.childyouth.2013.07.002

Mullins, J. L. (2011). A framework for cultivating and increasing child welfare workers' empathy toward parents. *Journal of Social Service Research, 37*(3), 242–253. https://doi.org/10.1080/01488376.2011.564030

Myers, J. E. B. (2011). A short history of child protection in the United States. In J. E. B. Myers (Ed.), *In the APSAC handbook on child maltreatment* (3rd ed.). Sage.

National Association of Social Workers. (2013). *NASW standards for social work practice in child welfare.* https://www.socialworkers.org/LinkClick.aspx?fileticket=zV1G_96nWoI%3d&portalid=0

National Conference of State Legislatures. (2020). *Family First Prevention and Services Act.* Retrieved from: https://www.ncsl.org/research/human-services/family-first-prevention-services-act-ffpsa.aspx

Peterson, C., Florence, C., & Klevens, J. (2018). The economic burden of child maltreatment in the United States, 2015. *Child Abuse & Neglect, 86*, 178–183. https://doi.org/10.1016/j.chiabu.2018.09.018

Segal, E. A., Gerdes, K. E., Lietz, C. A., Wagaman, M. A., & Geiger, J. M. (2017). *Assessing empathy.* University Press. https://doi.org/10.7312/kehr18115

UNICEF. (2020). *What we do.* https://www.unicef.org/what-we-do

U.S. Department of Health & Human Services. (2020). *The AFSCARS report.* https://www.acf.hhs.gov/sites/default/files/cb/afcarsreport27.pdf

Vermont Department for Children and Families. (n.d.). https://dcf.vermont.gov/fsd/career/characteristics

Wagaman, M. A., Geiger, J. M., Shockley, C., & Segal, E. A. (2015). The role of empathy in burnout, compassion satisfaction, and secondary traumatic stress among social workers. *Social Work, 60*(3), 201–209. https://doi.org/10.1093/sw/swv014

Wildeman, C., Emanuel, N., Leventhal, J. M., Putnam-Hornstein, E., Waldfogel, J., & Lee, H. (2014). The prevalence of confirmed maltreatment among US children, 2004 to 2011. *JAMA Pediatrics, 168*(8), 706–713. https://doi.org/10.1001/jamapediatrics.2014.410

World Health Organization. (2020). *Child maltreatment.* https://www.who.int/news-room/fact-sheets/detail/child-maltreatment

Chapter 2
How the Child Welfare System Works

Introduction

The child welfare system is simultaneously a simple and complex system. At the core, the system seeks to ensure the safety, permanency, and well-being of children. A child and family often enter the child welfare system when someone makes a report to child protective services about concerns about abuse or neglect. This begins a case in the system, which will follow a prescribed route based on assessments of risk and safety. There are different child welfare professionals who will be involved across the life of a case. These professionals work with other professional partners (e.g., law enforcement, mental health or substance abuse counselors, healthcare professionals) to best serve the child and family. The courts oversee cases and ensure that children's and parents' rights are protected.

Current Child Welfare System Description

There is a wide variety of ways child welfare systems are set up in the United States. At the most foundational level, there are child protective investigators and dependency case managers (also called ongoing case managers, foster care case managers, and permanency workers). Together, the child protection investigators and case managers are considered "frontline" workers. They are the ones interacting with children and families daily.

A child welfare agency becomes involved with a child and family because they are alerted through a report. This can be done through the hotline or an online reporting system. A concerned person, perhaps a teacher, nurse, neighbor, or family member, reports concerns about the safety of a child. In some cases, the caregiver may also contact a child welfare agency requesting assistance. The report includes basic information about the child and caregivers as well as the situation. At this

© Springer Nature Switzerland AG 2021
J. M. Geiger, L. Schelbe, *The Handbook on Child Welfare Practice*,
https://doi.org/10.1007/978-3-030-73912-6_2

point, the report may be "screened in" if there is enough information to investigate and the definitions of maltreatment have been met. Figure 2.1 explores how cases progress.

Child protection investigators are assigned cases that are "screened in" by the hotline. As their title suggests, they investigate the allegations of maltreatment. They interview the relevant people and assess the home environment. Along with their team and the courts, they make a determination of children's safety and of the substantiation of the report of maltreatment. After the determination of maltreatment has been determined, cases are assigned to dependency case managers, and the child protection investigator's role is complete. Dependency case managers work with children and families to work toward the case plan goals.

While cases are assigned to specific workers, a child welfare professional does not work in isolation. There is a team with a hierarchical structure that is in place to ensure the best decisions are made and multiple people sign off on cases. Supervisors review cases. Many child welfare agencies use a multidisciplinary team, sometimes called Child Protection Teams, to assess cases and conduct further investigation. These multidisciplinary teams are typically medically directed and work closely with law enforcement and the child welfare agency for assessment of maltreatment and psychological and medical evaluations. Members of the team conduct forensic interviews and as necessary provide expert court testimony. Multidisciplinary teams play a large role in providing perspectives from various experts, using a trauma-informed approach to court involvement, and improving outcomes (Bruns et al., 2012; Ezell et al., 2018; Herbert & Bromfield, 2019; Zinn & Orlebeke, 2017). Despite the benefits of across system collaboration among child welfare and the juvenile court, there is often a disconnect with values, purpose, and process (Ellett & Steib, 2005).

Special court processes and units have also been created to address specialized cases involving substance abuse (e.g., family drug court) and young children (e.g., Safe Baby Court Team). These specialized programs have been shown to be effective in improving permanency outcomes (i.e., reunification) and accessing services for children and caregivers (Bruns et al., 2012; Chuang et al, 2012).

With the knowledge that infants and young children are more vulnerable to child maltreatment and what is known about this age being an important period for development, variations of "Baby Court" have been implemented in states and jurisdictions across the United States. The approach typically uses one that minimizes trauma for parents and children by enhancing collaboration in the courts, child welfare, and community settings to reduce time in care and maximizing success in reunification and permanency (Casanueva et al., 2019; Zero to Three, 2017). These programs provide training, leadership development, and service coordination with community partners. Studies have shown these programs to be more effective in reducing costs, time, and improving child welfare and court process outcomes (Zero to Three, 2017).

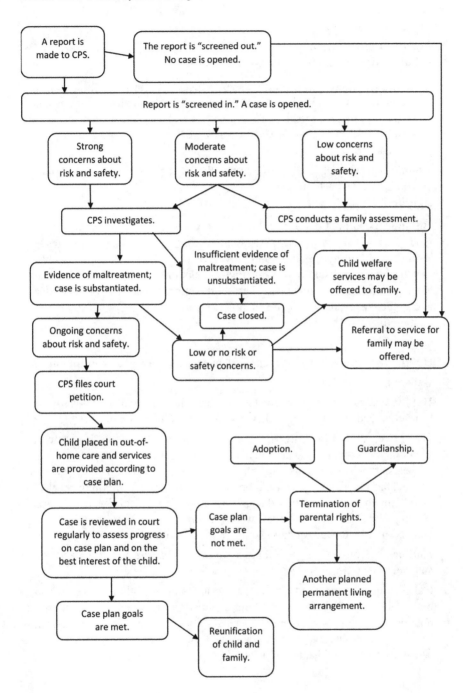

Fig. 2.1 Child protection services process

Practice Conversation
A Call to the Child Abuse and Neglect Hotline

As discussed, there are several reasons someone might call the hotline to report child abuse and neglect. Many of these reports come from teachers and other school officials, medical professional, neighbors, family members, and sometimes strangers. Here is an example an excerpt of a report made by a child's teacher.[1]

Hotline Operator: Thank you for calling the child abuse and neglect hotline, do you have a report to make?

Caller: Yes, I do.

Hotline Operator: First, I would like to tell you that you may remain anonymous on this call, however, it is important for you to ensure you honestly respond to all of my questions and provide as much information as possible. If you choose to disclose your identity or relationship with the child, your identity will remain confidential. The child welfare agency has protocol that allows them to evaluate this information to make a determination about investigating the report further.

Caller: OK.

Hotline Operator: Can you tell me first, in what capacity you know the child?

Caller: I am his teacher.

Hotline Operator: OK. Can you tell me about the child and what you saw or heard that leads you to believe there has been possible abuse or neglect?

Caller: Yes. Juwan is in my 2nd grade class. He is 8 years old. He came to school today with bruising around his wrists and upper arm. He was wearing a sweatshirt when he arrived to school, but took it off with a t-shirt underneath. That is when I noticed the bruising and at our mid-morning break, I asked him about what happened to cause the bruising. He told me that he was playing with his sister and they were making too much noise. His father grabbed him by the arm and dragged him to his room while he yelled at him.

Hotline Operator: Can you tell me more about what the bruises looked like and where they were located?

Caller: I noticed mostly dark red bruises on his upper right arm and around both of his wrists. When I asked him about what happened, at first he said nothing was wrong, that nothing happened. When I told him I was concerned, he started to cry and told me what happened. He said his father yells a lot and he is afraid what will happen if he tells.

---

[1] All names and other personal identifiers in cases and examples throughout this book have been changed to protect privacy and confidentiality.

> **Hotline Operator:** Can you tell me a bit more about the family – who lives in the home, about other children?
>
> **Caller:** The child lives with both of his parents and 2 younger siblings, ages 6 and 2.
>
> **Hotline Operator:** OK, thank you. We will follow up with additional questions as the investigator is assigned to the case. Before we get off the phone, I need some more information, including your contact information...

Intake

A report to child protection services is the beginning of the process. Reports can be made to the hotline or online and include basic information about the child and family as well as the allegations of maltreatment. The report is assessed by a child welfare professional and either screened out or screened in. Cases are screened out due to having insufficient information or not meeting the criteria of maltreatment. For cases that are screened in, the next step is an investigation by a child protection investigator. After the investigation process, maltreatment can be substantiated or unsubstantiated. When the maltreatment is unsubstantiated, families can be referred to voluntary services. With a substantiated case, the investigator's assessments of risk and safety determine if the child can remain in the home to receive in-home services or if the child should be removed from the home and placed in an out-of-home placement. For children who are removed from their caregivers, there is a shelter hearing where a judge determines the course of action for the child.

Case Management

Once the investigation is over and the children become legally dependent and involved with the child welfare system, the case is transferred to a case manager who will work with the child and family with the goals of safety, permanency, and well-being. This is done through development of a case plan which outlines what parents must accomplish before the case can be closed. Case plans are individualized to the circumstances of the family, taking in children's needs. Chapter 6 describes the processes of engagement children and families and details about how child welfare professionals work with children and families. Chapter 11 discusses how child welfare professionals can best serve special populations. The courts review the progress of the case plan on a regular basis. There are timelines determined by legislation that dictate the process.

A case is closed when a child is reunified with their caregivers, which happens in a majority of cases. When reunification is not possible, parental rights may be terminated and a child can be adopted or placed in a permanent guardianship. Occasionally, children are not reunified and do not achieve permanency through adoptions or guardianships and "age out" of the system. Details about these permanency outcomes are presented in Chap. 10.

Law Enforcement Investigations

In some instances of child maltreatment, law enforcement conducts investigations. This is a separate process from the child welfare system involvement, although ideally child welfare and law enforcement professionals collaborate. Not all cases reported to child protective services are investigated by law enforcement and criminally prosecuted. A recent study estimated that just over a quarter (28%) of cases reported to child protective services were investigated by law enforcement (Cross, Chuang, Helton & Lux, 2015). Variation in investigation was great due to type of maltreatment with more than half (54%) of the cases where sexual abuse was the primary alleged maltreatment as compared to 24% physical abuse and 11% of neglect. Likewise, there were differences across agencies, ranging from some agencies having no investigations by law enforcement to others having 70% of cases investigated.

Law enforcement and child protective services have different roles. Law enforcement's role is to ensure public safety and laws are followed, while child protective services are focusing on the child and family safety and well-being. When law enforcement is involved in a case, the role is to conduct an investigation through interviewing witnesses and collecting evidence. The case may be presented to a district attorney who will determine if there will be charges brought against the caregiver. Not all child maltreatment cases are prosecuted, even when law enforcement is involved.

Sometimes child protective services and law enforcement work incredibly together. In communities where there is a children's advocacy center, there may be coordination and teamwork among these systems as well as the prosecutor and community services providers   (e.g.,   mental   health,

Practice Highlight
Child Advocacy Centers
Child advocacy centers (CACs) are programs that are community-based, child-friendly that offer multidisciplinary services for children and families affected by or at risk for child maltreatment. CACs bring together professionals and resources from various areas of expertise, including child protective services investigators, law enforcement, attorneys, and medical and mental health professionals to offer specialized, coordinated, comprehensive services and supports to children and families (Herbert & Bromfield, 2016). Child advocacy centers can deliver programs that address the needs of children who have been sexual abused and their families to reduce children's symptoms and promote their well-being (Hubel et al., 2014).

medical). Even without a children's advocacy center, some child welfare agencies and law enforcement departments work well together and create a memorandum of understanding that documents how the systems will work together on cases. Unfortunately, sometimes the two systems do not work well together due to the different perspectives and fears. Law enforcement may be concerned that child protective services could potentially destroy evidence or interfere with their ability to create a case that will get a conviction. Child protective services may worry that law enforcement may not work with the parents and children in an appropriate manner. However, when the systems work together, there can be positive outcomes, and the goal should be to have the systems work together for the common goal of helping children.

Professional Partners

The child welfare system does not operate in isolation; there are multiple professionals who interact with the child welfare system. These professions include health care, law enforcement, legal services, and education. Professionals in mental health, substance misuse, and intimate partner violence are also involved with children and families involved in the child welfare system. In Chap. 6, more detailed information about collaborative practice is presented.

Doctors play a significant role in child welfare through their determining the likelihood that maltreatment occurred. They ultimately are the ones who determine if the injury or health concern was due to maltreatment. It must be stressed that healthcare professionals have a responsibility for identifying neglect and not just abuse (Keeshin & Dubowitz, 2013). Healthcare professionals' involvement in cases is not just about determining maltreatment; they also provide assessments and ongoing treatment for children in care. As will be discussed in Chap. 4, children who experience maltreatment have high rates of problems with their health. When a child enters foster care, they should receive a health screening evaluation. If it is determined that a child needs treatment, they should receive it while they are in care. In some communities, a medical home model is used. In this best practice, a child who enters foster care will be assessed and treated by the same team of healthcare professionals throughout their entire involvement in the child welfare system (Espeleta et al., 2020). Pediatricians have the opportunity to have parenting interventions delivered in their offices, and there is evidence that this is an effective strategy (Smith et al., 2020).

Law enforcement frequently collaborates with the child welfare system. As discussed above, sometimes there are parallel cases where law enforcement conducts investigations and prosecutes case of child maltreatment. Even when this does not occur, law enforcement may still be involved in the case. A sheriff's deputy or police officer is to be present when a child welfare professional is removing a child from their parents. Also, in many jurisdictions, child welfare professionals are encouraged to have a law enforcement escort when there are concerns about safety during home visits. This could be in cases where the caregivers have a documented history of violence and access to guns. (See Chap. 12 for more information about worker safety.)

The judicial system is an integral part of child protection. Children are only removed from their parents' care with the approval of judges. While the case plans may be developed by child welfare professionals and the interactions with the children and families are with the child welfare professionals, the decisions about children's removals are determined within the courts. As will be presented in Practice Highlight: Courtroom Players to Know, there are various professionals in legal services who play a role in child welfare cases.

The education system and child welfare system have not always worked well together, but with the passage of the federal legislation Every Student Succeeds Act in 2015, it became a requirement that school districts and child welfare agencies have agreements and points of contact to facilitate collaboration and best serving children. Even before this legislation was passed and there were requirements to work together, teachers, principals, and school personnel have played important roles in child welfare as they are frequent mandated reporters. With the growing awareness of the need for the educational and child welfare systems to work together, there are more collaborations. Additionally, there are more school systems that are adopting a trauma-informed approach to education. This is happening at all levels of school. There may be a particular interest in this at the preschool level as the beginning of a child's education is tremendously important (Loomis, 2018). In early childhood education, there is interest in addressing child mental health and ensuring optimal development early in life. Early childhood education is starting may incorporate mental health experts to assist in this process (e.g., Davis et al., 2020).

Mandatory Reporting

Under CAPTA, each state is required to have mandatory reporting legislation that outlines who is required to report suspected cases of child maltreatment to the authorities. Penalties for failure to report can be fines, jail time, or both. Statutes vary by state. In a few states, legislation specifies any person who believes that a child is being abused or neglected is required to make a report. In these states, the profession of the person is not taken into consideration. Other states require any person who believes that a child is being abused or neglected is required by state law to make a report but also identifies specific professions where there is a responsibility to report. The majority of states have mandatory reporting laws that identify specific professions responsible for reporting suspected child abuse or neglect. The professions are typically those where there is high contact with children. Common professions that are identified by state legislation as mandated reporters include social workers, school personnel (e.g., teachers, principals), doctors, nurses, healthcare workers, therapists, childcare providers, and law enforcement professionals.

Mandatory reporting laws extend beyond identifying who is responsible to report suspected cases of maltreatment. Many state laws also include requirement for "institutional reporting," which applies to circumstances when a mandated reporter works or volunteers at an institution (e.g., hospital, school) where they learn of suspected child maltreatment. These institutions are responsible to have a policy when someone suspects there is maltreatment. Typically, the policy includes notifying a specific person in the institution and a report being made to child protective services. State laws also determine if mandatory reporters may make a report anonymously or if they are required to provide their name. Most states' mandatory reporting statues prohibit the reporters' name from being released to the alleged perpetrator(s); however, in some states, reporters can waive their right to confidentiality. Because some of the professions listed in states' mandatory reporting laws have "privileged communication," which are interactions that are to remain confidential and legally the professional cannot disclose what was shared with them, most states' laws specifically address privileged communication. Some states' statutes require that mandatory reporters must report child maltreatment even if it was learned of during privileged communication; other states do not have such a requirement. In these states, a mandatory reporter learns of suspected maltreatment during privileged communication is not required to file a report with child protective services.

Services

There are a wide range of services provided to children and families within the child welfare system. Referrals can be made to various types of programs including those addressing employment, housing, mental health, substance misuse, and intimate partner violence. Details about working with families where there are concerns about mental health, substance misuse, and intimate partner violence are presented in Chap. 6. Services should be tailored to the needs of the caregivers, child, or the family. Some services are optional, while others are required of a case plan. Ideally services are provided to children and families soon after the maltreatment occurred, although it must be stressed that interventions can be effective later in life. For example, there are interventions for adults who were sexual abused as children (Wilen et al., 2017), which may occur years after the child welfare system was involved or even if the child sexual abuse had never been known about soon after it occurred. Regardless of when provided, services ideally will be evidence-based. Scholars have noted that the evidence-based programs and practices continue to need to be developed as they play an important role in child maltreatment prevention (Powell, et al., 2015).

One ongoing concern in child welfare is the availability and accessibility of services that children and families need. In some communities, especially rural settings, there may not be services. This means that families have to travel lengthy distances to access a service, which can add costs in transportation and in time. The costs can sometimes become prohibitive to someone accessing services. Fortunately, there are efforts to increase offering virtual services to children who have experience maltreatment (e.g., MacLoed et al., 2009). Even if services are available within the community, there may sometimes be long waiting lists because of the demand for services and limited number of providers. Sometimes services are sometimes provided in a way that is inconsistent with the needs of the person needing services. For example, a parent may be referred to anger management classes that only meet in the evenings, but the parent's work schedule conflicts with the time the class is offered. A parent not receiving services does not always mean that the parent does not want to receive services; there may be facing real challenges.

Privatization

Several states have privatized portions of the child welfare systems such that the child welfare professionals are not state employees. Rather they are employees of a company or nonprofit. Privatization is when the state contracts with agencies to provide specific services. In some cases, this could be providing case management, licensing foster care placements, and managing group homes. Reduction in costs and the ability to adapt to local communities' needs drove the movement toward privatization. Privatization has had varying levels of success across child welfare systems. Some have been less successful than others. For example, in the state of Nebraska, after child welfare services were privatized, there was a reduction in the availability and quality of services (Hubel et al., 2013). Although the motivation for the state had been to increase efficiency and cost savings, after privatization, the states' costs of child welfare services increased by 27%, and the private agencies spent over $21 million of their own funds as they tried to fulfill their contracts with the state. There were many factors that contributed to the problems of privatization in Nebraska including that there was inadequate planning in part due to a rushed timeline and the agencies had little experience providing child welfare services and coordinating contracts of the large scale. Lessons learned from Nebraska and other states who have had various levels of success can inform states privatizing their child welfare systems. The trend of privatization is continuing.

Note from the Field

The Power of Court Appointed Special Advocates
Brittany Mihalec-Adkins, M.S.Ed.

I started volunteering as a Court Appointed Special Advocate (CASA) when I was 23 years old. I had no experience parenting and no experience as a practitioner of any kind, and I was nervous that the parents of children on my caseload would glare at me from across the table and ask me what the heck I knew about parenting or how long I had been a CASA. And they did – and honestly: fair enough. I didn't have parenting stories to share in camaraderie; I couldn't tell them that I understood the difficulties of having a baby with colic, or a toddler who won't let me sleep, or a teenager who keeps running away. All I had was the binder I was given in training, and business cards with my name and email address that parents almost never wanted.

In CASA training, you are taught that your role is to be an unbiased advocate for the best interest of the child – without consideration for what others in the case (e.g., parents, relatives, caseworkers, etc.) want or think. You are supposed to be okay with saying things people don't want to hear, with the knowledge that you are doing what is best for a child in need. On the billboards that implore passersby to volunteer with CASA, there are pictures of sad-looking children that say something like "Be my voice," and indeed, newly minted CASAs walk into their first court hearings and home visits dead-set on doing just that – myself included. But the first time I walked into a parent's home to visit the first child I had been assigned to advocate for, I had such a hard time seeing the neglected child in a vacuum portrayed on those billboards. Yes, I saw the toddler who I knew had been exposed to methamphetamine and marijuana, but I also saw her finger paintings hanging on the refrigerator, and her pictures on every wall. I saw a toybox with her name painted on it, and grapes that had been cut in half like they're supposed to be. I saw her run to mom for comfort when she bumped her knee, and I saw mom kiss the bumped knee and say "all better!". I saw a mom who loved her daughter, but who was 14 when she became a mom, and who ended up in foster care shortly after when one parent relapsed and the other went back to prison for sexually abusing his own children. I saw a mom who needed (but never got) her own CASA. I saw a mom who genuinely tried not to miss any court-mandated appointments, but who also didn't have a car or a babysitter or money for a bus pass, if it wasn't paycheck week. Did I agree with all of mom's decisions – past and present? Of course not. But did I think she was the horrible person that she was sometimes made out to be in case conferences about her missed appointments or less-than-chipper attitude? Also, of course not. I felt for this mom. I was reminded by my supervisor no fewer than ten times that I was not mom's advocate.

But it is HARD to advocate for a child without considering the needs and the potential of the families in which these children are embedded, especially when there is NO ONE advocating for a mom that is only barely too old to qualify for a CASA herself. It is hard not to wonder whether you're a terrible CASA for not wanting this toddler to be adopted by the upper-middle-class foster parents who feed her organic foods, limit screen time, and keep a tight schedule – and instead wanting to give mom a chance to learn to be a mom who keeps a schedule, serves vegetables, and calls her sponsor when she's feeling the urge to use. It is HARD to testify in court that you agree with a petition to terminate parental rights after you've seen mom weep at every monthly home visit while asking you whether you're going to "let them keep her baby forever." But I know that it would be even HARDER to leave a court hearing after advocating for a child to be returned to a home where, yes, there was a mom who loved her child, but where there were other safety concerns mom was unable or unwilling to solve.

Now in my fourth year as a CASA, I think I have figured out how to reconcile all of these feelings, and that is to be open about the empathy I have for the parents of children I advocate for – open with caseworkers, with judges, with my supervisor, and most importantly, with parents. I hug moms. I give dads my cell phone number and text them updates when I visit their children in group homes. I make time to sit down with parents before court and explain that I am not going to recommend reunification today and explain WHY. The first time I did that, I was terrified that it was going to be awkward, but it wasn't any more awkward than any other part of the process. Parents have always been grateful that I take that time with them, in a system that often doesn't tell them much about what's happening – let alone the reasons behind it. I have come to terms with the fact that it is not my job to advocate for parents, and I tell parents as much. But I also make sure they understand that my job is to advocate for their child, to want the best for their child – just like they do. The vast majority of parents have responded surprisingly well to this. Now, when my cases end – and no matter how they end – I know that I treated parents with dignity and respect, that I stood firm in my role as a child advocate without demonizing or demoralizing parents, and that even when parents don't like or agree with me, they believe that I advocated for their child to the best of my ability. And that I can live with.

Roles in Child Protection and Foster Care

There are a number of roles within child welfare practice and depending on the state and/or jurisdiction, titles may be referred to differently. They typically fall into categories based on the responsibilities they primarily fulfill. See Table 2.1 for a

Table 2.1 Child welfare position and responsibilities

Child welfare position	Responsibilities	Example
Intake/investigator	• Conducts interviews and home assessments • Prepare documents and completes forms • Testifies in preliminary and protective hearings • May remove and place child in safe setting • Makes referrals for services (child/parent) • Participates in family group decision-making team meeting	A report of a 4-year-old being left alone at home for 2 hours while mother is shopping is received by the hotline. The investigator is assigned and visits the home immediately to determine the child's safety. The investigator hears the child inside the apartment and knocks on several neighbors' doors. The next-door neighbor offers a key to the apartment where the child is alone watching television. It is unclear how long the child has been home alone. He is wearing a diaper and no clothing. The neighbor provides the investigator with a number for the mother, who returns home after 30 min. The investigator conducts a thorough assessment of the home while asking the mother and neighbors several questions. The investigator decides to leave the child with a grandparent temporarily while they continue to investigate the case. The investigator writes the report and makes several referrals for services
Intact family specialist/family preservation specialist	• Develops and monitors family case plan • Makes referrals for services • Visits child and family in home regularly • Conducts home assessments • Participates in child and family team meetings • Prepares progress report	The intact family specialist was assigned to a case where the biological mother tested positive for marijuana when she gave birth to her child in the hospital. The intact family specialist assessed the family home to determine its safety for a newborn. The mother lives with her mother, who helps her care for the child. The intact specialist made referrals for home visitation services, substance abuse counseling, and parenting support. The intact specialist visits the home every 3–4 days unannounced to make sure the home is appropriate and the newborn is being cared for. They prepare a report for the court after 6 months of child welfare involvement and service engagement
Foster care specialist	• Monitors placement, services, and overall case progress • Develops and monitors family case plan • Prepares and distributes court progress report to case parties • Attends court • Visits child in setting • Participates in child and family team meetings	Following an investigation, 12-year-old Annette was placed with relatives after it was determined it was unsafe for her to stay with her biological parents. Her father was unable to care for her due to substance abuse and her mother received a 6-month jail sentence for assaulting her boyfriend. The foster care specialist completed an assessment of her aunt's home and asks them to commit to care for Annette until her mother is able to be reunified with her daughter. Annette's mother is released from jail after serving 4 months and begins to engage in services the foster care specialist has recommended: counseling, parenting classes, and substance abuse outpatient treatment. The foster care specialist receives regular updates regarding service engagement and progress. She visits with Annette and her aunt monthly

(continued)

Table 2.1 (continued)

Child welfare position	Responsibilities	Example
Adoption/ permanency specialist	• Assesses child's short- and long-term needs • Identifies adoption placement for child • Participates in child and family team meetings • Prepares necessary paperwork for court • Submits referrals for post-adoption subsidies and services	Tyler, a 9-year-old child had been in foster care for 2 years. After many attempts, his mother was not able to be reunified with her son. The case plan changed from foster care to severance and adoption. After a brief trial, the judge ordered that Tyler be free for adoption. Once an adoption specialist was assigned, they did not have to locate an appropriate family since his current family was willing to adopt him. They had not adopted a child before; therefore, they had to become certified to adopt, which include several forms and assessments to be completed by the adoption specialist. The specialist had to determine what services Tyler and his family were receiving and which would need to continue. The adoption specialist submitted all of the paperwork for any subsidies and services they were eligible for after adoption. The adoption date was set, and Tyler was legally adopted by his parents. His birth certificate was reissued with his adoptive parents being listed as his parents and his new last name

summary of child welfare professionals' positions, responsibilities, and examples of their work. For example, child protection investigators conduct investigations following a report of child maltreatment. These individuals will conduct interviews and home assessments, prepare documents and complete forms, and prepare for court testimony as necessary. If necessary, they will also remove a child from an unsafe home and make arrangements for alternative placement. Once a case has moved past the investigations stage and a child or children have been removed, an ongoing, foster care, or placement case manager is assigned to the case. Their role is to assist with assessing for services and supports and making the necessary referrals for them to be initiated. Child welfare professionals within this role will support the placement, attend court, monitor services for parents, children, and caregivers, and complete reports necessary for monitoring case progress. Placement, ongoing, or foster care child welfare professionals work closely with the family to promote permanency and may be assigned to specialty cases based on their experience and training (e.g., older youth, children with medical needs).

For cases where children are deemed safe to stay in the home but perhaps require support services, there may be a family preservation specialist or intact case manager that will also conduct assessments and make referrals for services and supports for children and families. These professionals will often have more frequent contact with the children and families and continue to assess for safety in the home.

When it is not possible for children to return to their family of origin safely and a case plan changes and is approved by the court to proceed with adoption, the case may be transferred to an adoption specialist. This professional role includes preparing documents related to adoption, finding an adoptive family that is a good fit for the child and their needs, assisting with the transition into a new home (if different from current placement), assessing and accessing services and supports following the finalization of the adoption, and attending court for the adoption hearing.

The majority of case manager positions in child welfare require some college, a bachelor's or master's degree and some experience working with children and/or families. Many of these positions are filled by trained social workers, which are those who have a bachelor's and/or master's degree in social work from an institution that is accredited by the Council on Social Work Education (CSWE) and who follow the National Association of Social Workers (NASW)'s Code of Ethics. Others may have related degrees (e.g., psychology, sociology, family studies) or combined education and experience with families and children. Requirements vary by state and agency, and some may require additional training and experience and/or licensure. Many child welfare professionals may have participated in one of the many Title IV-E funded training programs that helps students receive the necessary training experience in child welfare practice while they are in school. Although these programs vary, many will offer courses and internships/field placements in child welfare along with a financial stipend or tuition waiver. Once they have completed their program, they go on to seek employment at the local child welfare agency for a specific set of time. In addition to case manager positions, agencies will often also employ case aides or visitation specialists who supervise visits with children and their parents/caregivers, help with transportation, and conduct home visits. Chapter 12 further discusses supervisor positions and their responsibilities; however, many supervisors will have had extensive experience working in one or more of the positions mentioned above to be able to better understand the role, responsibilities, and expectations necessary to fulfill that position in child welfare practice.

Practice Highlight

Courtroom Players to Know

Judge: The judge presides over the courtroom and makes important decisions about the case, including placement, whether abuse and neglect has occurred, and permanency. The judge orders services and actions as part of the case.

Children's representatives: The court may appoint one or all of the following child representatives. Each serves a different role, depending on the case; however, all may be appointed as well depending on the need. Whether these individuals are a party to the case depends on state statues, which will dictate whether the child welfare professional is required to provide information about the case.

    Attorney: A child's attorney represents the child and advocates for their desires. The attorney also provides information about the case and the proceedings.

Guardian ad litem (GAL): A guardian ad litem (GAL) is an attorney or a layperson that represents the child's best interests, which may or may not be in line with the child's wishes.

Court Appointed Special Advocate (CASA): It is a trained volunteer appointed by the court to represent the best interests and advocate for the child's needs and desires. CASAs typically only have one to two cases at any given time and therefore can spend a greater amount of time with the child and on the case.

Parents' attorney is a legal representative that may be appointed to the parent to provide information and advocate for the parents' wishes at the beginning of a case. Even when parents are married or in a relationship, an attorney for each parent is often assigned.

Agency attorney is a legal representative for the child welfare agency. This attorney may be employed by a government agency such as the county, state, or city depending on the jurisdiction and how it is structured. This attorney represents the agency and therefore the child welfare professional as an employee of that agency.

Child welfare professional is the individual who has investigated a case of maltreatment or who is managing an ongoing case with the child welfare agency. The child welfare professional works closely with all of the key players in court as well as the child, their family, other professionals, and caregivers.

Bailiff or court staff may be law enforcement or security staff but may also serve in the role of scheduler and coordinator for the courtroom.

Navigating the Dependency Court System

One of the most challenging parts about being a child welfare professional is having to manage the legal requirements and maintaining relationships with individuals involved with the legal side of child welfare work. See Fig. 2.2 for an overview of the typical flow of a dependency case. For example, understanding the legal system, ensuring legal requirements, communicating with legal personnel, and testifying are some of the most difficult parts of being in child welfare as a caseworker. There are a number of lawyers, a judge, volunteers (e.g., Court Appointed Special Advocates [CASAs], mentors), and other individuals involved with each case and specific timelines, dates, and laws to adhere to. These individuals and legal statutes may

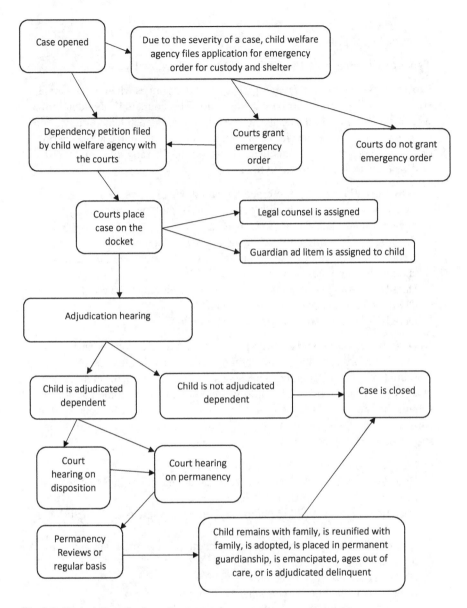

Fig. 2.2 Typical flow of a dependency case

vary by state and jurisdiction and child welfare professionals must understand where they practice. One way to better understand the individuals and statutes is to spend time at the dependency court to observe different types of hearings and different court personnel.

Practice Highlight

Types of Hearings and the Child Welfare Professional's Role

Protective/Dispositional Hearing: The court determines whether the parents are able, willing and fit to parent the child. The court will also determine whether it is in the child's best interest to be found "dependent" or a ward of the court, and whether the child can remain home, return home at the hearing, or placed under the care of another person. At this hearing, the child welfare professional should be prepared to discuss:

- Why the child cannot be returned home today
- Parameters for visitation with parents and/or siblings (no visitation, frequency, and duration) and recommendations
- Specific services offered to or engaged in by the parents
- Details concerning evaluations completed with parents, child, caretakers, and any recommendations
- Details regarding current and/or proposed placement of the child
- Child's special needs or need for service
- Details about concurrent permanency planning

Review or Permanency Hearings: The court reviews evidence on the progress made toward returning a child home. If it appears that the parents are not working to correct the conditions necessary for reunification, the court reviews other permanency options. The child welfare professional should prepare and submit the most recent court report and/or service plan to the court and all parties prior to the hearing. At these hearings, the child welfare professional should be prepared to discuss:

- Why the child cannot be returned home today
- How the services in the case plan are related to the conditions that required court intervention are being corrected
- Specific services offered to parents to correct conditions and whether services are being completed or not
- History of child's placement (number, length of time, provider, and reason for change)
- Child's special needs or need for service
- Details about concurrent permanency planning
- Parameters for visitation with parents and/or siblings (no visitation, frequency and duration) and recommendations
- Any recommendations regarding permanency and/or placement

Contested Hearings on Motions: The party making the motion has the burden of persuading the court to take action described in a motion between review hearings. The evidence needed might involve testimony. Some examples of such hearings include motions for visits, return home, motions to extend, or vacate an order of protection.

Status Reports: These reports are given at any state of the proceedings or hearings and typically involve a legal matter such as status on service progress, compliance with a court order, visitation, etc.

Termination of Parental Rights: This hearing occurs once a decision at a review hearing has been made to change the case plan goal to terminate parental rights and pursue adoption. This is done when it deemed that a child cannot return to their parents' care and a need for a permanent goal is in place. Termination is typically a multistep process. Although any party to the case can file for termination of parental rights, it is typically the attorneys representing the child welfare agency that will file the motion, once they have evidence that reunification is not possible, that the parents have not ameliorated the circumstances that brought the child into care (e.g., completed services, etc.), and determined that termination is in the best interest of the child. There must be "clear and convincing" evidence as the burden of proof in this case, and there may be stricter rules of evidence. Child welfare professionals should be prepared to provide documentation and testimony related to:

- What the circumstances were that brought the children into care, requiring court intervention and the impact it has had on the child's welfare
- Documentation of services offered and engaged in by each parent along with progress with such services
- Details concerning evaluations for parents and children and recommendations
- Details concerning visitations between parent and child
- Details concerning child's current placement
- Child's special needs and/or need for services
- Child's relationship with each parent

Family Conference: The family conference is more of a meeting than a hearing and is designed to save time with have all the parties gathering to review the case plan, problem solve, and discuss services. In addition to providing the most recent case/service plan, the child welfare professional should also be prepared to discuss:

- The reason the child cannot return home today
- Family strengths and needs and what services could be provided to improve circumstances that brought the child into care
- Efforts to locate parents and assessing their service needs
- Child's special needs and needs for services
- Details regarding visitation with parents and siblings

Preparing for and Testifying in Court

Testifying in court can be a stressful experience for anyone, under any circumstances. However, experts say that if witnesses are honest and prepared for the questions they will be asked, they will typically experience less stress during their testimony. Most child welfare agencies provide training on the dependency court process and how to testify for new child welfare professionals. Some also provide an opportunity to practice testifying in a mock court room or using language typically used in testifying.

There are often a number of individuals present in the courtroom during hearings. Depending on the type and purpose of the hearing, child welfare professionals may be required to provide testimony. Proceedings are not like they are on television or the movies. At the beginning of a hearing, the parties (those who are part of the case, such as attorneys, parents, etc.) and other attendees gather in the courtroom. When the judge enters the room, all parties must stand until the judge gives permission to sit. In most cases, the person who is talking will stand when talking to the judge or "the court." The person talking will address the court and not other parties when providing information or an argument. These are formal hearings and judges often have varying styles and rules for their courtroom. For example, some judges only allow the attorneys to answer questions, whereas others allow comments and questions from their clients and/or guests in the gallery. Typically, the judge will state the purpose for the hearing and allow the parties to offer information and/or evidence, such as reports. After everyone spoken, the judge may enter orders and set a follow-up hearing date. In the cases where a child welfare professional may need to testify includes preliminary hearings that require them to describe the reason a child removal from the home is necessary or during a trial. During a trial, a number of individuals may testify, including parents, family members, child welfare professionals and their supervisors, psychologists or other mental health professionals, and professionals who supervise visits or offer services to the parents, child, or caregivers.

> **Practice Tip**
> **Preparing for Court**
> Depending on their position, child welfare professionals will spend varying amounts of time in court. To prepare for court, child welfare professionals should:
> - Know the history of the case.
> - Review the service plan prior to the court date.
> - Know what services have been provided, completed, and in progress for each parent.
> - Bring extra copies of the report/service plan to the hearing.
> - Be aware of the purpose of the hearing.
> - Talk to the agency's attorneys about any issues or concerns.
> - Discuss the case with supervisor prior to the hearing.
> - Bring any necessary documents to court that might be relevant.
> - Communicate and share necessary reports with all parties prior to the hearing.

When preparing to provide testimony, it is helpful to meet with the child welfare agency's attorney (e.g., district attorney or state attorney) to review questions to prepare for and/or anticipate from a parent's attorney. It is helpful to review the case file and reports so that the child welfare worker can feel confident in providing accurate and thorough testimony.

Practice Highlight

Examples of Questions for Caseworkers in Dependency Court Hearings

Caseworkers may be asked questions like the following when they are in court:

- Was the family assessed for services?
- What services were offered?
- What services have been completed?
- Where is the child placed? How long have they been there? Which family members have been assessed for placement?
- What are the child's needs (medical, educational, and social-emotional)? What services are they receiving? Has the child been assessed?
- What is your recommendation regarding a) temporary custody? b) case plan? c) concurrent permanency plan?
- Are there visits with the parents and/or siblings? Please provide a report of these visits (e.g., frequency, duration).

Parents' Rights

The adults and children and involved in dependency court hearings have rights to protect them as outlined by the law. Parents and children involved in such cases have similar but different rights which differ by jurisdiction. States, courts, or child welfare agencies often publish literature for parents and children to better understand their rights at different points throughout a dependency case. This helps them to understand their responsibilities and what they are entitled to. When a child is removed from the care of their parent, the parent has the right to an attorney and if the parent cannot afford to hire an attorney, the judge in the case will appoint one to represent the parent. Biological/legal parents have the right

Reflection
Observations During Court Hearings
In many states, it is possible to observe court. This can help to learn about the process. When observing court, these questions can help to guide understanding of what is happening:

Who is asking the questions?
What types of questions are asked?
Who is in the courtroom and where are individuals seated?
Who is permitted in the court hearing?
Who is asked to offer their thoughts or concerns?
Was evidence submitted?
What type of hearing is it?
How long did the hearing take?
What, if any, orders were given?
How do the parties address each other and the judge?

to attend and participate in all conferences, meetings, and hearings, unless their parental rights have been legally terminated. For meetings outside of the court proceedings, parents may be excluded if it is deemed unsafe. Parents have a right to understand what is happening in court. It is their attorney's responsibility to explain the purpose of each hearing, what is expected of the parent during and outside of the hearing as it relates to the case, give sound advice to the client, and to be reasonably responsive to the parent as their client. Parents involved in dependency cases also have the right to an interpreter if necessary. If a parent speaks a language other than English and does not understand what is happening, they may request an interpreter for proceedings and discussions with their attorney and the child welfare agency representatives. Parents have the right to know what is required so that they may be reunited with their children and to be provided with the necessary services and supports in order to complete such tasks outlined by the judge.

Children's Rights

Similarly, children involved in dependency court cases have rights. They have the right to go to court, as deemed appropriate by the judge. Although it varies by state, children 10 years or older have the option to attend court, and their case worker should inform them of hearings and provide transportation for them to attend. Children have the right to be involved in their case and provide input on decisions about placement, services, case planning, and permanency. Children have the right to stay at their school. The child welfare agency should make arrangements as required by law to allow the child to remain in their school and arrange for transportation. Children have a right to visitation with their parents and their siblings. Some states have specific policies about the frequency and duration of such visits as well. If not automatically provided, children have the right to an attorney to advocate for their wishes in court. Some states provide a guardian ad litem, who could be an attorney or other professional to advocate for their best interests; however, an attorney appointed to them would advocate for what they would like with regard to things like placement, visitation, and services, especially if it differs from the guardian ad litem or the child welfare agency.

Conclusion

The child welfare system is often challenging to understand and navigate. It requires professionals and families to interact with multiple systems and is guided by federal and state policies. There are a number of key players that serve various roles in cases that are important in child welfare work. Part of child welfare work involves time preparing for and attending court hearings. The child welfare professional is a key player in hearings and ensuring that the case proceeds appropriately, which may involve testifying. These situations can often be undesirable, but necessary, and the more experience one has and the more prepared one is, can improve this experience.

Acknowledgments The authors thank Brittany Mihalec-Adkins, M.S.Ed, for the contribution to Chap. 2.

Discussion Questions

1. How are child maltreatment reports made? Who are the most common reporters of child maltreatment and why?
2. Without looking at the flowcharts in the chapter, describe the process in child protection services starting with a report to child protective services.
3. Name three different roles in child protection.
4. What are three ways child welfare professionals can prepare for court?
5. What types of questions might attorneys ask child welfare professionals in court?

Suggested Activities

1. Attend a dependency court hearing if they are open to the public in your community. Be sure to be aware and follow all of the rules of the court (e.g., confidentiality, respect, and appropriate dress). Write a reflection of your experience. Include observations of the type of hearing, who was in attendance and who was speaking, what decisions and findings that were made. Make note of your presence, who you spoke with, and what it was like to go through security, navigate the courtrooms and people.
2. Interview one of the identified courtroom key players (e.g., judge, GAL, CASA, attorney, etc.) about their role and work in the courtroom. Ask them about positive experiences and challenging cases. Ask about their relationships with child welfare professionals and how they work together.
3. Go online and find a flow chart or document that shows how the child welfare system in your state or jurisdiction is structured. Note the names of the departments/units, and the roles for those who work in the child welfare system, the types of hearings, and the typical case flow process. Compare to the description in this chapter.
4. Read Finno-Valasquez, He, Perrigo, and Hurlburt (2017) write a paper exploring why some communities that are demographically similar have different rates of maltreatment and different reporting rates of child maltreatment.
   Finno-Velasquez, M., He, A. S., Perrigo, J. L., & Hurlburt, M. S. (2017). Community informant explanations for unusual neighborhood rates of child maltreatment reports. *Child and Adolescent Social Work Journal, 34*(3), 191–204. (Available: https://rdcu.be/cb8Uh).

Additional Resources

American Professional Society on the Abuse of Children: https://www.apsac.org/
Badeau, S., & Gesiriech, S. (2003). *A child's journey through the child welfare system*. Washington, DC: The Pew Commission on Children in Foster Care. https://www.gascore.com/documents/AChildsJourneythrough the%20ChildWelfareSystem.pdf

Child Welfare Information Gateway. (2013). *How the child welfare system works.* Washington, DC: U.S. Department of Health and Human Services, Children's Bureau. https://www.childwelfare.gov/pubs/factsheets/cpswork/

Child Welfare Information Gateway. (2011). *Understanding child welfare and the courts.* Washington, DC: U.S. Department of Health and Human Services, Children's Bureau. https://www.childwelfare.gov/pubs/factsheets/cwandcourts/

National Center for State Courts, Dependency Courts Resource Guide: https://www.ncsc.org/topics/children-families-and-elders/dependency-court/resource-guide

National Drug Court Institute, Family Treatment Court Planning Guide: https://www.ndci.org/resources/family-treatment-court-planning-guide/

A family's guide to the child welfare system. Washington, DC: National Technical Assistance Partnership for Child and Family Mental Health at Georgetown University Center for Child and Human Development. https://cbexpress.acf.hhs.gov/index.cfm?event=website.viewArticles&issueid=53&sectionid=5&articleid=2072

References

Bruns, E. J., Pullmann, M. D., Weathers, E. S., Wirschem, M. L., & Murphy, J. K. (2012). Effects of a multidisciplinary family treatment drug court on child and family outcomes: Results of a quasi-experimental study. *Child Maltreatment, 17*(3), 218–230. https://doi.org/10.1177/1077559512454216

Casanueva, C., Harris, S., Carr, C., Burfend, C., & Smith, K. (2019). Evaluation in multiple sites of the Safe Babies Court Team approach. *Child Welfare, 97*(1), 85–107.

Chuang, E., Moore, K., Barrett, B., & Young, M. S. (2012). Effect of an integrated family dependency treatment court on child welfare reunification, time to permanency and re-entry rates. *Children and Youth Services Review, 34*(9), 1896–1902. https://doi.org/10.1016/j.childyouth.2012.06.001

Cross, T. P., Chuang, E., Helton, J. J., & Lux, E. A. (2015). Criminal investigations in child protective services cases: An empirical analysis. *Child Maltreatment, 20*(2), 104–114. https://doi.org/10.1177/1077559514562605

Davis, A. E., Barrueco, S., & Perry, D. F. (2020). The role of consultative alliance in infant and early childhood mental health consultation: Child, teacher, and classroom outcomes. *Infant Mental Health Journal.* https://doi.org/10.1002/imhj.21889

Ellet, A. J., & D. Steib, D. (2005). Child Welfare and the Courts: A Statewide Study with Implications for Professional Development, Practice and Change. *Research on Social Work Practice, 15*(5), 339–352. doi: https://doi.org/10.1177/1049731505276680.

Espeleta, H. C., Bakula, D. M., Sharkey, C. M., Reinink, J., Cherry, A., Lees, J., et al. (2020). Adapting pediatric medical homes for youth in foster care: Extensions of the American academy of pediatrics guidelines. *Clinical Pediatrics, 59*(4–5), 411–420. https://doi.org/10.1177/0009922820902438

Ezell, J. M., Richardson, M., Salari, S., & Henry, J. A. (2018). Implementing trauma-informed practice in juvenile justice systems: What can courts learn from child welfare interventions? *Journal of Child & Adolescent Trauma, 11*(4), 507–519. https://doi.org/10.1007/s40653-018-0223-y

Herbert, J. L., & Bromfield, L. (2019). Multi-disciplinary teams responding to child abuse: Common features and assumptions. *Children and Youth Services Review, 106*, 104,467. https://doi.org/10.1016/j.childyouth.2019.104467

Herbert, J. L., & Bromfield, L. (2016). Evidence for the efficacy of the Child Advocacy Center model: A systematic review. *Trauma, Violence, & Abuse, 17*(3), 341–357. https://doi.org/10.1177/1524838015585319

Hubel, G. S., Campbell, C., West, T., Friedenberg, S., Schreier, A., Flood, M. F., & Hansen, D. J. (2014). Child advocacy center based group treatment for child sexual abuse. *Journal of Child Sexual Abuse, 23*(3), 304–325. https://doi.org/10.1080/10538712.2014.888121

Hubel, G. S., Schreier, A., Hansen, D. J., & Wilcox, B. L. (2013). A case study of the effects of privatization of child welfare on services for children and families: The Nebraska experience. *Children and Youth Services Review, 35*(12), 2049–2058. https://doi.org/10.1016/j.childyouth.2013.10.011

Keeshin, B. R., & Dubowitz, H. (2013). Childhood neglect: The role of the paediatrician. *Paediatrics & Child Health, 18*(8), e39–e43. https://doi.org/10.1093/pch/18.8.e39

Loomis, A. M. (2018). The role of preschool as a point of intervention and prevention for trauma-exposed children: recommendations for practice, policy, and research. *Topics in Early Childhood Special Education, 38*(3), 134–145. https://doi.org/10.1177/0271121418789254

MacLeod, K. J., Marcin, J. P., Boyle, C., Miyamoto, S., Dimand, R. J., & Rogers, K. K. (2009). Using telemedicine to improve the care delivered to sexually abused children in rural, underserved hospitals. *Pediatrics, 123*(1), 223–228. https://doi.org/10.1542/peds.2007-1921

Powell B.J., Bosk E.A., Wilen J.S., Danko C.M., Van Scoyoc A., & Banman A. (2015) Evidence-based programs in "real world" settings: finding the best fit. In: Daro D., Cohn Donnelly A., Huang L., Powell B. (eds) Advances in child abuse prevention knowledge. child maltreatment (Vol. 5: Contemporary Issues in Research and Policy). : Springer. https://doi.org/10.1007/978-3-319-16327-7_7

Smith, J. D., Cruden, G. H., Rojas, L. M., Van Ryzin, M., Fu, E., Davis, M. M., et al. (2020). Parenting interventions in pediatric primary care: A systematic review. *Pediatrics, 146*(1). https://doi.org/10.1542/peds.2019-3548

Wilen, J. S., Littell, J. H., & Salanti, G. (2017). Psychosocial interventions for adults who were sexually abused as children. *The Cochrane Database of Systematic Reviews, 2017*(1) https://www.ncbi.nlm.nih.gov/pmc/articles/PMC6464780/

Zero to Three. (2017, December). *The evaluation is in: The Safe Babies Court Team™ approach is changing lives.* Washington DC.

Zinn, A., & Orlebeke, B. (2017). Juvenile court judicial expertise and children's permanency outcomes. *Children and Youth Services Review, 77*, 46–54. https://doi.org/10.1016/j.childyouth.2017.03.011

Chapter 3
Child Development and Well-Being

Introduction

For child welfare professionals to understand child maltreatment, it is important first to understand normative child development, family roles, relationships, and child and family well-being. In order to assess the needs of children and their families, child welfare professionals must understand basic patterns of human behavior and development, the family life cycle, how children develop attachments, and why these attachments are important for children's healthy development. This information also helps child welfare professionals understand how certain experiences can impede normal, healthy child and family development, and we can work alongside children and families in important prevention and intervention efforts in child welfare practice.

Domains of Child Development

Child development can be understood in five major domains: (1) physical, (2) cognitive, (3) emotional, (4) social, and (5) sexual. Physical development refers to the child's size and ability to perform physical tasks (e.g., lifting one's head, crawling, walking, running, etc.). Cognitive development refers to a child's ability to make sense of the world, understand speech, speak, read, write, and complete age-appropriate academic tasks. Emotional development is a child's ability to recognize, manage, and regulate emotions or feelings, while social development is how a child relates to other people, including their peers and adults. Sexual development refers to becoming sexually mature and experiencing specific physical changes associated with the body's ability to procreate.

Child development researchers have defined normative development, or what we should typically expect to observe among these domains for children in specific age groups (see Table 3.1 for details about normative development and areas of

© Springer Nature Switzerland AG 2021
J. M. Geiger, L. Schelbe, *The Handbook on Child Welfare Practice*,
https://doi.org/10.1007/978-3-030-73912-6_3

Table 3.1 Child development: normative observations and observations requiring attention

Stage	Age	Routine observations	Strengths and landmarks of development	Developmental issues (not problems)	Developmental observations requiring attention
Infancy	Birth–2 years	• Perceptual abilities • Reflexes • Weight gain and growth (height) • Sleep patterns • Rhythms and capacity for self-regulation • Temperament • Fit between infant temperament and parenting style • Attachment and strategies for maintaining relationships • Parents' nurturing capacities • Parental supports • Child-care resources	• Good health • Well-developed senses • Shows preferences • Recognizes primary caregivers • Demonstrates responsiveness to caregivers • Play develops within attachment relationships • Ability to entertain self for brief periods of time by 6 months • Flexible attention • Reaches physical milestones for fine motor, crawling, and grasping • Regular sleep, wakefulness, feeding, and elimination	• Some difficulties warming up • Sleep irregularities • Infant is perceived as fussy • Limited interest in eating • Object permanence • Limited vocalization • How infant sleeps (on stomach) • Teen parents • Poor parental preparation for the infant • Preparation of siblings for arrival of infant	• Lack of physical growth • Insecure attachment • Colicky • Over-arousal or under-arousal in the infant • Parent depressed or has other mental illness • Lack of supports and good child care • Serious health problems in the child • Serious parental healthcare concerns • Infant neglect or abuse • Poor fit between infant temperament and parenting styles
Early childhood	2–3 years (toddler) 3–5 years (preschool)	• Gross and fine motor skills • Toileting • Speech • Use of mental symbols • Peer relationships and siblings • Play preferences • Preschool • Limits, discipline, and daily routine • Dreams and night terrors, fears • Interest and skill development	• Parallel play (2.5) • Collateral peer play (3), cooperative play (3–4) • Bedtime ritual • Two- and three-word speed (2), creative use of speech (3–4) • Successful toilet training (2–3) • Accepts limits (2–3) • Development of special talents (e.g., music, dance) • Self-talk to guide behavior • Some leadership capacity in groups (3–4)	• Stuttering • Occasional soiling or wetting • Messy play • Won't put things away • Stubbornness • Aggressive and possessive play • Refuses new foods • Immature behavior when ill or sick • Asserts independence and fusses • Occasional temper tantrums • Unreasonable fears (short-lived)	• Persistent soiling and wetting • Persistent eating problems • Disturbed sleep patterns • Nonspeaking • Inappropriate play behavior • Excessive body rocking, finger sucking, or tics

Middle childhood	6–12 years	• Peer relationships and behavior • Adaptation to school • Family relationships • Interests and skills • Physical development (prepubertal changes), interests, and abilities • TV/ movie/computer viewing habits • Sleep and dreams • Daily routine established • Independent self-care • Academic achievement and classroom behavior • Reading/literacy skills • Reasoning abilities	• Enjoys reading • Comfortable away from home/ with peers • Development of moral thinking • Good at catching a ball • Can solve simple puzzles • Friendship development with same sex (8–10) • Participates in a peer group (9–11) • Physically active • Developing preferences for friends and activities (5–7) • Sexuality awareness	• Oversensitive to criticism • Prefers play to school and home responsibilities • Short-term fears • Noncompliance with parental request • Doesn't always share teacher-child conflicts • Poor table manners • Excessive aggressive behavior • Talking back • Moodiness • Temper outbursts • Secretiveness	• Persistent fearfulness • Lying • School failure • Language and speech problems • Victimized by bullies • Inappropriate sexual behavior • Overdependence • Running away • Fire setting • Persistent thumb sucking • Strange, bizarre, or withdrawn behavior • Lack of communication • Cruelty to animals • Lack of friends • Disturbed sleep patterns, enuresis • Persistently emotional over small things

(continued)

Table 3.1 (continued)

| Adolescence | Puberty–14 years (early) 15–17 years (middle) 18–22 years (late) | • Brain development and abstract thought
• Peer groups
• Body image
• Sense of morality
• Independence
• Sexual identity
• Romantic involvements
• Focus on physical appearance
• Increased caloric intake
• Hormonal changes
• Menstruation (girls) | • Increased resilience
• Development of autonomy and independence
• Increased influence of peers
• Enhancing parent-adolescent relationships
• Peer support
• Egocentrism | • Excessive concern with body image
• Spending too much time alone
• Negative peer influence
• Decreased interest in school
• Academic difficulties
• Moodiness
• Sexual behavior
• Transition to middle school
• Parent conflict
• Late maturing girls
• Risk behaviors | • Eating disorders
• Depression
• Pregnancy
• Sex abuse and rape
• Substance abuse
• Violent behaviors and exposure to violence
• Firearm exposure/use
• Conduct disorder and delinquency
• Anxiety |

development that might require attention). Developmental milestones are behaviors exhibited throughout the phases of development that are indicative of normal development that are based on average development. However, there is quite a bit of variability, and children may attain milestones at different rates. Milestones reached within a 6-month period are considered "within normal limits." Children are considered "delayed" in a developmental domain when 90% of other children are performing the task. Although it may vary, eligibility for early intervention services that address developmental delays requires at least a 30% delay.

Factors that Impede or Delay Normative Development

When humans are presented with the right conditions, they will progress through predictable stages of development. However, sometimes children face conditions that negatively affect or delay growth and development and, therefore, may later influence their ability to adjust later in childhood, adolescence, and adulthood. There are conditions that are out of the control of the child and at times, their parents. A child may face genetic or congenital conditions. A child could be at risk for development delays because the mother did not receive prenatal care or used drug or alcohol while pregnant. Children may experience environmental threats such as unsafe living conditions, poverty, crime, violence, or pollution. Various types of accidents or other experiences of trauma can lead to a delay or interruption in normative child development. Extensive research has shown that experiences of child maltreatment can interfere with child development (e.g., Cicchetti et al., 2000; Trickett & McBride-Chang, 1995; Zielinski & Bradshaw, 2006).

> **Research Brief**
> **Prenatal Drug Exposure and Its Impact on Development**
> In the United States, it is estimated that almost 15% of women use tobacco, 11.5% consume alcohol, and 8.5% use illicit substances while pregnant (Oh et al., 2017). Although states have different laws about child welfare and criminal regulations about prenatal alcohol and substance use, approximately 39% of child welfare agencies reported parental alcohol or other drug use as a contributing factor for removal of a child (AFCARS, 2020).
>
> Extensive research has been conducted on the impact of prenatal alcohol and substance exposure on child development. In the short term, children may experience birth anomalies (e.g., physical deformities), delayed fetal growth, withdrawal, and neurobehavioral problems. Long-term effects of prenatal substance exposure include delays and impairments in achievement, cognition, physical growth, and language development.

Consider the example of Layla,[1] a 13-year-old Caucasian girl who lives with both of her biological parents, who give her adequate love and support, in a safe neighborhood and who attends a local school. She lives in a fairly homogeneous community, where most of her peers and their families look the same as her and have similar average experiences. Like her peers and other children, she has a number of strengths and challenges. Her parents noticed at a young age that she presented with difficulties in her social development and sought out early intervention services in their community. At the age of 4, she was diagnosed with autism spectrum disorder and struggles with making friends and interacting with others. Since her diagnosis, she has received services in the community and at school. Her father works in the home and has a very flexible schedule that allows him to take her to appointments and attend meetings at school to ensure her needs are being met.

Research shows severe negative consequences for infants and children exposed to alcohol in particular. Estimates show that 6–9 per 1000 live births are infants exposed to alcohol with a diagnosis of fetal alcohol spectrum disorder (FASD; May et al., 2014). A number of factors influence the presentation of FASD in children, including pattern and timing of alcohol use, genetics, amount of alcohol consumed, the use of other substances, mother's health and nutrition, and the mother's age. Prenatal alcohol and drug use are often difficult to detect and are not routinely screened for biologically. The majority of prevention efforts focus on education, social support, counseling, and, for extreme cases, inpatient treatment, as appropriate.

Now, consider the example of Destiny, a 13-year-old child with similar qualities and experiences, with the exception of one factor: she and her family live in poverty. Her parents struggle to keep steady jobs. The family has moved several times and has been homeless on a few occasions. As a result of moving, Destiny has changed schools, creating an unstable environment. Destiny has been eligible for services at the same time Layla was; however, she did not begin to receive services until she was finishing the fourth grade due to the changes in schools and her parents being unaware of available support and the school not having the same resources as the one in Layla's more affluent neighborhood. Destiny's behavior was often perceived as negative and disruptive by teachers and caregivers and often attributed to the new environment and instability in housing and schools.

Clearly, there are multiple factors that mitigate the experiences of a child and lead to impaired and/or delayed development, particularly in the case where a child requires additional supports and services. Given what is known about trauma associated with community violence, natural disasters, and child maltreatment, for example, development should be viewed within the context of the child's and family's experiences in multiple developmental domains. (See Chap. 5 for more information about trauma.)

Human development is a dynamic process. It can be very predictable and also extremely variable. Developmental progress is based on various physical, emotional, and cognitive tasks that build upon each other. Table 3.2 outlines common

---

[1] All names and other personal identifiers in cases and examples throughout this book have been changed to protect privacy and confidentiality.

Table 3.2 Developmental tasks in first 24 months

Age	Physical	Cognitive	Language	Social/emotional
0–3 months	• Sucking and other reflexes • Can turn head to one side • Turns head to food source	• Learns to focus • Can discriminate some individual voices • Begins to follow things with eyes and recognize people at a distance • Can act bored (crying/fussiness) if activity doesn't change	• Coos • Develops differentiated cry • Turns head toward sounds	• Grasps fingers • Focuses on faces • Begins to smile at people • Can briefly calm self • Tries to look at caregiver
3–6 months	• Rolls over from stomach to back • Keeps head steady and does not fall back when pulled to sitting position • Beginning to reach for and grasp objects • Can lift shoulders or lift head to look around when on stomach • Can sit with support	• Lets people know if sad or happy • Responds to affection • Reaches for toy with one hand • Uses and hand and eyes together • Follows moving things with eyes • Watches faces closely • Recognizes familiar people at a distance	• Begins to babble • Babbles with expression and copies sounds heard • Cries in different ways to communicate different needs/emotions	• Smiles spontaneously at people • Likes to play with people and might cry when playing stops • Copies movements and facial expressions
6–9 months	• Rolls over in both directions • Begins to sit without support • When standing, supports weight on legs and might bounce • Rocks back and forth, sometimes crawling backward before moving forward	• Looks around at things nearby • Brings things to mouth • Shows curiosity about things and tries to get things that are out of reach • Begins to pass things from one hand to the other	• Responds to sounds by making sounds • Strings vowels together when babbling and likes taking turns with parent while making sounds • Responds to own name • Makes sounds to show joy and displeasure • Begins to say consonant sounds	• Knows familiar faces and begins to know if someone is a stranger • Likes to play with others, especially caregivers • Responds to other people's emotions and often seems happy • Likes to look at self in a mirror

(continued)

Table 3.2 (continued)

Age	Physical	Cognitive	Language	Social/emotional
9–12 months	• Stands, holding on • Can get into a sitting position • Sits without support • Pulls to stand • Crawls	• Watches the path of something as it falls • Looks for things they see someone hide • Plays peek-a-boo • Puts things in their mouth • Moves things smoothly from one hand to the other • Picks up things like cereal between thumb and index finger	• Understands "no" • Makes a lot of different sounds • Copies sounds and gestures of others • Uses fingers to point at things	• May be afraid of strangers • May be clingy with familiar caregivers • Has favorite toys
12 months	• Gets to a sitting position without help • Pulls up to stand, walks holding on to furniture (cruising) • May take a few steps without holding on • May stand alone	• Explores things in different ways (shaking, banging, throwing) • Finds hidden things easily • Looks at the right picture or thing when it's named • Copies gestures • Starts to use things correctly (e.g., brushing hair) • Bangs things together • Puts things in a container and takes them out • Lets things go without help • Pokes with finger • Follows simple directions	• Responds to simple spoken requests • Uses simple gestures (e.g., shaking head or waving) • Makes sounds with changes in tone • Says mama and dada • Tries to say words others say	• Is shy or nervous with strangers • Cries when caregiver leaves • Has favorite things and people • Shows fear at times • Hands someone a book when wants to hear a story • Repeats sounds or actions to get attention • Puts out arm or leg to help with dressing • Plays simple games

(continued)

Table 3.2 (continued)

Age	Physical	Cognitive	Language	Social/emotional
18 months	• Walks alone • May walk up steps and run • Pulls toys while walking • Can help undress self • Drinks from cup • Eats with a spoon	• Knows what ordinary things are • Points to get the attention of others • Shows interest in toy/doll by pretending to feed • Points to one body part • Scribbles on own • Can follow one-step verbal commands	• Says several single words • Says and shakes head "no" • Points to show someone what he wants	• Likes to hand things to others as play • May have temper tantrums • May be afraid of strangers • Shows affection to those they know • Plays simple pretend, such as feeding a doll • May cling to caregivers • Points to show others something interesting • Explores alone but with caregiver nearby
24 months	• Stands on tiptoe • Kicks a ball • Begins to run • Climbs onto and down from things without help • Walks up and down stairs while holding on	• Finds things even when hidden • Begins to sort shapes and colors • Completes sentences and rhymes in familiar books • Plays simple make-believe games • Builds towers of 4 or more blocks • Might use one hand more than the other • Follows 2-step instructions • Names items in a picture book	• Points to things when they are named • Knows names of people and body parts • Says sentences with 2–4 words • Follows simple instructions • Repeats words overheard in conversation • Points to things in a book	• Copies others • Gets excited when with other children • Shows more and more independence • Shows defiant behavior • Plays mainly beside other children but begins to include other children

Adapted from Centers for Disease Control and Prevention (CDC). Developmental Milestones. https://www.cdc.gov/ncbddd/actearly/milestones/index.html

developmental tasks in the first 24 months of life. These tasks create a foundation for future development to occur, leading to successful or challenging experiences as a result. Children's development occurs within the context of their relationships, particularly those with their caregivers, as well as the environment. All people learn how to behave in response to others, how to communicate effectively as it relates to their needs, as well as socially. These interactions are the foundation for humans to learn, adapt, and grow, and the development of skills is in response to the environment to ensure optimal functioning and adaptation.

Even before the birth of a child, the relationship between the parent and child is being developed. The circumstances and expectations related to the conception of the child can influence this relationship and the environment in which the child may enter. Although common for many women, pregnancy and birth can be a positive or negative experience in terms of physical comfort (or discomfort), illness, ability, and changes. The mother must adapt physically, emotionally, and psychologically to the changes resulting from pregnancy and birth. Culture, family, and past experiences influence the present experience. Prenatal exposure to drugs and alcohol can have a significantly negative effect on the developing fetus that lasts long after birth and throughout child development.

Supporting Healthy Child Development

Child welfare professionals can help to support healthy child development by first, being aware of appropriate physical, social, emotional, and cognitive development among children of all ages, particularly young children. For professionals working with families involved with the child welfare system and families who are at greater risk for child maltreatment, being able to identify a developmental delay or interruption in development can lead to early intervention for assessment and referral for any necessary services and supports for children and families. Early intervention programs can work with the child welfare system to ensure optimal child development (Allen et al., 2012). Early intervention is central for better outcomes, and ensuring children's access to services is a protective factor (Stepleton et al., 2010).

There are a number of assessment tools as well as activities and supports child welfare professionals can offer parents and caregivers to support their well-being. Child welfare professionals can encourage parents to track developmental milestones and seek appropriate well-checks with medical professionals. We can provide resources to promote healthy development and reduce the risk for child maltreatment. For example, there are applications parents/caregivers can download on their electronic devices to track child development or download a checklist of when to seek help. The Centers for Disease Control and Prevention (CDC, 2020) also has information about who to contact if a parent or caregiver is concerned a child is not meeting expected milestones.

Developmental Monitoring, Screening, and Evaluation

As child welfare professionals, it is important to understand not only normative child and human development but also what signs there are for non-normative development and signs of child maltreatment that may manifest in a child's behavior. Child welfare professionals should be aware of the latest recommendations for medical and dental routine assessments and know ways to make referrals if a child requires additional monitoring, screening, or evaluation for developmental concerns.

Like all experiences in one's life, trauma and adversity also shape one's development. Trauma is associated with a number of negative outcomes and impacts various developmental competencies related to one's interpersonal, intrapersonal, regulatory, and neurocognitive competencies (Blaustein & Kinniburgh, 2010) necessary for healthy development. We will discuss further how trauma is defined and manifested by age group and discuss the impact of various traumatic experiences, particularly complex and chronic trauma exposure for children who experience child maltreatment.

Recommendations for Child Developmental Monitoring, Screening, and Evaluation

Medical Examination: Well-child visits should occur regularly for children

Within first week (3–5 days)
1 month
2 months
4 months
6 months
9 months
12 months
15 months
18 months
24 months
2 ½ years
Every year between age 3 and 21

These visits serve various purposes, including children obtaining necessary immunizations to prevent illnesses, track child growth and development to ensure they are meeting necessary milestones, discuss any concerns a caregiver may have, and promote optimum health of the child over time (AAP, 2018).

Dental Examination
Ages 6 months to 1 year. The American Academy of Pediatric Dentistry (2020) recommends scheduling a child's first dental exam after the first tooth erupts and no later than the first birthday. Also expect the baby's teeth and gums to be examined at well-baby checkups.

Toddlers, school-age children, and adolescents. The American Academy of Pediatric Dentistry recommends scheduling regular dental checkups, with the most common interval being every 6 months. However, the dentist might recommend fewer or more-frequent visits depending on the child's risk factors for oral health problems.

Eye Examination

The American Optometric Association (2019) recommends the following schedule for eye examinations:

Once between 6 and 12 months old
At least once between age of 3 and 5 years
Once before first grade and annually thereafter

Attachment, Bonding, and Development

Attachment Theory

Attachment theory has been used to understand child development as well as child maltreatment. Research over the past several decades has established a clear relationship between the child-caregiver relationship and child development. Attachment begins at birth and is especially salient during the first 3 years of life (Bowlby, 2008). At birth and the early years, an infant relies completely on their caregiver, and the caregiver's response to meeting the child's needs is the foundation for the attachment relationship (Bowlby, 2008). For this attachment relationship to occur, caregivers must provide appropriate, consistent, and responsive care to the child. As needs are expressed and met, infants develop a sense of trust and attachment to their parents or caregivers even if their parents or caregivers do not adequately meet their needs.

The attachment relationship involves both the caregiver and the infant and is reciprocal. The caregiver acknowledges the infant's needs when communicated through crying and other means and consistently meets these needs appropriately and responsively. When needs are met, the infant and the caregiver are satisfied. Various factors can affect the attachment relationship such as culture, infant characteristics (i.e., temperament), caregiver characteristics (i.e., sensitivity, patience, responsive), and the environment (safety, support, relationships) in which the relationship and individuals exist. Cultural variations in attachment development may also exist. For example, some cultures value a multiple mother or multigenerational caregiving environment for children which can influence the infant-caregiver environment through support and parent's ability to care for the child.

From the research conducted by John Bowlby and Mary Ainsworth, four types of attachment styles have been identified within two types of attachment: secure and

Table 3.3 Attachment styles

Attachment style	Parenting approach	Adult characteristics and behavior
Secure	Aligned with the child; in tune with child's emotions	Ability to create and maintain healthy relationships; set and enforce appropriate boundaries; display appropriate emotions
Insecure-avoidant	Unavailable or rejecting	Avoids close relationships or emotional connections with others; critical; rigid, intolerant
Insecure-resistant/ ambivalent	Inconsistent and/or inappropriate communication	Anxious, insecure, controlling, blaming, erratic, unpredictable behaviors and emotions
Insecure-disorganized/ disoriented	Unresponsive to child's needs; frightening or traumatizing parental behaviors	Chaotic behaviors, insensitivity; abusive, distrustful; insecure

insecure (Belsky, 2002). Mary Ainsworth led research on attachment using the "strange situation" which involved the observation of various caregiver-child interactions following a series of separations and reunions (Ainsworth et al., 1978) in a laboratory setting. Attachment has continued to be studied in both laboratory and community settings, and there is evidence that childhood attachment may impact later life (e.g., Menon et al., 2020).

Table 3.3 describes the four types of attachment styles: secure, insecure-avoidant, insecure-resistant/ambivalent, and insecure-disorganized/disoriented. Secure attachments involve the child using the caregiver as a secure base. The child can explore freely, feels comfortable being away from the caregiver, but will check back or ensure that the caregiver is available and nearby. When separated from the caregiver, the secure child may react with little to extreme distress; however, when reunited, the child responds positively. Insecure-avoidant attachments are characterized by the child avoiding the caregiver, showing little to no interest in the caregiver as they explore their surroundings. When the caregiver leaves, the child shows little distress, and when reunited, the child does not show interest in the caregiver. Insecure-resistant/ambivalent child is preoccupied with the caregiver when they are present and has extreme difficulty separating from the caregiver. While in the presence of the caregiver, the child does not explore on their own but instead relies on the caregiver during this time. When separated, the child is extremely distressed and continues to be preoccupied with the caregiver when reunited. Insecure-disorganized/ disoriented attachment is characterized by a child who uses a disorganized or disoriented pattern of dealing with separation and displays odd behaviors with confusion or failure when approaching the caregiver. These children are the most distressed when they are separated from the caregiver.

Longitudinal research has shown that having a caring, responsive caregiver leads to more "organized" and "secure" attachment to the primary caregiver, which serves as a protective factor for infants and children, whereas attachment insecurity has been shown to be a risk factor for psychopathology and negative behavioral conditions. In summary, child welfare professionals should understand that (1) the quality of the infant/child-parent attachment is a powerful predictor of a child's later social and emotional development; (2) there is always an attachment relationship between a caregiver and child; however, what we assess for is the quality of the relationship; (3) children develop a hierarchy of attachments with different caregivers (mother, father, babysitter, grandparent) based on their relationship and needs being met by that individual; and (4) children can recover from negative or insecure attachment relationships through the development of secure, healthy attachment relationships (e.g., foster and adoptive parents). Figure 3.1 provides ways to assess parent-child attachment by developmental stage.

CHILD (Birth to One Year)		PARENT/CAREGIVER
Eye Contact Response to Caregiver Show Interest Effort to have Physical Contact Receive Comfort Vocalize Often Show Discomfort Regulate States Recognize Caregiver		Respond to Vocalization Adapt Voice Tone Uses Physical Touch Uses Face to Face Contact Respond to Child's Cues Able to Comfort Child Initiate Interactions with Child Identify Positive Qualities about Child

CHILD (One to Five Years)		PARENT/CAREGIVER
Environmental Exploration Check-in with Caregiver Respond to Caregiver Occupy Self Make eye contact with others Use appropriate emotions Response to Pain/Pleasure Speak to others Show normal fears Respond to separation Enjoy physical closeness		Aware of child's cues Respond to child's affection Set limits for child Use appropriate discipline Provide comfort as needed Promote autonomy Interact with child/play

CHILD (Five Years-Adolescent)		PARENT/CAREGIVER
Pride in Self Celebrate Accomplishments Awareness of Limits Try new Tasks Regulate and Show Emotions Show Confidence in Abilities React Appropriately to Physical Contact Positive Interactions with Peers and Siblings Show Guilt, Shame		Show interest in child's activities Understand child's range of emotions Provide Support when Needed Fairness among Siblings Appropriate Discipline Enjoy Time with Child Set Limits and Boundaries Provide Opportunities to Learn

Fig. 3.1 Assessing parent-child attachment

Parent-Child Bonding

Bonding refers to the initial tie that develops between newborn babies and their mothers. It is based on the innate physiological drive of mothers and their babies to recognize each other and be emotionally linked to each other. By recognizing and connecting with each other, parents (often the mother) develop a strong desire or need to provide care for the child. The child responds in ways that require the care from their parent and relies on their parent to give them what they need physically and emotionally. This bond will typically develop during pregnancy for mothers and possibly for babies and continue through the early stages of development and relationship. Immediately after birth and in the early stages, it involves close contact, feeding, holding, verbal sounds and words, and warmth. Mothers often describe this experience as an intense, extremely special relationship with their newborns. It is important to note that bonding is not attachment and they involve different circumstances. The presence of bonding is not necessarily predictive of any positive or negative outcomes.

Attachment Disorders

There are several short- and long-term consequences of an impaired attachment experience or relationship in infancy and early childhood, including challenges associated with interpersonal, emotional, social, and healthy relationship formation and maintenance (e.g., Baer & Martinez, 2006). Children who experience secure attachments feel as those the world can meet their needs and are able to form healthy relationships and can explore these relationships and the world around them comfortably. Children who experienced an insecure attachment relationship may interpret the world as hostile or unsafe, be fraught with anxiety, be aggressive or overly defensive, or ambivalent to those around them. In childhood, these children may be impulsive, have difficulty modulating their emotions and behaviors, or respond appropriately in various social situations (Fearon et al., 2010). Insecure children may form maladaptive coping behaviors such as substance abuse.

A severe form of an insecure attachment may result in reactive attachment disorder (RAD), a diagnosis in the *Diagnostic and Statistical Manual of Mental Disorders, fifth Edition* (DSM −5), when a child's normal attachment processes are disrupted. It usually results from extreme cases of maltreatment and multiple rejections. Children are often severely withdrawn and depressed, or may be extremely destructive or aggressive, or may vacillate between both extremes (usually requiring therapeutic intervention). Some children who have been abused/neglected and are in foster care have never formed secure attachment to caregivers. These children often behave in ways to compensate for their lack of attachment with manipulation, chronic anxiety, problems with authority, hostility, poor peer relationships, poor self-esteem, and self-isolation. Parents and caregivers can promote attachment and reduce behavior problems through positive interactions, strong nurturing and engagement, allowing children to grieve and mourn, providing structure in the home, and appropriately touching the child.

Family Roles

Each family is different, with different members, experiences, traditions, and roles that are determined by the family members themselves. As families grow and learn from each other, each member often will serve a specific role in the family. These roles include positive and negative characteristics, including but not limited to behaviors, mood, financial support, food preparers, etc. Typically, parents provide more of a caretaker role, and children learn to be responsible to the family in other ways, such as through chores, caring for younger children, and self-care. These roles are dependent on age, resources, and culture. Understanding these roles helps us as child welfare professionals to understand family dynamics, how families operate, and the expectations of each family member.

Parenting Styles

With parents having such an important role and influence on child development, it is important to understand what is known about the ways in which parents serve within the role and the impact on child's behavior, growth, and development. Extensive research has been conducted on parenting styles and child development and outcomes. However, despite examining the relationship between these variables, it is difficult to make actual cause-and-effect links between a parent's style of parenting and child's behavior in adolescence and adulthood. Some children with similar upbringings with the same parents in the same household can have very different outcomes, and children who grow up in different households can have very similar personalities.

In the 1960s, psychologist Diana Baumrind (1967) conducted a study with more than 100 preschool-age children and their parents and identified 4 important dimensions of parenting which are (1) disciplinary strategies, (2) warmth and nurturance, (3) communication styles, and (4) expectations of maturity and control. Based on these dimensions, Baumrind determined that the majority of parents display one of three parenting styles. Further research by Maccoby and Martin (1983) added a fourth parenting style.

Practice Highlight

Overview of Parenting Styles

Authoritarian Parenting

Parents displaying this type of parenting style expect children to follow strict rules and failure to do so often results in punishment. Authoritarian parents typically do not provide reasons for the rules, have high, often unrealistic demands, and are not responsive to their children.

Authoritative Parenting

Similar to authoritarian parents, those with an authoritative parenting style have rules and consequences for their children but involve their children more in establishing the rules and consequences. They are more responsive and provide a rationale for rules and consequences, while listening to the child's perspective. When rules are not followed, authoritative parents are more nurturing and forgiving rather than punitive.

Permissive Parenting

Permissive parents have very few demands of their children. These parents rarely establish rules or discipline their children. They have no to low expectations of children and do not require responsible behavior of their children. Permissive parents are nurturing; however, they do not provide structure that involves learning and discipline.

Uninvolved Parenting

An uninvolved parenting style is characterized by few demands, low responsiveness, and little communication. While these parents may fulfill the child's basic needs, they are generally detached from their child's life. In extreme cases, these parents may even reject or neglect the needs of their children.

Since Baumrind's studies, researchers have conducted a number of studies to determine what impact the different parenting styles have on children's personality, emotions, and behaviors. Findings suggest that authoritarian parenting styles generally lead to children who are obedient and proficient but lack in areas of happiness, social competence, and self-esteem. Authoritative parenting styles often result in happy, capable, confident, and successful children, whereas children with permissive parents have shown to be unhappy, struggle with self-regulation, and may have difficulty with authority. Uninvolved parenting styles rank lowest in that children often lack self-control, self-esteem, and are less competent than their peers. These findings may be grossly overgeneralized, when we know that many social circumstances can mediate these relationships. Further, the majority of these studies are correlational, and a number of factors can contribute to these outcomes. There is no one "best" way to parent, and parents make these decisions and have behaviors that reflect their generation, experiences, culture, and education.

Child Discipline

Child discipline is conceptualized as training that is expected to elicit specific behaviors. The American College of Pediatricians presents child discipline as central to the success of child-rearing. The process and practices are often controlled by caregivers, typically parents, and are dependent on multiple factors, including parenting style, parents' experiences of discipline as a child, culture, and public norms and expectations.

Earlier, the chapter discussed the roles within a family and how these roles serve a key role in child development. A fundamental goal of parenting is to teach and support a child in developing character traits such as respectfulness, self-regulation, integrity, and honesty. Child discipline and parental guidance evolve over time and are highly dependent on a child's developmental stage and ability. Discipline often involves training through teaching, enforcement, reinforcement, and modeling of acceptable patterns of behaviors. Discipline should also include healthy caregiver-child interactions involving encouragement and correction. The purpose of child discipline is to ensure healthy moral, emotional, and physical development as well as safety.

Acceptable means of child discipline have varied greatly in the past centuries, and the "best" way to discipline a child can be quite controversial. For example, the Old Testament eluded to strict corporal punishment, which was accepted by many cultures across the world for many centuries. Further, much of how children were disciplined stems from society's view of the child's role and use to a family. Until the twentieth century, children were often viewed as "less than" adults, and children were therefore dissuaded from challenging, questioning, or rebelling against authority – their parents and other adults. This harsh, physical discipline often took place in school settings in addition to the home and some public spaces.

Over time, research has shown that harsh physical punishment is not effective in changing children's negative behavior in the long term (Gershoff, 2008). Further, other means such as positive reinforcement, treating children more respectfully, and granting more freedom to learn appropriate behavior along with natural consequences has become more popular in recent decades. For example, in the 1940s, Dr. Benjamin Spock encouraged parents to more "open, understanding, reasonable, and consistent because children are driven from within themselves to grow, explore, experience, learn, and build relationships with other people" (Spock, 1946).

Society in the United States continues to have a divided attitude toward spanking and corporal punishment among children, while it is illegal in more than 50 countries worldwide. Despite not having national policy that outlaws corporal punishment, the American Academy of Pediatrics (Sege & Siegel, 2018) issued a position against spanking and harsh words. Research shows that spanking, slapping, and other forms of physical and verbal punishment are not effective in reducing negative child behavior and can in fact damage a child's long-term physical and mental health. The American Academy of Pediatrics (2020) offers guidelines about appropriate discipline techniques that correspond to child development stage and age, which include using positive reinforcement rather than punishments, positive modeling of desired behaviors, assigning responsibilities for self-care and chores, and educating children about appropriate emotion identification and expression.

Challenging Child Behaviors

There are several difficult developmental phases that can exacerbate caregivers' frustrations and difficulties managing child behavior, which can lead to physical or emotional abuse. These difficult phases can provoke anger, distress, confrontation, and can become dangerous or deadly for the child living in a high-risk family. The majority of these behaviors are out of the child's conscious control and are developmentally appropriate and variable. Child welfare professionals should be prepared to discuss this with parents and caregivers and offer practical alternatives and support to avoid violent responses. These alternatives include using behavior modification, setting clear boundaries and rules, appropriate child discipline, and offering rewards for desirable behavior, for example, having a discussion with parents about how behavioral patterns emerge and how caregivers can help to modify a child's behavior. Parents can be counseled and supported on how behavior is learned and shaped by consequences (i.e., depending on whether consequence is positive or negative, it will be repeated or not). Many parents have not been provided with adequate parenting education about child development along with strategies to managing difficult circumstances, especially new, first-time parents. Child welfare professionals can serve as a support by providing education regarding normative development, information about attachment and bonding, resources for supportive programs and groups, and empathy in lieu of criticism and judgment. It is also important to realize that many caregivers parent children as they were parented. Therefore, when a parent has been shown love and support from a caregiver, they learn to do this with their children. Conversely, those who have been shown harsh punishment, abuse, and neglect often learn these contexts for caregiving. It is very important, however, to note that if a parent experienced maltreatment as a child that is not to say they will also be an abusive parent; most children who were maltreated do not grow up to abuse and neglect their children (Schelbe & Geiger, 2017).

Difficult Developmental Phases

Examples of difficult developmental phases include colic, night crying, separation anxiety, normal negativism, normal exploratory behavior, poor appetite, and toilet training resistance. There are specific strategies that parents can use to reduce the stress associated with these difficult developmental phases, including education, behavior modification, and accessing support from other adults. Child welfare professionals can be supportive of parents and caregivers experiencing these phases with their child by being knowledgeable of these strategies and providing resources and information to parents and caregivers.

Colic is described as fussy, unexplained crying with an infant. Colic occurs one or more times a day and lasts anywhere from 20 min to 2 h and begins in the first month of life, usually within the first week of life. The cause is unknown, and it resolves spontaneously within 3 months (or sooner). Parents have difficulty soothing their baby and will often bring the child to a healthcare professional for help. Colic or excessive crying that a parent is unable to resolve with holding, rocking, feeding, or other means of soothing is the most common precipitant of serious physical abuse. It is one of the most challenging parenting experiences of newborns and is one of the most common reasons for parents seeking medical advice in the child's first 3 months of life. Colic can also impact the parents' ability to bond with the child because of feelings of inadequacy and anger, leading to developing behavioral problems as the child grows (Krugman, 1993). Physicians and other helping professionals often recommend rhythmic calming techniques are effective in calming colicky babies which forms the core of the 5 S's approach.

Experts have developed various strategies to help calm babies, such as using the "5 S's" (e.g., swaddling, shushing, swinging), which if used at night they can improve sleep or reduce crying; and, when the "5 S's" are done correctly and in combination, they offer significant potential to promptly reducing infant crying and promote sleep (Karp, 2015). It is important to also remind parents about the importance of feeding a hungry baby, changing wet diapers, and comforting a baby who is cold and crying as a result of these factors. Soothing music accompanied with parental attention (including eye contact, talking, touching, rocking, walking, and playing) may be effective in some infants and is never harmful. Child welfare professionals can encourage parents to discuss their feelings and concerns with each other to obtain support as well as emphasize the responsibility of the whole family in the care of a baby with colic.

Similar to colic is night crying. A common myth is that infants should be able to sleep through the night by 3–4 months of age. Research suggests that the average age for infants to sleep through the night is 3–6 months and in fact sleeping through the night (at least 5–6 h). Many babies do not sleep for more than 6 hours at a time at night until later. Infants not sleeping for extended periods of time (5–6 h) at night can have a profound effect on caregivers and can lead to diminished judgment, abuse, and/or neglect. Professionals recommend that parents keep a regular daytime and bedtime routine for babies (e.g., bath, reading a book, etc.); create a comfortable, safe, quiet, and dark space for the child to sleep; be consistent; encourage self-soothing; and acknowledge that there may be setbacks. It is also reassuring for parents to know that babies will eventually sleep through the night.

Toilet training can also be an extremely frustrating experience for parents/caregivers if there is resistance from the child, failure, or regression in toilet training. Parents and caregivers often have expectations for children in terms of when a child *should* achieve a particular developmental task, such as toilet training. When a child does not achieve this task easily and/or promptly, parents can become frustrated. With toilet training failure, children usually resist when parents try to toilet train their child too quickly or in too forceful a manner. Children can become daytime wetters, daytime soilers, or stool holders if the parents continue a harsh approach to toilet training. Children are at risk of becoming injured if parents are forceful in their attempts (e.g., injuries to the genital area, burns). Child development experts recommend that parents assess readiness. Although early toilet training is ideal, child readiness is a more common measure of success than timing (i.e., age). Most children are ready by 24–30 months; however, some children are ready earlier and some later. Parents should be encouraged to help the child practice using the potty, establishing a routine for using the toilet, reward the child for cooperation and success, and respond supportively to accidents.

Other difficult developmental phases include separation anxiety, normal exploratory behavior (approximately 1 year when children begin to walk and explore their surroundings easier but could hurt themselves or become injured if the environment is not safe), normal negativism, and normal poor appetite. People often refer to the "terrible twos" with toddlers who are experiencing a lot of cognitive, physical, and emotional growth. Children begin to communicate verbally during this stage and learn how to respond to others, which is often negatively. The word "no" is many children's first word, and they often respond negatively to requests and other questions at this stage. In response, parents can provide the child with choices to increase the sense of freedom and control (i.e., what they will wear that day, what they want to play with, or eat). Children between the ages of 18 months and 3 years old experience a decrease of appetite in between physical growth spurts. They often prefer one to two meals a day, versus a family's typical four meals a day and tend to eat more at one of those meals. It's important to note that for young children in particular, abuse often occurs when a caregiver or parent has an expectation for how a child should behave and when he/she does not comply or learn quickly enough.

Research Brief

Maltreatment Prevention Through Early Care and Education Programming

Christina Mondi-Rago, PhD.

Child maltreatment most commonly occurs during infancy and early childhood and is overwhelmingly perpetrated by caregivers (AFCARS, 2020). There is a critical need for interventions that will prevent child maltreatment and enhance caregiver capacities, and that can be feasibly implemented at large scales with high-risk populations. *Early care and education (ECE) programs* represent a particularly promising venue for accomplishing these aims. ECE programs offer comprehensive educational and family support services to young children and families in institutional settings (e.g., public schools, childcare centers). Many ECE programs (e.g., Project Head Start, the Child-Parent Center Program) were originally developed during the "War on Poverty" of the 1960s, with the goal of enhancing the well-being and school

(continued)

readiness of low-income children. Decades later, these programs serve millions of young children and families across the country.

A number of studies have reported that ECE program graduates experience lower rates of physical discipline (e.g., spanking) and child maltreatment than children who did not participate in such programming (Love et al., 2005; Magnuson & Waldfogel, 2005; Pratt et al., 2016; Zhai et al., 2013). For example, participation in Early Head Start has been linked to small but significant reductions in child welfare system involvement over time. These long-term impacts appear to be driven by other positive post-program outcomes in the domains of parenting (e.g., emotional responsiveness, warmth, supportiveness), family conflict, and child development (e.g., cognitive and self-regulation skills; Green et al., 2014). Participation in the Child-Parent Center preschool program has also been linked to lower rates of child maltreatment and child welfare system involvement over time. These effects are partially explained by increased parental involvement, reduced school mobility, and increased enrollment in supportive school environments following early intervention (Mersky et al., 2011; Reynolds & Robertson, 2003). Overall, these findings indicate that ECE programs may reduce rates of child maltreatment by increasing parenting skills, enhancing child development, reducing conflict around children's behaviors and academic achievement, and building networks of support for vulnerable families (Klein et al., 2016).

ECE programs hold great promise to reduce rates of child maltreatment; however, there is a critical need to expand access among high-risk populations. According to a recent study, less than one-third of young children (ages 5 and younger) who are under the supervision of the US child welfare system are enrolled in center-based ECE programs. Among child welfare system supervisees, young children with physical abuse histories are half as likely to be enrolled in ECE programs (Klein et al., 2016). Thus, ECE programs should make concerted efforts to recruit and children who are involved in the child welfare system.

Supporting Healthy Parent-Child Relationships

Parenting is a challenging and rewarding. It requires effort and hard work but also provides joy, happiness, and a sense of purpose for many. It is important for child welfare professionals to acknowledge both the challenges and the rewards, as well as the differences in experiences, feelings, and styles of parenting among caregivers and families. By acknowledging and normalizing emotions and thoughts that may differ from what is typically expected of parents allows parents to feel seen, heard, and understood, especially in times of difficulties in their parenting journey. For example, it is common for parents to feel inadequate, disappointed, imperfect at times, or to not feel loved or love for their children or other family members. Some parents feel as though they might be judged if they ask for help or for a break from their daily responsibilities and duties. Some parents feel shame and guilt when they overreact or respond negatively to their child, when this is very common. As child welfare professionals, it is important for us to listen and provide the support caregivers need, while also offering some ideas and advice, as appropriate to help guide toward healthy parent-child interactions and relationships. It is also important to note that these interactions and relationships change over time, particularly through children's developmental stages.

A positive parent-child relationship is important because it nurtures the physical, emotional, and social development of the child. It is a unique bond that involves trust, understanding, and safety. Our knowledge about attachment and bonding tells us that it lays the foundation for the child's personality, life choices, and behaviors. Healthy parent-child relationships help children to exhibit positive and confident social behaviors, improves social and academic skills, and problem-solving skills. There are many ways that parents can form a lasting connection with their children, for example, telling a child "I love you" regularly, in different scenarios, and at every age. Parents can also show their love and care by playing and spending time with their children, being available, eating meals together, and acknowledging their children's individual qualities through one-on-one time. Parents should also be encouraged to care for themselves so that they can be the best parents they are able to be.

Tips for Positive Parenting

Foster warm, loving interactions: Treat every interaction as an opportunity to show love and connect through eye contact, smiles, physical contact, and kind words.

Provide boundaries, rules, and consequences: Ensure consistent and appropriate structure. Communicate expectations and follow-through.

Listen and show understanding and empathy: Teach, model, and acknowledge appropriate emotions. Teach emotional self-regulation and be available when they need a parent.

Model and help with problem-solving: Be a role model for working through difficult times, provide and practice effective problem-solving skills and building solutions.

Note from the Field

Giving Advice to Parents

When I first started my career in child welfare, I was in my mid-20s and I didn't have children. Sure, I had a lot of experience with nieces and nephews and with babysitting, but I had not given birth and not had to parent a child on my own. I remember feeling nervous about giving advice about parenting and worrying that I would inadvertently pass judgment about someone else's parenting. How could I really know what it was like to be a parent? How could I

(continued)

understand how challenging it could be to have enough money and support to provide good care to a child? What I learned over time was that I could learn as much as I could about child development, positive parenting techniques, and community resources available to best support children and their caregivers. By supporting the parents, you could improve outcomes for the kids. Most importantly, I had to listen to the parents, show empathy and understanding, and give them the opportunity to also learn and improve. It takes time to get better and to recover from the trauma often experienced by parents who become involved with the child welfare system. It takes support and guidance, understanding, and compassion. Many of the parents we work with don't have the positive role models in their lives and have to unlearn what they know about parenting and how to show love. Once I prioritized this approach, it didn't matter that I didn't have kids of my own yet. The parents and children I worked with didn't care if I had kids – they just wanted to be heard, respected, and cared for.

Conclusion

Child welfare professionals serve an important role in the lives of children and families. They are often a critical resource when a family is struggling or facing challenges related to child development, parenting, or family roles. Child welfare professionals must have a clear understanding of how families may operate, what healthy and unhealthy child development may look like, parenting styles and behaviors, and how to provide the support and guidance caregivers may need across child development. This knowledge and support can oftentimes ensure safety for children and families during difficult times.

Acknowledgments The authors thank Christina Mondi-Rago, PhD, for the contribution to Chap. 3.

Discussion Questions

1. Why is it important for child welfare professionals to understand stages of child development?
2. What are three healthy discipline techniques?
3. In what ways can a child welfare worker assess parent-child attachment and relationship?
4. At what age are children most at risk for child maltreatment? Why?
5. What are two ways child welfare professionals best support new parents?

Suggested Activities

1. Arrange to spend time with a friend or family member who has young children. If you do not know anyone with young children, consider observing children and

parent interactions in public such as at a grocery store, mall, playground, or public event. Especially when observing in public, remember to respect privacy and to be safe. Observe their interactions (e.g., physical, emotional, verbal) and how the parent meets the child's needs. How do they speak to each other? How do they show affection and emotions?

2. Choose a stage of development (infancy, toddler, pre-school, elementary age, adolescence) and outline the ways they present emotionally, physically, cognitively, and socially. Explain to a friend, peer, or field instructor.

3. Explore early intervention programs in your state and region that promote healthy development for young children. Find pamphlets and/or other forms of media (website, handouts, etc.) that talk about the program's goals and focus. Look for ways they promote family engagement and offer resources. Explore how they address diversity.

4. Read Corr and Santos (2017) and discuss potential barriers to collaboration across child welfare and early intervention systems. Identify reasons why these barriers exist and solutions to reducing any potential barriers.

   Corr, C., & Santos, R. M. (2017). "Not in the same sandbox": Cross-systems collaborations between early intervention and child welfare systems. *Child and Adolescent Social Work Journal, 34*(1), 9–22. (Available: https://rdcu. be/cb8T8).

Additional Resources

Kids Health, A Guide for First-time Parents: https://kidshealth.org/en/parents/ guide-parents.html

Baby Navigator—what every parent needs to know: https://babynavigator.com/

Centers for Disease Control and Prevention, Developmental Milestones: https:// www.cdc.gov/ncbddd/actearly/milestones/index.html

Center on the Developing Child at Harvard University, Applying the Science of Child Development in Child Welfare Systems: https://developingchild.harvard. edu/resources/child-welfare-systems/

Child Welfare Information Gateway, Early Childcare and Childhood Services: https://www.childwelfare.gov/topics/preventing/prevention-programs/ earlychildhood/

Child Welfare Information Gateway, Impact on Child Development: https://www. childwelfare.gov/topics/can/impact/development/

March of Dimes, Caring for your Baby: https://www.marchofdimes.org/baby/ caring-for-your-baby.aspx?gclid=CjwKCAiA-_L9BRBQEiwA-bm5ftrgfobcja_ 76T6MOgXrfBNpiIU1svXcELAH5pMtVPWaa-nbB1u8ShoCVmwQAvD_BwE

National Center on Substance Abuse and Child Welfare, Children and Families Affected by Parental Substance Use Disorder (SUDs): https://ncsacw.samhsa. gov/topics/parental-substance-use-disorder.aspx

References

Ainsworth, M. D., Blehar, M., Waters, E., & Wall, S. (1978). *Patterns of attachment*. Erlbaum.

Allen, A. D., Hyde, J., & Leslie, L. K. (2012). "I don't know what they know": Knowledge transfer in mandated referral from child welfare to early intervention. *Children and Youth Services Review, 34*(5), 1050–1059. https://doi.org/10.1016/j.childyouth.2012.02.008

American Academy of Pediatric Dentistry. (2020). *Oral health policies & recommendations (The reference manual of pediatric dentistry)*. https://www.aapd.org/research/oral-health-policies%2D%2Drecommendations/

American Academy of Pediatrics. (2020). *What's the best way to discipline my child?* https://www.healthychildren.org/English/family-life/family-dynamics/communication-discipline/Pages/Disciplining-Your-Child.aspx

American Academy of Pediatrics. (2018). *AAP schedule of well-child care visits*. https://www.healthychildren.org/English/family-life/health-management/Pages/Well-Child-Care-A-Check-Up-for-Success.aspx

American Optometric Association. (2019). *Championing children's eye care*. https://www.aoa.org/news/inside-optometry/aoa-news/championing-childrens-eye-care?sso=y

Baer, J. C., & Martinez, C. D. (2006). Child maltreatment and insecure attachment: A meta-analysis. *Journal of Reproductive and Infant Psychology, 24*(3), 187–197. https://doi.org/10.1080/02646830600821231

Baumrind, D. (1967). Child-care practices anteceding three patterns of preschool behavior. *Genetic Psychology Monographs, 75*, 43–88.

Belsky, J. (2002). Developmental origins of attachment styles. *Attachment & Human Development, 4*(2), 166–170. https://doi.org/10.1080/14616730210157510

Blaustein, M., & Kinniburgh, K. (2010). Treating traumatic stress in children and adolescents: How to foster resilience through attachment. In *Self-regulation, and competency*. Guilford.

Bowlby, J. (2008). *A secure base: Parent-child attachment and healthy human development*. Basic Books.

Centers for Disease Control and Prevention. (2020). *Concerned about your child's development*. https://www.cdc.gov/ncbddd/actearly/concerned.html

Cicchetti, D., Toth, S. L., & Maughan, A. (2000). *An ecological-transactional model of child maltreatment*. https://doi.org/10.1007/978-1-4615-4163-9_37

Fearon, R. P., Bakermans-Kranenburg, M. J., Van IJzendoorn, M. H., Lapsley, A. M., & Roisman, G. I. (2010). The significance of insecure attachment and disorganization in the development of children's externalizing behavior: A meta-analytic study. *Child Development, 81*(2), 435–456. https://doi.org/10.1111/j.1467-8624.2009.01405.x

Gershoff, E. T. (2008). *Report on physical punishment in the United States: What research tells us about its effects on children*. Center for Effective Discipline.

Green, B. L., Ayoub, C., Bartlett, J. D., Von Ende, A., Furrer, C., Chazan-Cohen, R., et al. (2014). The effect of early head start on child welfare system involvement: A first look at longitudinal child maltreatment outcomes. *Children and Youth Services Review, 42*, 127–135. https://doi.org/10.1016/j.childyouth.2014.03.044

Karp, H. (2015). *The happiest baby on the block; fully revised and updated second edition: The new way to calm crying and help your newborn baby sleep longer*. Bantam.

Klein, S., Merritt, D. H., & Snyder, S. M. (2016). Child welfare supervised children's participation in center-based early care and education. *Children and Youth Services Review, 68*, 80–91. https://doi.org/10.1016/j.childyouth.2016.06.021

Krugman, R. (1993). Child abuse and neglect. *World Health, 46*(1), 22–23. https://doi.org/10.1001/archpedi.1993.02160290023009

Love, J. M., Kisker, E. E., Ross, C., Raikes, H., Constantine, J., Boller, K., et al. (2005). The effectiveness of early head start for 3-year-old children and their parents: Lessons for policy and programs. *Developmental Psychology, 41*(6), 885–901. https://doi.org/10.1037/0012-1649.41.6.885

Maccoby, E. E., & Martin, J. (1983). Socialization in the context of the family: Parent-child interaction. In Mussen (series ed.) & Hetherington (vol. ed.), *Handbook of child psychology: Socialization, personality and social development* (Vol. 4, pp. 1–101).

Magnuson, K. A., & Waldfogel, J. (2005). Preschool child care and parents' use of physical discipline. *Infant and Child Development, 14*(2), 177–198. https://doi.org/10.1002/icd.387

May, P. A., Baete, A., Russo, J., Elliott, A. J., Blankenship, J., Kalberg, W. O., et al. (2014). Prevalence and characteristics of fetal alcohol spectrum disorders. *Pediatrics, 134*(5), 855–866. https://doi.org/10.1542/peds.2013-3319

Menon, M., Katz, R. C., & Easterbrooks, M. A. (2020). Linking attachment and executive function systems: Exploring associations in a sample of children of young mothers. *Journal of Child and Family Studies, 29*(8), 2314–2329. https://doi.org/10.1007/s10826-020-01759-5

Mersky, J. P., Topitzes, J. D., & Reynolds, A. J. (2011). Maltreatment prevention through early childhood intervention: A confirmatory evaluation of the Chicago child-parent center preschool program. *Children and Youth Services Review, 33*(8), 1454–1463. https://doi.org/10.1016/j.childyouth.2011.04.022

Oh, S., Gonzalez, J. M. R., Salas-Wright, C. P., Vaughn, M. G., & DiNitto, D. M. (2017). Prevalence and correlates of alcohol and tobacco use among pregnant women in the United States: Evidence from the NSDUH 2005-2014. *Preventive Medicine, 97*, 93–99. https://doi.org/10.1016/j.ypmed.2017.01.006

Pratt, M. E., Lipscomb, S. T., & Schmitt, S. A. (2016). The effect of head start on parenting outcomes for children living in non-parental care. *Journal of Child and Family Studies, 24*, 2944–2956. https://doi.org/10.1007/s10826-014-0098-y

Reynolds, A. J., & Robertson, D. L. (2003). School-based early intervention and later child maltreatment in the Chicago longitudinal study. *Child Development, 74*(1), 3–26. https://doi.org/10.1111/1467-8624.00518

Schelbe, & Geiger. (2017). *Intergenerational transmission of child maltreatment.* Springer. https://doi.org/10.1007/978-3-319-43824-5

Sege, R. D., & Siegel, B. S. (2018). Effective discipline to raise healthy children. *Pediatrics, 142*(6). https://doi.org/10.1542/peds.2018-3112

Spock, B. (1946). *The common sense book of baby and child care* (pp. 258–259). Duell, Sloan and Pearce.

Stepleton, K., McIntosh, J., & Corrington, B. (2010). *Allied for better outcomes: Child welfare and early childhood.* Center for the Study of Social Policy.

Trickett, P. K., & McBride-Chang, C. (1995). The developmental impact of different forms of child abuse and neglect. *Developmental Review, 15*(3), 311–337. https://doi.org/10.1006/drev.1995.1012

Zhai, F., Waldfogel, J., & Brooks-Gunn, J. (2013). Estimating the effects of head start on parenting and child maltreatment. *Children and Youth Services Review, 35*(7), 1119–1129. https://doi.org/10.1016/j.childyouth.2011.03.008

Zielinski, D. S., & Bradshaw, C. P. (2006). Ecological influences on the sequelae of child maltreatment: A review of the literature. *Child Maltreatment, 11*(1), 49–62. https://doi.org/10.1177/1077559505283591

Chapter 4
Identifying Child Maltreatment

Introduction

Child maltreatment is comprised of multiple types of abuse and neglect. Abuse is purposeful, specific, and repeated mistreatment from a caregiver. Neglect is the failure of a caregiver to meet the child's basic needs, such as food, shelter, security, clothing, and hygiene. Conceptually, the types of maltreatment can be divided into physical abuse, sexual abuse, psychological and emotional abuse, and neglect. The definition of maltreatment within Child Abuse Prevention and Treatment Act (CAPTA) Reauthorization Act of 2010 is "Any recent act or failure to act on the part of a parent or caretaker which results in death, serious physical or emotional harm, sexual abuse or exploitation"; or "An act or failure to act which presents an imminent risk of serious harm."

The key elements of child maltreatment definition include the following: 1) the victim is a child, a person under age 18; 2) the perpetrator is a caregiver who has care, custody, or control of the child; 3) risk of harm must be sufficient; 4) actual harm does not necessarily need to occur; and 5) acts of omission are considered. The legal definitions of maltreatment vary slightly by state. Likewise, research operationalizes maltreatment differently. For example, in some studies maltreatment may be measured by adult retrospectively reporting maltreatment as a child and include any physical punishment including spanking, whereas other research may rely only upon official court records of substantiated maltreatment. These different definitions have implications as they can greatly impact the prevalence of maltreatment. There are calls to think of maltreatment holistically and incorporate more issues of child adversity when addressing maltreatment (e.g., Van Scoyoc et al., 2015). The sections below describe types of maltreatment broadly, although it must be stressed that states have different definitions.

Child maltreatment has a wide range of short- and long-term consequences. These will look different in children across their life span depending on many factors at different levels (i.e., the child, the parent, the family, and the community).

© Springer Nature Switzerland AG 2021
J. M. Geiger, L. Schelbe, *The Handbook on Child Welfare Practice*,
https://doi.org/10.1007/978-3-030-73912-6_4

The various risk and protective factors can help to understand how to work with children and families as well as how to prevent child maltreatment. It is important to remember that both risk and protective factors are not static; child welfare professionals can work with families to reduce risks factors and increase protective factors.

Physical Abuse

About one in five cases reported to child protection services includes physical abuse (US DHHS, 2020). Physical abuse is any non-accidental injury inflicted on a child which causes or poses a substantial risk of death, disfigurement, impairment of physical or emotional health, or loss or impairment of any bodily function. The intent of the caregiver is not considered in the definition of physical abuse. For example, if a caregiver grabs a child's arms forcefully and twists giving the child a spiral fraction in her arm, it is irrelevant if the caregiver intended to break the child's arm. Therefore, excessive corporal punishment may be considered physical abuse. Physical abuse also includes acts of torture where caregivers deliberately and/or systematically inflict cruel or unusual treatment which results in the child's physical or mental suffering.

The lists of activities of injuries resulting from physical maltreatment are practically inexhaustive. Caregivers may physically abuse a child through biting, pinching, hitting, choking, smothering, shaking, throwing, violently pushing, or shoving into fixed objects. Injuries may include bruises, cuts, bites, bone fractures, and burns. One type of injury worth specific mention is abusive head trauma. Fatalities due to abusive head trauma are estimated to be greater than 20%, and two-thirds of survivors experience significant disability (Duhaime, 2008; Chiesa & Duhaime, 2009). Another common cause of fatal child abuse is abdominal injuries, which are most frequently caused by punching or kicking. Female genital mutilation and giving controlled substances are considered physical abuse in some jurisdictions.

Practice Highlight

Factors Related to Increased Concern of Abuse for Fractures
- Absence of credible history explaining fracture
- Child is young age
- Additional injuries in addition to fracture
- Delay in seeking medical treatment
- Caregiver's explanation does not make medical or physical sense
- Specific types of fractures
- Specific fractures raise concern
- Multiple fractures (especially bilaterally)
- Repetitive fractures
- Hands and feet fractures
- Posterior (rear) rib fractures
- Certain clavicle fractures
- Should blade (scapula) fractures
- Fractures in various stages of healing
- Spine fractures
- Breastbone (sternum) fractures
- Skull fractures

Signs and Symptoms of Physical Abuse

There are multiple indicators of physical abuse. The physical indicators include injuries to the child including bruises, lacerations, fractures, burns, head injuries, and internal injuries. While an injury alone is insufficient to determine if maltreatment occurred, there are several things to consider that make the injury more likely to be more non-accidental.

The way that parents present the child's injuries can also be indicative of maltreatment. Delay in treatment is one red flag that the injury may be due to maltreatment. An explanation of what caused the injury that is inconsistent with the injury is another indicator. For example, a parent may say that the child sustained injuries when falling off a bicycle, but the child has bruises on the back of their legs that likely would not have occurred from a bike accident. Likewise, an explanation that is not plausible could raise concerns that a child was abused or neglected. Going back to the parents stating the child was hurt in a bike accident, it may not be plausible for a young child who lacks the motor skills to be on a bicycle. There are specific patterns of bruising that are indicators of maltreatment. Sometimes it is possible to see what caused the bruise as is in the case when an outline of a hand or shoe is

> **Practice Tip: Understanding Non-accidental Bruises**
>
> Bruises are a natural consequence of injury to our body; however, not all are accidental. To determine whether a bruise is accidental is to understand the physical indicators based on several factors such as the age of the child, location of the injury, seriousness of the injury, and the explanation for the injury. Often bruising on an infant who is not ambulatory (not crawling or walking yet), on the posterior side of the body or non-bony areas can be concerning and possibly not accidental. Investigators must look for patterns in bruises – does it reflect an instrument (e.g., iron)? Or does it have a certain color that shows healing?
>
> When dating a bruise, consider the following guidelines (these vary by individual):
>
> Less than 1 day – red, red/blue
> 1–2 days – black/blue to blue/brown, purple
> 3–5 days – yellow/green to brown
> 5–7 days – yellow and fading
> Over one week – yellow/brown and fading

present. Bruises that are bilateral (on both sides of the body) are more likely to be non-accidental. This could be bruises on each arm that come from being forcefully grabbed or on the backs of thighs from being hit with a switch. Injuries on certain parts of the body are more likely to be intentional. For example, bruises on the ear are nearly always intentional due to being struck; a child hitting their head rarely causes bruising to the ears. Another indicator is when there are multiple injuries in various stages of healing.

Behavioral indicators fall into two categories. Children who are physically abused may be extremely passive, accommodating, and engaging in submissive behaviors. Alternatively, children experiencing physical abuse may have notably aggressive behaviors and express hostility toward others. Another indicator of physical abuse is there may be developmental delays in children who have been physically abused.

Practice Tip

Common Indicators Mistaken for Abuse

Coining or Cupping: A common healing remedy used by several Asian cultures. The child's skin is rubbed with a coin or cup, which may be heated that causes blood to rise to the surface and resemble a bruise or burn.

Impetigo: A rash caused by bacteria that forms round, crusted spots that appear typically on hands and face. The rash may resemble cigarette burns; however, impetigo wounds are concave, where cigarette burns are convex.

Sexual Abuse

Approximately 10% of reports to child protective services involve sexual abuse (US DHHS, 2020); however, it is estimated that 1 in 4 girls will be sexually abused before they turn 18 as well as between 1 in 6 or 1 in 13 boys (Finkelhor et al., 1990; Pereda et al., 2009). Sexual abuse includes all sexual contact and activities between an adult responsible for a child and a child. It may include activities of sexual penetration, sexual touching, oral sex, exposure, voyeurism, pornographic photography, or sexual gestures. Sexual abuse can be categorized as sexual battery, sexual molestation, and sexual exploitation.

Sexual battery involves the oral, anal, or vaginal penetration by, or union with, the sexual organ of a child; the forcing or allowing a child to perform oral, anal, or vaginal penetration on another person; or the anal or vaginal penetration of another person by any object. This includes digital penetration, oral sex (cunnilingus, fellatio), coitus, and copulation.

Sexual molestation involves sexual conduct with a child when such contact, touching, or interaction is used for the caregiver's arousal or gratification of sexual needs or desires. Sexual molestation is when either the caregiver or child intentionally touches genitals or intimate parts, including the breasts, genital area, groin, inner thighs, and buttocks, or the clothing covering them. Exceptions are if the touching is considered a normal caregiver responsibility or action or if the touching intended for a valid medical purpose. Thus, changing a diaper would not be considered sexual molestation, although the caregiver is intentionally touching the child's genitals and intimate parts.

Sexual exploitation is the caregiver's sexual use of a child for sexual arousal, gratification, advantage, or profit. It also includes any other sexual acts intentionally conducted in the presence of a child. Commercial sexual exploitation of children

(CSEC), a form of human trafficking, is also considered sexual exploitation, although some states have a separate category for this type of abuse. Chapter 11 provides information about working with children who have experienced human trafficking.

Sexual Abuse Disclosure

A child's disclosure of sexual abuse should be taken seriously, regardless of when and how it is made. Sexual abuse can take place for years before a child discloses. Rarely do children make false disclosures about child sexual abuse. Children may recant their disclosures of sexual abuse. They may do so for various reasons including pressure from the perpetrator or others. They may change their disclosure and say the abuse did not occur because they perceive negative consequences (e.g., a stepfather moving out of the house, not being allowed to spend time with a family member, family members being upset). In many regards, the recanting may be the child's attempt to restore the status quo in the family and return to "normal." Children can be conflicted about sexual abuse because it often occurs in the context of a relationship with someone they care about, and they may enjoy the attention from the perpetrator or the gifts that the perpetrator gives as bribes to keep the secret. A child's recanting of the abuse does not mean that it did not occur.

Understanding Child Sexual Abuse

In most sexual abuse, there is a predictable pattern that involves five stages: engagement, sexual interactions, secrecy, disclosure, and suppression. The initial stage, engagement, is when the perpetrator selects and "grooms" the child. As time progresses, the perpetrator will engage the child in sexual activity, typically starting with a lesser behavior and escalating to a more serious behavior. Once there is sexual behavior, the perpetrator focuses on secrecy and ensuring that the child keeps the activities secret. This allows the sexual abuse to continue. Secrecy can be facilitated through rewards and threats. The period can last for weeks, months, or years. The next stage is disclosure which occurs when either accidentally or intentionally the child or perpetrator lets someone know the sexual activity is occurring. Following disclosure there is often a period of suppression during which time the sexual abuse is minimized or denied. The suppression can be from the perpetrator, the child, or family members. There may be pressure from the perpetrator for the child and family to suppress the information.

Signs and Symptoms of Sexual Abuse

There are multiple indicators of sexual abuse. The physical indicators include the child having a sexually transmitted infection/disease; early, unexplained pregnancy; problems with urination, including bladder or urinary tract infections; painful bowel movements; suspicious stains, blood, or semen on a child's underwear, clothing, or body; and bruising or injuries of the genitals or genital area. Children may also express behavioral indicators including acting out sexually or engaging in sexual activity. They may have knowledge about sex that is inappropriate for their age. Children who are sexually abused may exhibit general indicators of emotional distress and be withdrawn and express a fear of being touched. The psychological indicators of sexual abuse also include low self-esteem, anger, fear, anxiety, and depression.

Emotional Abuse

Approximately 10% of cases reported to child protective services are emotional abuse (US DHHS, 2020), although it is widely understood that there is underreporting of this type of maltreatment. Emotional abuse often occurs with other forms of maltreatment; children who have been physically abused or neglected frequently also experience emotional abuse. Emotional abuse, also called psychological abuse, occurs when the caregiver is belittling, humiliating, rejecting, undermining a child's self-esteem, and generally not creating a positive atmosphere for the child. Emotional abuse falls into several basic categories: spurning, terrorizing, exploiting/corrupting, isolating, and ignoring.

Spurning is a caregiver's verbal and nonverbal acts that reject and degrade a child. This may include belittling, degrading, ridiculing, and other verbal tactics that demean a child. Spurning can occur when a caregiver constantly shames a child or singles the child out to criticize or punish. It also includes humiliating a child in public.

Myths About Emotional Abuse

Children may say, "Sticks and stones may break my bones, but words will never hurt me" in response to name calling and mean things said about them. The thought is pervasive in regard to emotional abuse. However, it is a myth that emotional abuse does not hurt children. Words can hurt.

Attacking a child's self-worth and undermining her through verbal assaults can be damaging. There are many deeply held myths about emotional abuse including the child deserves the verbal abuse because of his behavior, including being noncompliant or disagreeing with the caregiver. This is related to the belief that the abuse only occurs because the caregiver is angry due to the child making him angry.

Emotional abuse extends beyond a pattern of name-calling, belittling, insulting, or criticizing a child. It includes rejecting, isolating, terrorizing, ignoring, corrupting, and over-pressuring a child. It is a myth that emotional abuse is not as bad as hitting a child.

Caregivers terrorize a child through actions or comments that threaten or scare a child. Examples could include caregiver's threats to physically hurt, kill, abandon, or place the child or child's loved ones/objects in recognizable dangerous situations. Terrorizing also includes placing a child in dangerous, unpredictable, or chaotic circumstances or threatening to do so, for example, leaving or threatening to leave a child along the roadside or dangling a child over the edge of a bridge. The threats or actions do not always need to be toward the child as directing the threats or actions toward a loved one (e.g., sibling, parent, friend, pet) or a favorite possession (e.g., toy, doll) can also serve to terrorize a child.

> Emotional abuse can negatively impact a child's development. Research suggests that emotional abuse is as damaging as violent abuse in terms of mental and behavioral health outcomes.
>
> Children who experience emotional abuse may experience negative long-term outcomes including depression, anxiety, low self-esteem, and problems in relationships. Emotional abuse can greatly impact a child even if it does not cause broken bones.

Exploiting or corrupting is when a caregiver encourages or supports the child engaging in illegal or deviant behaviors or developing inappropriate or maladaptive behaviors. The behaviors could include those which are self-destructive, antisocial, criminal, or deviant, for example, prostitution, substance abuse, violence, stealing, or fighting. The caregiver may encourage or support these behaviors through the caregiver's modeling, permitting, or encouraging. Exploiting or corrupting also occurs when a caregiver facilitates developmentally inappropriate behavior (e.g., parentification or infantilization) that is damaging to a child.

Another form of emotional maltreatment is isolation. A caregiver isolates a child through keeping a child away from other appropriate relationships and denying the child opportunities to connect with others outside the home. Isolating may include a caregiver confining a child or restricting the child's movement. It may also include placing rigid limitations on a child's interactions with peers and others in the community.

Ignoring broadly defined is a caregiver denying emotional responsiveness and failing to express affection, caring, and love for the child. It may be a caregiver ignoring the child or pretending the child is not there. The caregiver's failure to respond and detached involvement can be intentional, lack of motivation, or an incapacity.

Signs and Symptoms of Emotional Abuse

Children can have a range of reactions to emotional abuse, and likewise there are a range of signs and symptoms. There interactions with others may be outside typical behaviors; they may be withdrawn and not engage with other or alternatively may desperately seek affection. They may have developmental emotional development and/or act inappropriately emotionally. Children who are emotionally abused may be depressed and have low self-esteem or self-confidence. They may avoid certain settings or interactions. School-aged children who are emotionally abused may perform poorly in school.

Neglect

Approximately 75% of all reports of child maltreatment are neglected (US DHHS, 2020). Other types of abuse may occur with neglect. Sixty-five percent of neglected children suffer from another form of maltreatment, and 45% suffer from three or more forms (US DHHS, 2020). Neglect occurs when a caregiver deprives or fails to provide a child with basic needs. This includes depriving a child of physical, emotional, medical, mental health, or educational needs. Neglect also includes when a caregiver provides inadequate supervision of a child where a child is either unsupervised or under the care of someone unable to supervise due to his or her condition. Neglect can be considered failure to meet "minimal parenting standards" for providing supervision, food, clothing, shelter, medical care, or other basic needs. Neglect consists of caregiver acts of omission, the failure to do something, rather than acts of commission, where caregivers do something. Neglect includes when a child is in an environment that increases the child's likelihood of harm to the health or well-being of the child. It includes physical neglect, inadequate supervision, abandonment, educational neglect, and medical neglect.

Neglect tends to be a persistent chronic condition with families often being referred multiple times to child protection. It does not require a "critical event" to be present even though a "critical event" usually triggers a report and investigation. Repetitive "subthreshold events" may harm a child more than isolated "critical events." A critical event could be a toddler found wandering in the street wearing only a diaper that needed to be changed. Prior to this critical event, the child may have been routinely experiencing subthreshold events in the home such as not having their diaper changed, not being adequately fed, not being supervised. These ongoing subthreshold events may not have been known to others as the toddler was in the home and not visible to others; however, the impact of the neglect remains the same.

Poverty or Neglect?

Consider the following examples that Jerry Milner, the Associate Commissioner at the Children's Bureau, and David Kelly (2020) present:

- "The children of a young, single mother were removed solely due to an eviction. She had hoped that the system would rally to help her find decent, safe housing only to be told 'you must comply with this or that in your case plan in order to regain custody.'"
- "Parents were required to pay for certain services or drug testing they could not afford and had that inability to pay used against them as failure to comply with a case plan, preventing them from regaining custody of their children."

In these cases, the parents' lack of resources interfered with their ability to meet the goals of the case plan. Poverty was the underlying reason that the children were removed from their parents' care and contributed to their remaining in out-of-home placement.

Consider how the following examples compare to those above:

- "A judge ordered a child welfare agency to pay for a necessary repair to a septic tank that would otherwise leave a home uninhabitable and a family separated."
- "A parent attorney successfully argued that supplemental security income death and disability payments be made to a mother positioning herself for reunification instead of the child welfare agency so that she would not lose her apartment."
- "A community adoption agency took on the prevention mantle by rallying around a family at risk of losing its children by lining up safe child care, bringing meals to the family, and securing rent to head off an impending eviction."

In these examples, there is a recognition that helping parents address poverty-related needs, it may be possible to help reduce child welfare system involvement and if (and how long) children are in out-of-home placements. The issue of housing is paramount, and child welfare should collaborate with programs addressing family housing stability (e.g., Gubits et al., 2018).

Milner and Kelly (2020) conclude, "If we truly care about children and families, it's time to stop confusing poverty with neglect and devote ourselves to doing something about it."

Neglect can be either situational or chronic. In situational situations, the caregiver fundamentally can provide and care for the child yet due to temporary circumstances is unable to, in many cases due to being overwhelmed. This could be due to a divorce, death, disability, or other set of conditions that interfere with the caregiver providing for the child. In chronic neglect, there are enduring issues where the parent has serious and continuous difficulties that interfere with providing for a child. There may be ongoing issues related to substance misuse, mental health, or cognitive ability issues that contribute to the caregiver not providing for the child. With situational neglect, short-term interventions may be adequate for ensuring the neglect ends, and the caregiver can provide for the child. With chronic neglect, longer interventions may be necessary to change the complex issues that are contributing to the neglect.

Most children who live in poverty are not neglected; however, neglect is strongly associated with poverty. Children who live in homes where there is low income, unemployment, use of public assistance, or housing instability are more likely to experience neglect. A recent study found that children living in households that file for a foreclosure have a higher probability of being involved in the child welfare system (Berger et al., 2015). In addition to these family-level economic risks, neglect is also associated with neighborhood poverty and higher neighborhood rate of unemployment (Morris et al., 2019) meaning a child living in a neighborhood with high levels of poverty is at risk for maltreatment. The contexts of neighborhoods are associated with parenting practices; lower affluence is associated with more parental aggression (Shuey & Leventhal, 2017). Social cohesion within a neighborhood is also related to neglect (Maguire-Jack & Showalter, 2016).

The risks and dangers of neglect have frequently been minimized and over-looked, yet it is a serious form of maltreatment. Indeed, the long-term outcomes of neglect are more severe than other types of maltreatment. There are multiple risks of harm associated with neglect. There are increased risks of physical injury and poisoning due to inadequate supervision. Children who are neglected may have health problems due to untreated medical issues. This is not surprising due to family instability being associated with poorer children's health (Smith et al., 2017). They may also experience cognitive and psychosocial developmental delays due to their environment. Annually many child fatalities related to neglect occur due to drowning and unsafe sleeping. There is a need to better understand how best to address neglect and understand the macro-level forces that contribute to it (Bullinger, Feely, Raissian, & Schneider, 2019).

Physical neglect is the caregiver's failure to protect from harm or danger and provide for the child's basic physical needs, including shelter, food, and clothing. Physical neglect excludes these failures caused primarily by financial inability unless relief services had been offered and refused. A child experiences physical neglect when their caregiver does not provide a safe environment that is free from violence and hazards, for example, a young child living in a home where there is a swimming pool without any fencing preventing the child's access or a home environment where a child is exposed to dangerous toxins. It could also be a home that is unhygienic and has feces or trash throughout the house. Physical neglect is the most widely recognized and commonly identified form of neglect.

Inadequate supervision refers to situations in which the child is without a caretaker or caretaker is inattentive or unsuitable and the child is in danger of harming self or others. It includes placing a child or failing to remove a child from a situation that requires judgment or actions beyond the child's level of maturity, and that results in bodily injury or a substantial risk of immediate harm. As such, the child's maturity and ability to respond to a crisis are relevant. The lack of supervision can occur due to different circumstances. For example, the parent could be physically absent because of working and leaving a child who is too young to care for themselves home alone. Alternatively, the parent could be in the home but not able to appropriately supervise because of their substance abuse. For example, they could be using substances or hung over and not attending to the child's needs.

Abandonment is when a caregiver leaves a child in a situation where the child would be exposed to a substantial risk of physical or mental harm, without arranging for necessary care for the child, and demonstrates an intention not to return. It should be noted that some states have "safe-haven" laws that allow a parent to surrender an infant at certain places (i.e., hospitals, police station, or fire station) sometimes referred to as "safe surrender sites." In most laws, there is an age limit for the child to be surrendered. In these states, a parent surrenders their child who is under the age limit outlined in the statute at a safe surrender site would not be considered as having abandoned their child by state policies.

Educational neglect is when a parent fails to provide a child with access to education. This could include not enrolling a child in school, allowing a child to go to school or not facilitating the child's attendance at school when children are younger. Caregivers may not want their child to attend school because the child could report the abuse or neglect experienced at home. Educational neglect can occur in the homeschool settings when the caregiver fails to meet the standards set by the state. Educational neglect can also include a caregiver not addressing the educational issues or needs of a child. For example, a caregiver of a child who has been diagnosed with a learning disorder refuses to have the child receive treatment recommended by professionals.

Medical neglect occurs when a parent or caregiver who does not ensure a child receives necessary medical care, especially when it is needed to treat a serious illness or injury, such that the child is a risk for death, injury, or disfigurement or the child's development and functioning will be impaired. The caregiver may refuse to have the child receive treatment or may ignore medical recommendations for treatment. Examples include a caregiver not following physician orders for a child to undergo chemotherapy, a caregiver not giving the child with diabetes the needed insulin, or a caregiver not taking a child in need of medical attention to see a healthcare provider. Some definitions of medical neglect also include meeting the mental health needs of a child and withholding necessary mental health treatment falls into the category of medical neglect.

Signs and Symptoms of Neglect

There are multiple indicators of neglect. Children who are neglected may be unresponsive and uninterested in their surroundings. They may have difficulty relating to others. They may not interact with others and when they do may be withdrawn. Conversely, some children who experience neglect may be aggressive and have temper tantrums. Due to not having a caregiver provide limits and boundaries, a child may exhibit "out of control" behavior. A child may be unable to concentrate and appear to be hyperactive with a short attention span. The child may engage in various behavior problems and display signs of anxiety and emotional distress. Additionally, physical indicators of stress, such as physical illness or regressive behaviors, may be present in children who are neglected.

In homes where neglect is present, some children assume adult roles and responsibilities related to caring for themselves and siblings. In this role reversal, the child may take on a parent role in the family, where the child rather than the parent is making adult decisions and responsible for the household, including caring for the parent. This is called parentification. A child experiencing neglect may feel responsible for the parent, although in some cases, a child may express fear of the parent. Neglect may cause children to be hungry. To try to feed themselves, older children may steal food or hoard food. As children may have a hard time concentrating and engaging, children may not do well in school.

Children who are neglected may experience physical health or mental health issues. They may have problems in school, which may stem from not attending school or not being able to focus while in school due to a range of issues (e.g., having poor nutrition impacting their ability to think, living in a chaotic home environment which disrupts sleep, not having an adult enforce a bedtime, having responsibilities to care for younger siblings, or having developmental delays cognitively which impacts learning). Children who are neglected may have mental health problems or emotional and behavioral problems. They may be withdrawn or act out. They may have problems connecting with peers and adults. Children who are neglected may not be properly supervised and may live in an environment where there are hazards and problems with sanitation. Children may have poor personal hygiene and be unbathed. They may wear clothing that is dirty or inappropriate for the season. Children may exhibit signs of hunger.

Practice Highlight

How Do Doctors Decide if the Injury Was due to Maltreatment?

Doctors conduct a physical exanimation and may run labs and testing (e.g., blood work, MRI, X-rays). They will talk with the caregivers and child. They rely on their medical training and take multiple factors into consideration including:

- Age and developmental status of the child
- Caregiver's presentation of the child's medical history
- Changes in report or history provided by caregivers
- Inconsistencies among information provided by caregivers
- Social context where injury occurred
- Likely biases and motivations of witnesses
- Likelihood the injuries could be accidental
- Investigation conducted by CPS and law enforcement

Polyvictimization

Approximately 15.5% of children who experience abuse and neglect experience two or more types of child maltreatment (U.S. DHHS, 2020). David Finkelhor and colleagues at the Crimes Against Children Research Center (CCRC) have conducted numerous studies to understand the pathways, consequences, and prevalence of violence against children, including maltreatment. Studies have shown that victims of polyvictimization or multiple forms of violence are often more symptomatic than those who experience one type of abuse (Finkelhor et al., 2007). Research using the Developmental Victimization Survey (DVS), a 3-wave longitudinal study of children in the United States showed that 59% of polyvictims were abused by family and non-family members, 50% were abused by adults and peers, and 40% were sexually abused (Finkelhor et al., 2009). Further examination showed that several risk factors predisposed children to polyvictimization, including living in a dangerous community, residing with family experiencing a higher level of violence and conflict, and families that were experiencing issues such as unemployment, financial problems, and substance abuse (Finkelhor et al., 2009). Polyvictims are also overrepresented among certain groups, including boys, African American children, and children in single-parent, stepparent, and other adult caregiver families. As described throughout this chapter, different forms of maltreatment can elicit similar and different manifestations in symptomology among children. Knowledge about the potential for increased symptomology among children who experience multiple forms of violence points to the importance of intervention from professionals in schools, child welfare systems, and the community to be aware of the individual and collective impact of maltreatment experiences.

Research Brief

Implementation Science for Child Welfare
Leah Bartley, PhD.

As child welfare professionals consider the best approaches for working with a child, family, or focus population, they often consider the evidence behind an intervention or approach. Evidence-based practice in child welfare requires the combination of best research evidence, best clinical experience, and alignment with a child's or family's values and assets (IOM, 2001). We cannot underestimate the importance of a match between an evidence-based program's intention and the unique needs and assets of the families and communities we serve. But focusing solely on the program or best intervention will not lead to the positive and improved outcomes we hope to achieve; it requires care and attention to the program's implementation and the context in which it is implemented (Metz & Bartley, 2012; Mildon & Shlonsky, 2011).

The field of implementation science studies the "methods to promote the systematic uptake of research findings and other evidence-based program into routine practice…" (Eccles & Mittman, 2006, p. 1), and the fundamental goal of implementation science is to integrate research and practice in way that improve outcomes (Estabrooks et al., 2018). Implementation science includes both research and practice; implementation research aims at identifying what approaches work best in translating research into practice settings and implementation practice aims at adapting and applying implementation strategies based on the context and settings to achieve and sustain positive outcomes (Ramaswamy et al., 2019).

There are key concepts that have emerged from implementation science. Implementation frameworks are organizing models that detail factors likely to influence the implementation process (Nilsen, 2015). Common components

(continued)

across frameworks include recognizing the developmental or phased process of implementation, identifying needs and understanding current practice, assessing evidence and fit of a potential outcome, and considering relevant implementation outcomes (Meyers et al., 2012). An implementation strategy is a systematic process to adopt and integrate evidence-based programs into the real world (Powell et al., 2012). Strategies can represent discrete (i.e., a single strategy, such as supervision) multifaceted (i.e., combination of more than one strategy, such as training and knowledge assessments) and blended (i.e., comprehensive and multilevel, such as community development teams that lead implementation overtime). Practitioners and leaders can use implementation frameworks to consider what strategies (e.g., coaching or learning communities) to use when considering implementation of evidence-based programs. They can also use frameworks to identify structures such as teams or leader groups to support implementation. They can also use frameworks to consider relevant stage-based activities and identify the appropriate outputs and outcomes that are developmentally appropriate for the given implementation phase (Birken et al., 2018).

There are also emerging competencies for implementation science researchers and practitioners. Researcher competencies focus on the knowledge and skills required to carrying out rigorous dissemination and implementation research and include activities such as identify and apply implementation theories and approaches or identify and describe practice-based considerations (Padek et al., 2015). Implementation practitioner competencies reflect the skills and abilities of those developing the capacity of practitioners and organizations to effectively use and integrate evidence-based programs. Implementation practitioner competencies may include skills and knowledge related to co-creation, ongoing improvement, and sustaining change (Metz et al., 2020). Implementation science offers child welfare professionals the strategies and potential to ensure programs meet the needs of vulnerable children and families so that ultimately they benefit.

Understanding Maltreatment

While a lot is known about maltreatment, the etiology—what causes maltreatment—remains unclear. Research has yet to pinpoint the mechanisms that lead to abuse and neglect, although risk factors and protective factors have been identified.

Risk Factors

Risk factors for child maltreatment occur at the individual, family, and community level. These risk factors often occur together. See Fig. 4.1 for visual representation of the relationship among levels of risk factors. Even in the presence of multiple risk

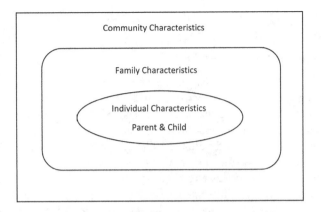

Fig. 4.1 Risk factors may be at individual, family, and community levels

factors, maltreatment may not occur; risk factors may increase the likelihood of maltreatment, yet they are not deterministic. Risk factors can be present without maltreatment occurring. Nor are risk factors fixed; characteristics can change over time, often with interventions. Additionally, protective factors can buffer or mitigate the risks present.

At the individual level, there are characteristics of the child as well as the parent that function as risk factors. It must be stressed that though there are child characteristics that increase the risk for maltreatment, children are never to be blamed for causing maltreatment. Children do not cause abuse or neglect. There are several characteristics of children that make them more vulnerable to child maltreatment including their age and having a disability or medical needs. Young children are more at risk for child maltreatment due to their inability to care for themselves, developmental stages that are stressors to parents, as well as the fact that young children may be out of the public's view as they are not in school. Most children entering child welfare are ages 0–5. Children younger than 1 year have the highest rates of victimization. The majority of child fatalities occur in children under the age of 3. Children with disabilities are more likely to experience maltreatment as well.

There are a range of parental characteristics that are risk factors. Parental substance misuse and mental illness are two risk factors commonly associated with child maltreatment. Parental substance misuse can interfere with a parent's ability to care for a child and provide a safe environment. The use of drugs and alcohol can negatively impact a parent's decision-making and lower inhibition. The money and time that is spent to obtain and use the substances can also create circumstances where children are neglected and placed in dangerous situations, including being unsupervised. The presence of drugs and alcohol also can be dangerous, especially with young children who could ingest substances that are poisonous.

Practice Highlight

Understanding Surveillance Bias

Kaela[1] was in foster care when she became pregnant. After giving birth, her foster mom helped her raise her son. Kaela loved her son deeply and was committed to give him the life that she never had. She wanted him to be able to have a stable life, full of opportunities, and above all, she desired for him never to be involved with the child welfare system. Kaela often felt her foster mom and caseworker did not think that she was a good parent. As she approached age 18 and was eligible to leave foster care, she was torn about what to do. If she went into extended foster care, she would be able to continue living with her foster mom and have some support from the foster care system including get a clothing allotment, a monthly bus pass, and a stipend to continue her education. However, staying in care also meant that she would not be completely autonomous because she would still have a caseworker, whom was critical of her parenting her son. Ultimately, Kaela decided that she would prefer to be on her own as she was concerned that if she stayed in foster care, her caseworker would have her son taken away from her. At age 18, Kaela left foster care with her young son and moved in with one of her aunts. After a conflict arose, she moved among other family members. Despite being homeless, Kaela attempted to go to school so she could get a better paying job. A few months after leaving foster care, Kaela was reported to child protective services. She suspected that it was her caseworker or former foster mom who made the report, which she felt was punishment for her leaving care when they had wanted her to go into extended foster care. Kaela's son was placed in foster care with her former foster mom. While she never used the term "surveillance bias," Kaela vehemently felt that had she never been in foster care or if she had stayed in extended foster care, she would have never been reported to child protective services.

---

[1] All names and other personal identifiers in cases and examples throughout this book have been changed to protect privacy and confidentiality.

Research on the role of parental mental illness in causing child maltreatment is inconclusive, although it is seen as a risk factor. The strongest evidence exists that maternal depression contributes to child maltreatment. Early childbearing is a known risk factor for maltreatment; young parents are more likely to abuse or neglect their children. A parental history of child maltreatment is another risk factor for maltreatment. While it is widely believed that parents who abuse or neglect their children were always abused or neglected as children, research has found this not to be the case (e.g., Thornberry et al., 2012; Stith et al., 2009), although a recent study found that a maternal history of child maltreatment was associated with increased risks of child maltreatment, especially when the mother experienced multiple types of child maltreatment (Bartlett et al., 2017). It must be stressed that most children who were maltreated do not grow up and maltreat their children. Having experienced maltreatment is a risk factor, but it is not inevitable that someone who was abused or neglected will continue the cycle of violence when they have children.

The context of the family plays a role in child maltreatment. There are multiple family characteristics that are risk factors for child maltreatment. The presence of intimate partner violence increases the likelihood of a child being abused or neglected.

It should be noted that witnessing intimate partner violence is also considered a form of maltreatment in some states. Poverty is another family-level risk factor. Children who live in low socioeconomic status household experience higher rates of child maltreatment. As described below, some of this may be related to surveillance biases. The relationship between poverty and maltreatment is complicated as both share multiple risk factors. It is further complicated as both can be intergenerational (e.g., Robertson & O'Brien, 2018). Housing insecurity (Warren & Font, 2015) and economic insecurity (e.g., income losses, housing hardship, and cumulative material hardship) have been found as a predictor of child maltreatment (Conrad-Hiebner & Byram, 2020). Job loss in economically disadvantaged communities is associated with reports for child maltreatment (Schenck-Fontaine et al., 2017). Thus, providing concrete economic supports may be an effective strategy in decreasing child maltreatment (Rostad et al., 2017). When a family has high levels of social isolation, there is a great risk of child maltreatment. Family structure has been identified as important in understanding child maltreatment. Children in households categorized as single parent headed or households with nonbiological parents (e.g., stepparents, paramours) experience higher rates of child maltreatment. There are lower rates of child maltreatment within households with two biological parents present.

Child maltreatment can occur in any community, yet there are some communities where it is more prevalent. Some of this may be due to surveillance bias, which means that there is a higher likelihood of something being detected because of observation or surveillance. In child welfare, there are concerns that surveillance bias occurs in some neighborhoods, specifically lower-income neighborhoods, because families are receiving public assistance or because there are more social service providers who make more reports to child protective services. Neighborhoods where there are higher rates of poverty and unemployment can be considered a risk factor for maltreatment (Morris et al., 2019). Likewise, there is a relationship between child maltreatment reports and eviction; as eviction notices increase in a neighborhood, reports of child maltreatment increase (Bullinger & Fong, 2020). Lower social capital in neighborhoods appears to be related to child maltreatment (Abner, 2014).

Protective Factors

The presence of protective factors can mitigate negative effects of risk factors, disrupt the cumulative effect of risk factors, and avoid the consequence of risk factors. Protective factors reduce the risk of maltreatment and increase child and family well-being. The five protective factors at the family level that the Center for the Study of Social Policy identified through a rigorous process including a review of research are referred to as "Strengthening Families" and include the following: parental resilience, social connections, concrete support in times of need, knowledge of parenting and child development, and social and emotional competence of children (Center for the Study of Social Policy, n.d.). (See Chap. 7 for details about Strengthening Families.) Parental resilience is the ability for a parent to "bounce back" from challenges. Those with higher resilience can problem solve and build relationships with others. Social connection is the connection with others (e.g., family, friends, community members) who can provide support through giving advice or tangible assistance. Positive friendships, connections, and networks are important to the protective factor of concrete support in times of need. This factor is based on a family's ability to meet basic living needs (i.e., food, clothing, shelter), and if there is a crisis, the family can access services to avoid a disruption in their needs being met. Knowledge of parenting and child development is when parents have accurate information about their children's behaviors and needs at each age and promote their children's well-being and development. Social and emotional competence of children is when children communicate emotions effectively, interact positively with others, and self-regulate.

Protective factors strengthen family and can be integrated into work with all families in various ways. Most states in the United States use a Strengthening Families framework to prevent abuse and neglect. It is important to note that there are other models based on protective factors that also are used throughout the country. For example, the Essentials for Childhood, developed by the CDC, focuses on safe, stable, and nurturing relationships and environments (CDC, 2014). More information about Essentials for Childhood is provided in Chap. 7. The Administration on Children, Youth and Families identified protective factors based on research for specific populations they serve (e.g., youth in or aging out of foster care, children exposed to domestic violence, victims of child maltreatment, pregnant and parenting youth, and runaway and homeless youth; Development Services Group 2013). These models of protective factors incorporate individual- and community-level factors that can contribute to reducing child maltreatment.

Research Brief

Youth in Care with Disabilities

Leah Cheatham, PhD, JD

Youth with disabilities are notably overrepresented within the child welfare system. Estimates suggest that over half of youth in the child welfare system carry a physical, cognitive, or emotional disability diagnosis (Slayter, 2016) — a rate of disability *five times higher* than within the general population (Brault, 2012). Yet, understanding the reason for this overrepresentation is complicated. Some suggest youth with disabilities are at increased risk for abuse and neglect (Sullivan & Knutson, 2000), while others point out that the experiences of abuse and neglect leading youth into the child welfare system may impose serious challenges to their mental health (Salazar et al., 2013), increasing the likelihood that youth will experience mental health disability during or after their time in care. Both propositions may, unfortunately, be correct.

Further complicating this issue is the fact that many youth with disabilities in the child welfare system carry more than one disability diagnosis. Complex medical diagnoses, which often include emotional challenges, require specialized care and can pose a barrier to youth achieving permanency within the child welfare system. Hence, many youth with disabilities find themselves among those "aging out" of the foster care system. While many youth aging out of foster care face challenges during the transition to adulthood (e.g., Okpych et al., 2017), youth aging out with disabilities—particularly emotional disabilities—are less likely to be successful during this transition period than their peers without disabilities (Cheatham et al., 2020).

Given the challenges faced by youth with disabilities in the child welfare system (and beyond), it is imperative that child welfare practitioners develop competencies to support youth with disabilities. These competencies could include developing familiarity with federal laws protecting the rights and opportunities of youth with disabilities (e.g., IDEIA, 2004 & Section 504 of the Rehabilitation Act, 1973); understanding and applying principles of trauma-informed care; and gaining comfort coordinating with parents, teachers, and other support systems to make needed accommodations for youth with disabilities during their time in care. Through continued attention to the needs of this sizeable population, we can ensure that all child welfare-involved youth, regardless of disability diagnoses, have the ability to thrive.

Consequences of Maltreatment

Maltreatment has both short- and long-term consequences for children. Consequences fall within the categories of development, health, mental health, and behaviors and can vary with the different types of maltreatment. Maltreatment is a form of trauma or toxic stress that is often chronic. It can impact a child's neurobiology. Specifically, the brain structure and functioning can be changed (e.g., Gold et al., 2016; Xerxa et al., 2020). A recent study demonstrated that child maltreatment can impact the prefrontal lobe of the brain (Jedd et al., 2015), and the changes can continue through adolescence (Hein et al., 2020). Childhood violence exposure and social deprivation are linked to adolescent threat and reward neural function. Likewise, gene expression can change. The entire nervous system can be put in a state of overdrive with high levels of cortisol release. The allostatic load of a child who is maltreated is frequently increased. With the elevated stress, the body's stress response system goes into overdrive. The higher levels of stress-related chemicals flooding the body impact children in both the short and long term.

Research has clearly identified that child maltreatment can impact children's behaviors, health, and well-being in the short term. For example, it may be related to experiencing bullying (Kennedy, 2018). While there is a significant amount of knowledge about this, new ideas and the mechanisms are still being explored. For example, an innovative recent study looked at sleep in children who had been maltreated and found that less sleep predicted increased internalizing and externalizing behaviors (e.g., Zajac et al., 2020).

Long-term child maltreatment increases the likelihood of chronic disease and various other issues including mental health problems and substance misuse. With mental health, there are countless studies looking at the impact of childhood maltreatment. For example, a recent systematic review of 35 studies found child maltreatment predicted perinatal depression as well as post-traumatic stress disorder, both of which can be considered risk factors for child maltreatment (Choi & Sikkema, 2016). Child maltreatment is also a predictor of intimate partner violence (e.g., Street, 2015). These long-term outcomes highlight how consequences of maltreatment potentially can span generations.

Factors that influence the consequence of maltreatment include severity, frequency, duration, and timing of the maltreatment. Maltreatment that is more severe, frequent, and lasts for a longer period of time has been found to have more damaging results on children both in the short and long term. For example, greater severity of child abuse has been found to be related to more PTSD symptomology, and higher levels of attachment anxiety and attachment avoidance (Busuito et al., 2014). When maltreatment occurs in a developmental period also affects the consequences. Maltreatment in early childhood during the critical periods of brain development can have serious consequences. See Chap. 5 about the negative consequences of adverse childhood experiences broadly on development and well-being. Children under the age of 3 may be most susceptible to maltreatment both from a developmental perspective because of the critical developmental period and their vulnerability as they are unable to care for themselves. Additionally, the reality that young children may be absent from the public eye and maltreatment may occur longer as it is not coming to the attention of authorities. There are also differences in the consequences by maltreatment type. Of all the types of maltreatment, the long-term consequences of neglect are the most severe.

Consequences of Physical Abuse

The short-term consequences of physical abuse are evident in physical injuries as well as emotional and behavioral issues. However, physical abuse can have long-term consequences. Specifically, abuse can result in physical disabilities. For example, a head injury could cause permanent cognitive damage, or an injury to the spine could cause paralysis. In addition to the physical consequences, those who have experienced physical maltreatment may have problems with relationships in the future, specifically around trusting others or intimate partner violence. Another long-term consequence is drug and alcohol use and potentially mental health concerns such as depression or low self-esteem.

Consequences of Sexual Abuse

Children who have experienced sexual abuse may experience a range of negative outcomes. They may engage in problematic sexual behavior. In the long term, children who were sexually abused may have mental health problems including depression and anxiety. They may experience feelings of guilt, shame, and self-blame and often experience dissociation or repression of the memories. They may have eating disorders. Children who experienced sexual abuse may have sexual problems and problems with intimacy and relationships. Survivors of sexual abuse may experience difficulty in establishing and maintaining interpersonal relationships due to issues related to trust, fear of intimacy, fear of being different, establishing healthy boundaries, or becoming involved with abusive relationships.

Note from the Field

Familial Consequences After Child Sexual Abuse

Kesha was sexually abused by her father and reported the abuse to her teacher. During the investigation and after the abuse was substantiated, the child welfare agency required her father to move out of the home. A criminal investigation was also underway. Kesha's mother had a difficult time believing what her daughter had reported. During her therapy sessions, Kesha also disclosed that her teenage brother had also been sexually abusing her for some time. Her mother was then asked to decide whether her son or her daughter would move so that they could be separated and receive treatment. She asked that Kesha be placed in foster care during the case. Her mother continued to deny the abuse and refuse any treatment. Kesha struggled emotionally and behaviorally. She had a hard time focusing in school and just wanted to go home. She could not understand why her brother could stay at home and that she had to leave. Her mother continued to refuse treatment and refuse to comply with the child welfare agency. Her brother was mandated to receive treatment, and her father was charged with sexual abuse and was incarcerated. Therapists had a very difficult time engaging Kesha's mother in family therapy, which was so desperately needed to begin to heal this family. This case illustrates how damaging not only the abuse experienced can be but also how complex and challenging the associated emotions, family ties, and relationships can be when sexual abuse occurs within a family.

Consequences of Emotional Abuse

Consequences of emotional abuse span a child's physical, behavioral, emotional, developmental domains. Emotional or psychological abuse may be seen by some as insignificant, but it has serious consequences. The saying "sticks and stones may break my bones, but names will never hurt me" is wrong. Being called names and other forms of emotional abuse can be damaging to children. The short- and long-term consequences of emotional abuse are significant and lasting. Children who were emotionally abused may experience mental health problems such as depression and anxiety and may have low self-esteem. Research has found that women who experienced emotional abuse may have prolonged emotional arousal and poor physiological regulation of emotion (Bernstein et al., 2013). Children who experience emotional abuse also may have problematic relationships and a difficulty expressing empathy.

Consequences of Neglect

Neglected children often experience worse outcomes than physically or sexually abused children over a range of developmental, psychological, and physical parameters. Many child fatalities due to maltreatment are the result of neglect. Specifically, deaths may be related to inadequate supervision where a child dies due to something that could have been avoided (e.g., drowning, poisoning, falling). They may also die because of being in a hazardous environment (e.g., drugs, unhygienic environment). Especially for young children, failure to thrive could be a cause of death related to neglect as well. Failure to thrive is a serious medical condition where a child does not grow as she or he should. The insufficient weight gain or inappropriate weight loss is accompanied with delayed development. For infants, failure to thrive is associated with chronic neglect.

Neglect impacts brain development. Of great concern is when neglect occurs early in a child's life. As much of brain development happens in the first 3 years of a child's life, neglect during this time can be especially damaging. Neglect can cause developmental and cognitive delays. The lack of adequate nutrition and stimulation within the environment can stunt multiple types of child's development. Children who are neglected are often smaller in size and have poorer motor skills and language delays. They may have poor social skills, passive, and a lack of emotions.

Neglect has different impacts with children of different developmental periods, and it can be especially harmful to young children. Children who are neglected may not have attachment to caregivers and may develop anxious, insecure attachments in other relationships. With attachment issues, children may be less likely to explore their environment, which is central to their development, and development of self-efficacy. Thus, children may experience problems with brain, motor, and physical development. Other effects include serious health problems and malnutrition. Toddlers who experience neglect may have impaired cognitive and physical development. They may experience malnutrition and significant health problems. Behaviorally, toddlers may be withdrawn and passive. They may have limited coping skills where they become easily frustrated and angry. They may be noncompliant and undisciplined. They may also indiscriminately seek attention and affection from adults.

Neglect impacts older children as well. School-aged children may experience multiple various types of consequences of neglect. Like younger children, they may experience developmental delays and health problems as well as attachment problems. They may have delayed or impaired speech and have significant learning deficits and delays. Related to this is children may have problems concentrating and limited curiosity. Children experiencing neglect may be severely withdrawn or may act out violently. They often have low self-esteem. Neglected adolescents may exhibit low self-esteem and are at high risk for truancy, running away, and substance use. They may work and learn at levels below average and have poor attendance at school.

Note from the Field

Why Lack of Supervision is so Dangerous

When I worked in child welfare, methamphetamine abuse was rampant where I lived. If I could guess, meth abuse by parents was the most common reason a child was removed from their parent's care. It wasn't always a case of a parent using drugs in the same room as their child or using meth during pregnancy, or living in a home where meth was being manufactured (all of which are dangerous, of course), but parents leaving their kids unattended (physically, by leaving them alone) or by being high and unaware of the child's needs and safety. When approached, most parents would argue that their drug use was not harming their children because they were using in another room or going to a friend's house to use substances or drink alcohol. What was occurring was that young children were put at risk because they were unsupervised. There were cases of children not being fed, diapers not being changed, dirty homes, and lack of clothing. There were also situations where young children were left alone at home or left under the care of others who abused or also neglected the child. I saw babies abandoned minutes after their birth because their mother needed to leave the hospital to use again. I saw families broken because of the addictive nature of drugs and alcohol.

One case I remember clearly was the case of Angela, a 3-year-old toddler who was left alone at the motel where they were staying while her biological mother went to use meth with her neighbor. The motel was located on a busy street only a few hundred yards from a freeway entrance. It is unknown how long the toddler was left alone, but she was able to open the front door and climb down the stairs. She made her way to the busy street and walked along until she almost reached the freeway. A motorist about to enter the freeway saw the child on the side of the road with only a shirt and a diaper on and pulled over to see where her caregiver might be. It was amazing that she had not been struck by a car or stepped on something sharp.

Another case involved a 5-year-old child who walked out the back door and climbed the gate to the pool at the apartment complex where the family lived. He did not know how to swim but wanted to get in the pool. When his brother went to look for him to play, he noticed a splash in the water and screamed for help. He couldn't get in to the pool area, but a neighbor heard him and rushed over to help.

Neglect can have serious long-term effects in adolescence and adulthood. In adolescence, there may be engagement in non-prosocial behavior such as delinquent behavior, crime, violence, and drug use and abuse. Adolescents may have academic issues including poor performance, truancy, suspension, and not graduating. The problems may continue into adulthood with increased criminal behavior and lower occupational levels. Likewise, adults may have ongoing issues with criminal behaviors and lower occupational levels. They may also have cognitive issues with lower IQ and reading problems.

Multiple factors influence the severity of the impact of neglect. The age at which the neglect occurs can influence the extent to which a child is impacted. Neglect in early childhood is the most damaging, as children at that age are unable to care for themselves. When neglect occurs in infancy, children are especially at risk for death and serious consequences. The length of time that the neglect occurred as well as the frequency of the neglect occurred are also factors which influence the impact of neglect on children, with longer periods of time and more frequent neglect creating more damage and more negative outcomes. The relationship that the child has with the caregiver impacts the severity of outcomes. A positive relationship with the caregiver can mitigate some of the negative outcomes. For example, a parent could be attentive, caring, and attached to a child, yet they live in a hazardous environment where the child is not always appropriately supervised. In general, having support can serve as a protective factor and decrease the likelihood of poor outcomes due to neglect. There is evidence that a child's personality also factors into the impact the neglect has on a child. This is not to say that a child is responsible for the outcomes; rather it is to acknowledge there are individual characteristics that contribute to resilience.

Societal Consequences

It is estimated that each victim of child maltreatment will incur more than $830,000 in costs over their lifetime to treat the consequences of their maltreatment (Peterson et al., 2018). The consequences of child maltreatment extend beyond individual children who experience abuse and neglect. Society is impacted economically and socially. There is a significant economic burden to states with the overall costs varying in each state due to the number of cases of maltreatment a state has (Klika et al., 2020). The most recent estimate is the costs each child who is maltreatment will incur over the lifetime to $830,928 (in 2015 dollars; Peterson et al., 2018). The cost of a child fatality due to maltreatment is over $16.6 billion per child. With these estimates, the economic burden of the lifetime costs of child maltreatment that occurred in 2015 was $428 billion (Peterson et al., 2018). When these recent costs of maltreatment were applied to the number of child maltreatment cases substantiated in 2018 as well as the child fatalities that occurred in the same year, the costs were approximately $592 billion (Klika et al., 2020).

While the financial cost of maltreatment is astounding, there are costs that extend beyond the economic burden. Child abuse and neglect is a violation of children's basic human rights, and when a society condones the violation of human rights, all citizens are potentially jeopardized. Human rights are the foundation of strong, healthy communities. When children's rights are violated, it not only impacts current society but also the future as the children potentially grow up with ongoing problems due to the maltreatment inflicted upon them.

Prevention

Considering the costs to children, families, and communities, investing in prevention of child maltreatment is important. Chapter 7 explores prevention in depth. Prevention not only includes stopping maltreatment from happening but also mitigating the impact of maltreatment and ensuring that does not reoccur. It is cost-effective to focus on prevention as the costs—both financial and personal—are tremendous. There is growing recognition in federal policy, specifically the Family First Prevention Services Act, about the need to prioritize child maltreatment prevention. While child welfare professionals are often seen only as working in the aftermath of abuse and neglect, they also play an important role in prevention.

Cultural Considerations

Throughout all of child welfare, the issues of culture need to be considered. Especially considering the longstanding history of racial disparities (see Chap. 1), child welfare professionals should make cultural considerations in the identification and assessment of various types of maltreatment. For example, several cultural healing practices may leave markings on children that could be perceived to be from maltreatment. "Coining," an ancient healing practice used in several Southeast Asian cultures, involves an intense rubbing of the skin, which can leave red marks or abrasions. Another ancient healing practice of multiple cultures that has increasingly been used in the United States by natural healers is "cupping" which can leave circular bruising, typically on a person's back. It is important that culturally healing practices are not mistaken for child maltreatment.

Each culture has specific understandings of what child maltreatment is. Different cultures interpret caregivers striking a child differently. For example, in some cultures, it is never appropriate for a child to be hit, whereas in other cultures, striking a child with an open hand or with specific objects is perceived to be a form of discipline. Even within cultures, there may be variation and context that should be taken into consideration, as a recent study of Black families in the United States emphasized (Scott & Pinderhughes, 2019). While physical discipline, also called corporal punishment, is accepted in many countries around the world, the World Health

Organization (2015) launched a Global Initiative to End All Corporal Punishment of Children in 2015 citing that corporal punishment was the most common form of violence against children, and it "violates children's right to respect for their human dignity and physical integrity, as well as their rights to health, development and education, and is associated with a wide range of negative health, developmental and behavioral outcomes for children that can follow them into adulthood" (p.1). The American Academy of Pediatrics has issued a statement that spanking is harmful and recommends that caregivers do not use any forms of physical discipline (Sege, Seigel, Council on Child Abuse and Neglect, & Committee on Psychological Aspects of Child and Family Health, 2018).

Ongoing Debates in Child Welfare

There are many ongoing debates and hot topics within child maltreatment and child welfare besides how to handle caregivers physically disciplining their children. Specifically, the debates are often about if a behavior constitutes maltreatment and at what point can and should the child welfare system get involved as well as what is the appropriate course of action. It is clear that it is a debate when different states respond differently. One current ongoing debate is about prenatal exposure to substances such as opioids. While some states see this is maltreatment, other states argue that if mothers' substance use during pregnancy is criminalized, then women who are using drugs may not disclose to their doctors their drug use or may avoid prenatal care out of fear of their healthcare providers reporting them to child welfare. Another debate is around children witnessing intimate partner violence and to what extent it constitutes child maltreatment, who is held responsible, and how to respond. While it is widely recognized that a child's exposure to intimate partner violence can be damaging, states respond differently. An ongoing debate related to neglect is the religious exemption for seeking medical treatment. In some states, caregivers may withhold necessary medical treatment of their children for religious reasons. In these cases, if a caregiver holds views from a recognized religious group that does not support a medical treatment, then it is not recognized as medical neglect if the caregiver does seek treatment. Not all states grant this exemption, and there are concerns that in the states where exemptions are granted, there are higher rates of child fatalities due to not receiving necessary medical care.

At the center of these debates are research, values, and rights. There is often ample research that indicates that something is not optimal and in fact damaging (e.g., witnessing intimate partner violence); yet, the value of allowing the autonomy of the family and rights of the parents is protected. Social norms and deep-seeded beliefs, sometimes within different cultures, may be counter to what the research supports (i.e., spanking is harmful). Additionally, some of the logistics of how the child welfare system can respond and where to "draw the line" as many of the behavior occur on a continuum or there are complicated interrelated issues. For example, there are many things a woman can do during a pregnancy that could be harmful to a child (i.e., smoking, drinking alcohol, not getting prenatal care), and these are not considered child maltreatment yet in many states prenatal exposure to substances is. At what point does the child welfare system have the right to intervene when children are being harmed by the mother's actions or inactions? The understanding of children's safety and well-being continues to evolve and so will the child welfare system.

Conclusion

Child maltreatment consists of different types of child abuse and neglect: physical abuse, sexual abuse, psychological and emotional abuse, and neglect (physical, educational, emotional, and medical). While what causes child maltreatment remains unknown, research has identified risk and protective factors. The consequences of child maltreatment are great and impact a person's well-being both in the short and long term. Additionally, child maltreatment is costly to society. In addition to prioritizing the response to child maltreatment, child welfare professionals should emphasize prevention efforts.

Acknowledgments The authors thank Leah Bartley, PhD, and Leah Cheatham, PhD, JD, for their contributions to Chap. 4.

Discussion Questions

1. What are the four types of child maltreatment? Briefly describe how prevalent are they, what are the signs and symptoms, and what are the consequences.
2. When assessing for child physical abuse, how do you know when a fracture or bruise is accidental?
3. In what ways does child neglect present? What makes child neglect so challenging to assess and address?
4. What are three risk factors for child maltreatment?
5. In what ways does culture play a role in child maltreatment assessment and treatment?

Suggested Activities

1. Sign up for a listserv or alerts to keep up to date on issues related to child maltreatment, prevention, and treatment:
   APSAC Alerts: https://www.apsac.org/apsacpublications
   Children's Bureau Listserv: https://www.acf.hhs.gov/cb/get-updates
2. Visit Prevent Child Abuse America's website and read about new initiatives, research, and updates: https://preventchildabuse.org/latest-activity/
3. Choose a controversial topic about child maltreatment (spanking, witnessing intimate partner violence, prenatal drug exposure, child marriage, religious exemptions for medical neglect) and write a narrative about how different states

and countries handle these types of cases. Discuss recommendations and thoughts with a peer or field instructor.

4. Read Bulllinger et al. (2019) and write a reflection paper about the importance of understanding neglect and incorporating macro-level forces into both research and prevention efforts.

> Bullinger, L. R., Feely, M., Raissian, K. M., & Schneider, W. (2019). Heed Neglect, Disrupt Child Maltreatment: a Call to Action for Researchers. *International Journal on Child Maltreatment: Research, Policy and Practice*, 1–12. (Available: https://rdcu.be/cb8VP).

Additional Resources

American Professional Society on the Abuse of Children: https://www.apsac.org/
Childhelp. https://www.childhelp.org/
Child Welfare Information Gateway, Recognizing Child Abuse and Neglect: https://www.childwelfare.gov/pubPDFs/signs.pdf
Child Welfare Information Gateway, Definitions of Child Abuse and Neglect https://www.childwelfare.gov/topics/systemwide/laws-policies/statutes/define/
Child Welfare Information Gateway, How you Can Help Someone Who is Being Abused or Neglected: https://www.childwelfare.gov/pubs/kids-tipsheet/
Child Abuse Medical Provider Program, Documenting Child Abuse and Neglect with Photographs: https://champprogram.com/pdf/photo-documentation-pocket-guide-dec-2008.pdf
HelpGuide, Child abuse and neglect: https://www.helpguide.org/articles/abuse/child-abuse-and-neglect.htm
Prevent Child Abuse America: preventchildabuse.org

References

Abner, K. S. (2014). Dimensions of structural disadvantage: A latent class analysis of a neighborhood measure in Child Welfare data. *Journal of Social Service Research, 40*(1), 121–134. https://doi.org/10.1080/01488376.2013.852651

Bartlett, J. D., Kotake, C., Fauth, R., & Easterbrooks, M. A. (2017). Intergenerational transmission of child abuse and neglect: Do maltreatment type, perpetrator, and substantiation status matter? *Child Abuse & Neglect, 63*, 84–94. https://doi.org/10.1016/j.chiabu.2016.11.021

Berger, L. M., Collins, J. M., Font, S. A., Gjertson, L., Slack, K. S., & Smeeding, T. (2015). Home foreclosure and child protective services involvement. *Pediatrics, 136*(2), 299–307. https://doi.org/10.1542/peds.2014-2832

Bernstein, R. E., Measelle, J. R., Laurent, H. K., Musser, E. D., & Ablow, J. C. (2013). Sticks and stones may break my bones but words relate to adult physiology? Child abuse experience and women's sympathetic nervous system response while self-reporting trauma. *Journal of Aggression, Maltreatment & Trauma, 22*(10), 1117–1136. https://doi.org/10.1080/10926771.2013.850138

Birken, S. A., Rohweder, C. L., Powell, B. J., Shea, C. M., Scott, J., Leeman, J., Grewe, M. E., Kirk, M. A., Damschroder, L., Aldridge, W. A., II, Haines, E. R., Straus, S., & Presseau, J. (2018). T-CaST: An implementation comparison and selection tool. *Implementation*

Science, 13. Retrieved from: https://implementationscience.biomedcentral.com/articles/10.1186/s13012-018-0836-4#citeas. https://doi.org/10.1186/s13012-018-0836-4

Brault, M. W. (2012). Americans with disabilities: 2010. *Current Population Reports*, 70–131. http://www.census.gov/prod/2012pubs/p70-131.pdf

Bullinger, L. R., Feely, M., Raissian, K. M., & Schneider, W. (2019). Heed neglect, disrupt child maltreatment: a call to action for researchers. International journal on child maltreatment: research, policy and practice, 1–12.

Bullinger, L. R., & Fong, K. (2020). Evictions and Neighborhood Child Maltreatment Reports. *Housing Policy Debate*, 1–26. https://doi.org/10.1080/10511482.2020.1822902

Busuito, A., Huth-Bocks, A., & Puro, E. (2014). Romantic attachment as a moderator of the association between childhood abuse and posttraumatic stress disorder symptoms. *Journal of Family Violence, 29*(5), 567–577. https://doi.org/10.1007/s10896-014-9611-8

Centers for Disease Control and Prevention. (2014). Essentials for childhood: Creating safe, stable, nurturing relationships and environments for all children. Retrieved from: https://www.cdc.gov/violenceprevention/childabuseandneglect/essentials.html

Cheatham, L. P., Randolph, K. A., & Boltz, L. D. (2020). Youth with disabilities transitioning from foster care: Examining prevalence and predicting positive outcomes. *Children and Youth Services Review, 110*. https://doi.org/10.1016/j.childyouth.2020.104777

Chiesa, A., & Duhaime, A. C. (2009). Abusive head trauma. *Pediatric Clinics, 56*(2), 317–331. https://doi.org/10.1016/j.pcl.2009.02.001

Choi, K. W., & Sikkema, K. J. (2016). Childhood maltreatment and perinatal mood and anxiety disorders: A systematic review. *Trauma, Violence & Abuse, 17*(5), 427–453. https://doi.org/10.1177/1524838015584369

Conrad-Hiebner, A., & Byram, E. (2020). The temporal impact of economic insecurity on child maltreatment: A systematic review. *Trauma, Violence & Abuse, 21*(1), 157–178. https://doi.org/10.1177/1524838018756122

Development Services Group. (2013). *Protective factors for populations served by the Administration on Children, Youth, and Families: A literature review and theoretical summary*. Administration on Children, Youth and Families.

Duhaime, A. C. (2008). Demographics of abusive head trauma. *Journal of Neurosurgery: Pediatrics, 1*(5), 349–350. https://doi.org/10.3171/PED/2008/1/5/349

Eccles, M. P., & Mittman, B. S. (2006). Welcome to implementation science. *Implementation Science, 1*. https://doi.org/10.1186/1748-5908-1-1

Estabrooks, P. A., Brownson, R. C., & Pronk, N. C. (2018). Dissemination and implementation science for public health professionals: An overview and call to action. *Preventing Chronic Disease, 15*, retrieved from: https://www.ncbi.nlm.nih.gov/pmc/articles/PMC6307829/pdf/PCD-15-E162.pdf. https://doi.org/10.5888/pcd15.180525

Finkelhor, D., Hotaling, G., Lewis, I. A., & Smith, C. (1990). Sexual abuse in a national survey of adult men and women: Prevalence, characteristics, and risk factors. *Child Abuse & Neglect, 14*(1), 19–28. https://doi.org/10.1016/0145-2134(90)90077-7

Finkelhor, D., Ormrod, R., Turner, H., & Holt, M. (2009). Pathways to poly-victimization. *Child Maltreatment, 14*(4), 316–329. https://doi.org/10.1177/1077559509347012

Finkelhor, D., Ormrod, R. K., & Turner, H. A. (2007). Polyvictimization and trauma in a national longitudinal cohort. *Development and Psychopathology, 19*(1), 149–166. https://doi.org/10.1017/S0954579407070083

Gold, A. L., Sheridan, M. A., Peverill, M., Busso, D. S., Lambert, H. K., Alves, S., Pine, D. S., & McLaughlin, K. A. (2016). Childhood abuse and reduced cortical thickness in brain regions involved in emotional processing. *Journal of Child Psychology and Psychiatry, 57*(10), 1154–1164. https://doi.org/10.1111/jcpp.12630

Gubits, D., Shinn, M., Wood, M., Brown, S. R., Dastrup, S. R., & Bell, S. H. (2018). What interventions work best for families who experience homelessness? Impact estimates from the family options study. *Journal of Policy Analysis and Management, 37*(4), 835–866. https://doi.org/10.1002/pam.22071

Hein, T. C., Goetschius, L. G., McLoyd, V. C., Brooks-Gunn, J., McLanahan, S. S., Mitchell, C., Lopez-Duran, N. L., Hyde, L. W., & Monk, C. S. (2020). Childhood violence exposure and social deprivation are linked to adolescent threat and reward neural function. *Social Cognitive and Affective Neuroscience.* https://doi.org/10.1093/scan/nsaa144

Individual with Disabilities Education Improvement Act of 2004 (IDEIA), [Amending 20 U.S.C. §1400 et seq.].

Institute of Medicine (US), Committee on Quality of Health Care in America. (2001). Crossing the quality chasm: A new health system for the 21st century. Retrieved from: https://www.iom.edu/~/media/Files/Report%20Files/2001/Crossing-the-Quality-Chasm/Quality%20Chasm%202001%20%20report%20brief.pdf

Jedd, K., Hunt, R. H., Cicchetti, D., Hunt, E., Cowell, R., Rogosch, F., Toth, S. L., & Thomas, K. M. (2015). Long-term consequences of childhood maltreatment: Altered amygdala functional connectivity. *Development and Psychopathology, 27*(402), 1577. https://doi.org/10.1017/S0954579415000954

Kennedy, R. S. (2018). Bully-victims: An analysis of subtypes and risk characteristics. *Journal of Interpersonal Violence.* https://doi.org/10.1177/0886260517741213

Klika, J. B., Rosenzweig, J., & Merrick, M. (2020). Economic burden of known cases of child maltreatment from 2018 in each state. *Child and Adolescent Social Work Journal, 37*, 227–234. https://doi.org/10.1007/s10560-020-00665-5

Maguire-Jack, K., & Showalter, K. (2016). The protective effect of neighborhood social cohesion in child abuse and neglect. *Child Abuse & Neglect, 52*, 29–37. https://doi.org/10.1016/j.chiabu.2015.12.011

Metz, A., & Bartley, L. (2012). Active implementation frameworks for program success: How to use implementation science to improve outcomes for children. *Zero to Three, 32*, 11–18.

Metz, A., Louison, L., Ward, C., Burke., K. (2020). Implementation support practitioner profile: Guiding principles and Core competencies for implementation practice. University of North Carolina Chapel Hill, Frank Porter Graham Child Development Institute. Retrieved from: https://nirn.fpg.unc.edu/sites/nirn.fpg.unc.edu/files/resources/IS%20Practice%20Profile-single%20page%20printing-v6-2.20.20.pdf

Meyers, D. C., Durlak, J. A., & Wandersman, A. (2012). The quality implementation framework: A synthesis of critical steps in the implementation process. *American Journal of Community Psychology, 50*, 462–480. https://doi.org/10.1007/s10464-012-9522-x

Mildon, R., & Shlonsky, A. (2011). Bridge over troubled water: Using implementation science to facilitate effective services in child welfare. *Child Abuse and Neglect, 35*, 753–756. https://doi.org/10.1016/j.chiabu.2011.07.001

Milner, J., & Kelly, D. (2020). It's time to stop confusing poverty with neglect. *Children's Bureau Express, 20*(10) Available: https://cbexpress.acf.hhs.gov/index.cfm?event=website.viewArticles&issueid=212&sectionid=2&articleid=547

Morris, M. C., Marco, M., Maguire-Jack, K., Kouros, C. D., Bailey, B., Ruiz, E., & Im, W. (2019). Connecting child maltreatment risk with crime and neighborhood disadvantage across time and place: A Bayesian spatiotemporal analysis. *Child Maltreatment, 24*(2), 181–192. https://doi.org/10.1177/1077559518814364

Nilsen, P. (2015). Making sense of implementation theories, models and frameworks. *Implementation Science, 10*(1), 1–13. https://doi.org/10.1186/s13012-015-0242-0

Okpych, N. J., Courtney, M., & Dennis, K. (2017). *Memo from CalYOUTH: Predictors of high school completion and college entry at ages 19/20.* Chapin Hall at the University of Chicago.

Padek, M., Colditz, G., Dobbins, M., Koscielniak, N., Proctor, E. K., Sales, A. E., & Brownson, R. C. (2015). Developing educational competencies for dissemination and implementation research training programs: An exploratory analysis using card sorts. *Implementation Science, 10*(1), 114. https://doi.org/10.1186/s13012-015-0304-3

Pereda, N., Guilera, G., Forns, M., & Gómez-Benito, J. (2009). The prevalence of child sexual abuse in community and student samples: A meta-analysis. *Clinical Psychology Review, 29*(4), 328–338.

Peterson, C., Florence, C., & Klevens, J. (2018). The economic burden of child maltreatment in the United States, 2015. *Child Abuse & Neglect, 86*, 178–183. https://doi.org/10.1016/j.cpr.2009.02.007

Powell, B. J., McMillen, C., Proctor, E. K., Carpenter, C., et al. (2012). A compilation of strategies for implementing clinical innovations in health and mental health. *Medical Care Research and Review, 69*, 123–157. https://doi.org/10.1177/1077558711430690

Ramaswamy, R., Mosnier, J., Reed, K., Powell, B. J., & Schenck, A. P. (2019). Build capacity for public health 3.0: Introducing implementation science to MPH curriculum. *Implementation Science, 14*. https://doi.org/10.1186/s13012-019-0866-6

Robertson, C., & O'Brien, R. (2018). Health endowment at birth and variation in intergenerational economic mobility: Evidence from US county birth cohorts. *Demography, 55*(1), 249–269. https://doi.org/10.1007/s13524-017-0646-3

Rostad, W. L., Rogers, T. M., & Chaffin, M. J. (2017). The influence of concrete support on child welfare program engagement, progress, and recurrence. *Children and Youth Services Review, 72*, 26–33. https://doi.org/10.1016/j.childyouth.2016.10.014

Salazar, A. M., Keller, T. E., Gowen, L. K., & Courtney, M. E. (2013). Trauma exposure and PTSD among older adolescents in foster care. *Social Psychiatry and Psychiatric Epidemiology, 48*, 545–551. https://doi.org/10.1007/s00127-012-0563-0

Schenck-Fontaine, A., Gassman-Pines, A., Gibson-Davis, C. M., & Ananat, E. O. (2017). Local job losses and child maltreatment: The importance of community context. *Social Service Review, 91*(2), 233–263. https://doi.org/10.1086/692075

Scott, J. C., & Pinderhughes, E. E. (2019). Distinguishing between demographic and contextual factors linked to early childhood physical discipline and physical maltreatment among Black families. *Child Abuse & Neglect, 94*. https://doi.org/10.1016/j.chiabu.2019.05.013

Section 504 of the Rehabilitation Act of 1973, 34 C.F.R. Part 104.

Sege, R. D., Seigel, B. S., & Council on Child Abuse and Neglect, & Committee on Psychological Aspects of Child and Family Health. (2018). Effective discipline to raise healthy children. *Pediatrics, 142*(6). https://doi.org/10.1542/peds.2018-3112

Shuey, E. A., & Leventhal, T. (2017). Pathways of risk and resilience between neighborhood socioeconomic conditions and parenting. *Children and Youth Services Review, 72*, 52–59. https://doi.org/10.1016/j.childyouth.2016.09.031

Slayter, E. (2016). Youth with disabilities in the United States child welfare system. *Children and Youth Services Review, 64*, 165–175. https://doi.org/10.1016/j.childyouth.2016.03.012

Smith, C., Crosnoe, R., & Cavanagh, S. E. (2017). Family instability and children's health. *Family Relations, 66*(4), 601–613. https://doi.org/10.1111/fare.12272

Stith, S. M., Liu, T., Davies, L. C., Boykin, E. L., Alder, M. C., Harris, J. M., Som, A., McPherson, M., & Dees, J. E. M. E. G. (2009). Risk factors in child maltreatment: A meta-analytic review of the literature. *Aggression and Violent Behavior, 14*(1), 13–29. https://doi.org/10.1016/j.avb.2006.03.006

Street, J. C. (2015). Childhood maltreatment and revictimization by an intimate partner: The role of Africultural coping for at-risk African American women. Available: https://scholarworks.gsu.edu/psych_diss/135/

Sullivan, P., & Knutson, J. (2000). Maltreatment and disabilities: A population-based epidemiological study. *Child Abuse & Neglect, 24*(10), 1257–1273. https://doi.org/10.1016/S0145-2134(00)00190-3

Thornberry, T. P., Knight, K. E., & Lovegrove, P. J. (2012). Does maltreatment beget maltreatment? A systematic review of the intergenerational literature. *Trauma, Violence & Abuse, 13*(3), 135–152. https://doi.org/10.1177/1524838012447697

U.S. Department of Health & Human Services, Administration for Children and Families, Administration on Children, Youth and Families, Children's Bureau. (2020). Child Maltreatment 2018. Available from: https://www.acf.hhs.gov/sites/default/files/cb/cm2018.pdf

Van Scoyoc, A., Wilen, J. S., Daderko, K., & Miyamoto, S. (2015). Multiple aspects of maltreatment: Moving toward a holistic framework. In D. Daro, A. Cohn Donnelly, L. Huang, & B. Powell

(Eds.), *Advances in child abuse prevention knowledge. Child maltreatment (contemporary issues in research and policy)* (Vol. 5). Springer. https://doi.org/10.1007/978-3-319-16327-7_2

Warren, E. J., & Font, S. A. (2015). Housing insecurity, maternal stress, and child maltreatment: An application of the family stress model. *Social Service Review, 89*(1), 9–39. https://doi.org/10.1086/680043

World Health Organization (2015). https://www.who.int/topics/violence/Global-Initiative-End-All-Corporal-Punishment-children.pdf

Xerxa, Y., Delaney, S. W., Rescorla, L. A., Hillegers, M. H., White, T., Verhulst, F. C., Muetzel R. L & Tiemeier, H. (2020). Association of poor family functioning from pregnancy onward with preadolescent behavior and subcortical brain development. *JAMA Psychiatry*. https://doi.org/10.1001/jamapsychiatry.2020.2862.

Zajac, L., Prendergast, S., Feder, K. A., Cho, B., Kuhns, C., & Dozier, M. (2020). Trajectories of sleep in child protective services (CPS)-referred children predict externalizing and internalizing symptoms in early childhood. *Child Abuse & Neglect, 103*, 104433. https://doi.org/10.1016/j.chiabu.2020.104433

Chapter 5
Trauma-Informed Child Welfare Practice

Introduction

There is no doubt children who experience child abuse and neglect and who experience child welfare system involvement and possibly removal from their caregivers
are impacted by these traumatic events. Traumatic events such as child abuse and
neglect can impact people in a variety of ways and can be manifested in different
ways. Trauma and traumatic experiences are extremely complex as they occur in a
context that includes individuals' personal characteristics, life experiences, and current circumstances. These factors influence people's experience of trauma, how they
understand and make sense of it, how they interpret and process the experience, and
how they adjust following the traumatic experience. As child welfare professionals,
it is critical to understand this dynamic and very individualized experience and how
to use an appropriate, ethical, and holistic approach in our practice with children
and families involved with the child welfare system.

What Is a Traumatic Event?

A traumatic event is one that is dangerous and frightening and that poses a threat to
a person's life or body. Experiencing and witnessing such an event can be traumatic
as well as incidences where one fears for their life or where one believes they might
be hurt or injured. A number of experiences can be traumatic for an adult and/or
child, such as physical, sexual, or psychological abuse and neglect; family or community violence; war and refugee experiences; serious accidents; illnesses; military
experiences; sudden loss and/or death of a loved one; substance use disorder or
exposure to someone with substance use disorder; and natural disasters. Trauma
also results from experiences related to economic stress and poverty, homelessness,
and crime. Adults and children often feel helpless, confused, and afraid during and

© Springer Nature Switzerland AG 2021
J. M. Geiger, L. Schelbe, *The Handbook on Child Welfare Practice*,
https://doi.org/10.1007/978-3-030-73912-6_5

after a traumatic event has occurred. They may feel unable to stop the event from occurring or to protect themselves or others from it, resulting in their inability to process the event(s) without support from others.

How Does Trauma Affect Individuals?

Trauma affects individuals in different ways, depending on various factors, including the severity, exposure, chronicity, reactions of others, developmental stage, incidence of multiple traumatic events, and previous experiences. A traumatic response is also impacted by one's experience with and ability to use various means of healthy processing and coping strategies.

For children, any one or more traumatic events and the events that follow can continue to affect their lives long after the event(s) have ended. Child traumatic stress is characterized by a series of events, similar or different in nature, related or unrelated that when experienced over time can have a significant impact on a child's physical, emotional, social, and cognitive development. The traumatic stress response is often manifested by depression, anxiousness, behavior changes (e.g., sleeping, eating), physical complaints, issues related to school performance, social relationships, withdrawal or isolation, and/or risky behaviors (e.g., substance use or sexual).

Signs of Traumatic Stress

Given the diverse experiences of trauma and response, there is also a range of signs and signals that indicate traumatic stress in children. As discussed in Chap. 3, it is critical for child welfare professionals to understand normative development in childhood and across the life span in order to be able to recognize the signs and respond appropriately with services and support.

Infants and Toddlers

Infants and toddlers rely exclusively on their caregivers to provide for their most basic needs as well as emotional and physical nurturing and care. Despite their rapid growth – physically, cognitively, and emotionally – they are also unable to process many of the interactions they experience, including trauma, without the support and guidance of adults, primarily their caregivers. Even with support, children may still experience a variety of signs of traumatic stress response. These behavioral indicators include changes in sleeping and eating patterns; increased tantrums and/or inappropriate emotional reactions to various circumstances; difficulty with self-soothing and/or being soothed by others; excessive crying; and/or easily startled.

Preschool and Elementary School-Age Children

Young children have improved agency with some aspects of their lives, including improved ability to care for themselves (e.g., dressing, washing hands, feeding, using the toilet, etc.), improved social and cognitive ability to manage relationships and problem solving, and have more physical control over their own bodies in general. However, most preschool and elementary school-age children rely on their caregivers to guide them through these scenarios. When children ages 3 to 10 years old experience prolonged trauma or traumatic stress, they may demonstrate feelings of helplessness and uncertainty; fear and anxiety when separating from caregiver; excessive screaming or crying; eating poorly; toileting regression or bedwetting (that did not occur before); using baby talk; arrested development; rapid changes in behavior; anxiety and fearfulness; excessive worrying; displaying guilt and shame; overreaction to bumps and bruises or falls; difficulty sleeping or concentrating; changes in school performance; easily startled; and the recreation and retelling of the traumatic event(s). Many children this age who have experienced trauma experience nightmares regularly and have difficulty self-regulating.

Middle School- and High School-Age Children

Middle school- and high school-age children have developed more mastery in their ability to care for themselves, navigate social relationships, and manage their bodies and behavior. When children and youth ages 11–18 years old experience trauma, their behavior can be manifested in internalized and externalized ways due to their ability to cognitively process trauma differently, their physical development (hormones, etc.), and reliance placed on social relationships – romantic and platonic. Signs of traumatic stress in youth include feeling depressed and alone; developing eating disorders and/or self-harming behaviors (e.g., cutting); use and abuse or alcohol and/or other drugs; becoming sexually active; feeling out of control emotionally; experiencing feelings of being different; taking risks; having sleep disturbances; avoiding places that remind them of a traumatic experience or event; having changes in school performance; being isolated or avoidant; and discussing the traumatic event in detail, often repeatedly.

Triggers and Trauma Reminders

Those who experience trauma have a variety of immediate and long-term reactions in the aftermath of trauma, and as described earlier, many factors impact how one might experience and cope with trauma. Coping styles can vary from emotional expression to action oriented. These responses can be healthy and unhealthy for the individual, but they are almost always effective for them in that they allow the individual to manage the emotions and thoughts associated with the trauma experience. Measuring these responses tends to be related to how they impact the individual's ability to go about their daily life and responsibilities. As children experience such variation in development, this can often be shielded by shifting developmental task navigation. Initial reactions to trauma can include sadness, anger, anxiety, agitation, numbness, dissociation, confusion, physiological response, and exhaustion. This is the body's response to a traumatic event, and it is appropriate to respond in this way. More severe responses tend to persist and include more distress without one's ability to calm, rest, or manage those symptoms. Delayed responses to trauma can include fatigue, sleeping and eating interruptions, nightmares, fear, flashbacks, and depression. Trauma can also affect how someone thinks and feels about the future, about hope, and expectations. It can negatively impact positivity, which has an impact on relationships and one's ability to focus.

Another unique feature of traumatic stress includes the presence of "triggers" or "trauma reminders." Triggers are experiences that remind a person of the trauma experienced through their senses – touch, smell, sound, sight, and taste. These triggers can bring back strong memories of the traumatic event and can feel as though it is happening again. For example, anxiousness, nervousness, or fear when they encounter places, people, sights, sounds, smells, and feelings that remind them of past traumatic experiences, even years afterwards. Individuals also experience distressing mental images, thoughts, and emotional/physical reactions, as well as responses to sudden loud noises, destroyed buildings, the smell of fire, ambulance or police sirens, locations where they experienced the trauma, funerals, anniversaries of the trauma, and television or radio news about the event.

Triggers, as a result of a traumatic experience or traumatic stress, develop when a person's body has a response when they are faced with danger. In response to a dangerous event (e.g., car accident, abuse, etc.), a person's bodies must respond quickly in a way to protect themselves and initiates the fight, flight, or freeze response. People have a physiological response with sweating and fast heartbeat, and their senses are on high alert. Their brain stops some of its normal functions, such as short-term memory, in order to face the danger. The brain then associates details (e.g.,

> **Practice Highlight**
>
> **Examples of Triggers and Trauma Reminders**
>
> - Anxiousness, nervousness, or scared when they encounter places, people, sights, sounds, smells, and feelings that remind them of past traumatic experiences, even years afterward
> - Distressing mental images, thoughts, and emotional/physical reactions
> - Sudden loud noises, destroyed buildings, the smell of fire, ambulance or police sirens, locations where they experienced the trauma, encountering people with disabilities, funerals, anniversaries of the trauma, and television or radio news about the event

smells, sights, or sounds) of the experience to the memory. This is what becomes the trigger. When these experiences occur in the future, it triggers a person's body's response system or alarm system. Events that remind someone of what happened right before or during a trauma can be a potential trigger. They are typically tied to their senses and when the person sees, feels, smells, touches, or tastes something that reminds them of the event, it can bring on symptoms associated with the danger response. While triggers themselves are usually harmless, they cause the person's body to react as if the person is in danger because the body may not be able to distinguish the events and determine safety in that moment.

Impact of Trauma

In the past several decades, researchers have begun to document the impact of trauma on individuals, families, and communities. Earlier in the chapter, there is discussion about how children, in particular, manifest trauma through emotions and behaviors. When left untreated, complex trauma or traumatic stress can have long-term effects on a child's current and future relationships, academic performance, thinking and cognition, physical health, and overall stability. See Fig. 5.1 describing the impact of childhood trauma. Early childhood trauma such as child maltreatment can impact a person in adolescence (e.g., Heleniak et al., 2016).

When children do not form healthy attachment relationships as a result of a traumatic experience in that relationship or outside of that relationship, they often struggle with forming healthy relationships with peers, caregivers, teachers, and family members. As children mature into adults, they may continue to struggle forming and maintaining those relationships in addition to romantic relationships. When individuals experience trauma, whether it is related to child maltreatment, many experience disruptions in those relationships, regardless of whether they were healthy or not prior to the experience. See Chap. 3 for more information about the importance of the attachment relationships formed between a child and their caregiver and the impact of having a strained and/or abusive caregiving relationship for a child.

Children and adults can also experience a negative impact on their physical health as a result of trauma. Earlier, this chapter presented the stress response and the development of triggers. For children who are exposed to chronic stress, their bodies may not be able to self-regulate or respond appropriately when there is no danger present. Their body is always on alert and ready to respond with "fight, flight, or freeze." Because of the hormones associated with this response, their bodies cannot physically manage the constant state of alertness. Regular states of stress can impair the development of the brain and nervous system. Research involving scans of the brain shows that childhood adversity impacts neurodevelopment (Hoffman et al., 2019). Childhood stress can prevent mental stimulation required for normal growth. Children with a history of trauma may also have difficulty self-regulating physically and emotionally. They might be oversensitive or

Impact of Childhood Trauma

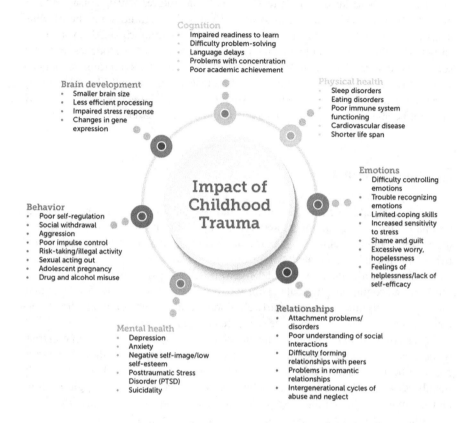

Cognition
- Impaired readiness to learn
- Difficulty problem-solving
- Language delays
- Problems with concentration
- Poor academic achievement

Brain development
- Smaller brain size
- Less efficient processing
- Impaired stress response
- Changes in gene expression

Physical health
- Sleep disorders
- Eating disorders
- Poor immune system functioning
- Cardiovascular disease
- Shorter life span

Impact of Childhood Trauma

Behavior
- Poor self-regulation
- Social withdrawal
- Aggression
- Poor impulse control
- Risk-taking/illegal activity
- Sexual acting out
- Adolescent pregnancy
- Drug and alcohol misuse

Emotions
- Difficulty controlling emotions
- Trouble recognizing emotions
- Limited coping skills
- Increased sensitivity to stress
- Shame and guilt
- Excessive worry, hopelessness
- Feelings of helplessness/lack of self-efficacy

Mental health
- Depression
- Anxiety
- Negative self-image/low self-esteem
- Posttraumatic Stress Disorder (PTSD)
- Suicidality

Relationships
- Attachment problems/ disorders
- Poor understanding of social interactions
- Difficulty forming relationships with peers
- Problems in romantic relationships
- Intergenerational cycles of abuse and neglect

Child TRENDS

Fig. 5.1 Impact of Childhood Trauma. (Source: Child Trends (2019); https://www.childtrends.org/publications/how-to-implement-trauma-informed-care-to-build-resilience-to-childhood-trauma)

under-respond to sensory stimuli, such as sounds, smells, touch, or light. They may respond unusually to pain or touch, which may lead to injuries. Children with a history of complex trauma can also develop chronic or recurrent physical complaints such as headaches and stomachaches. Adults also experience similar physical impairments in addition to engaging in risky behaviors that may lead to other physical conditions (e.g., smoking, risky sexual behaviors, overeating).

Trauma can also have an impact on a person's emotional identification and expression. Children learn how to appropriately identify how they are feeling and express emotions in a way that is congruent with how they feel, the circumstances, and can learn to self-regulate through modeling others' behaviors, social-emotional growth through interactions with others, and learning about emotions with peers in a school setting. Children who experience trauma will often have difficulty in identifying, expressing, and regulating emotions. They may not know how to accurately verbalize their feelings or the reasons for those feelings. As a result, they may internalize their emotions and show symptoms of depression and anxiety, or they may inappropriately externalize their feelings through acting out, disruptive behavior, or aggression. Children with repeated exposure to trauma or complex trauma experiences may experience triggers at unpredictable times, may react powerfully, and/or have trouble calming down in certain situations that remind them of the trauma. They learn that the world is a dangerous place and may lack the ability to trust and display hypervigilant behaviors. They may be guarded and may not respond well to interventions and/or expressions of care from others.

Experiencing complex trauma can also cause a child (or an adult) to be more likely to have highly intense reactions or a lack of reaction when

> **Practice Highlight**
>
> **Trauma Impact of Investigation, Removal, and Out-of-Home Placement**
>
> Children may have a number of behavioral, emotional, and cognitive experiences to child welfare investigation, removal, and out-of-home placement. Here is some possible responses to these circumstances:
>
> - Surprise, shock, confusion
> - Feelings of loss of control, powerlessness, helplessness
> - Betrayal, loss of trust
> - Negative view of law enforcement or child welfare agency representatives
> - Fear of unknown
> - Sense of guilt
> - Abrupt and overwhelming feelings of loss
> - Attachment disruption from caregiver
> - Confused and conflicted about new caregiver and surroundings

one would have been appropriate. When a child struggles with self-regulation, they may lack impulse control which can lead to unpredictable and volatile behaviors. This may also lead to engaging in risky behaviors, aggression, or becoming involved with the juvenile justice system as a result of such behaviors.

Children with a history of trauma may have trouble thinking clearly, reasoning, or problem solving. They may have difficulties with thinking about the future, planning, and responding appropriately. When a child is faced with chronic stress and trauma, they are often only able to focus and consider their actions in the moment and/or near future instead of looking forward and considering consequences. Decision-making can also be challenging when presented with multiple options. Children with a history of trauma may also have difficulty focusing and concentrating and may show delays in language development. Children exposed to trauma may also struggle with establishing self-esteem and self-worth. In cases of child maltreatment, many children will blame themselves and feel shame and guilt. When children do not feel safe, they lack a sense of hope and purpose and positive thoughts about the future. With that, they do not plan for the future and may feel as though they do not have agency over their actions or circumstances around them.

Trauma has a significant economic impact as well. Childhood trauma, especially that related to interpersonal violence, has a major impact on public health (e.g., Lambert et al., 2017). It is estimated that the cumulative economic impact is close to $100 billion, which includes the cost of child maltreatment, meeting the needs of children in various systems (mental health care, child welfare, law enforcement, etc.) and secondary and long-term effects with regard to education, legal systems, mental and health care, and intergenerational effects (Peterson et al., 2018).

> **Practice Highlight**
>
> **Impact of Trauma**
> The impact of trauma depends on many factors including:
>
> - Age and development
> - Perception of danger
> - Experience of trauma as victim or witness
> - Relationship to perpetrator
> - History of trauma
> - Post-trauma experiences and support

Adverse Childhood Experiences (ACEs)

Adverse childhood experiences are described as potentially traumatic childhood experiences such as experiencing violence, abuse, or neglect, witnessing violence, or growing up in a household where there was substance abuse, mental health problems, or parental separation. The Adverse Childhood Experiences (ACE) Study was a groundbreaking longitudinal study examining the long-term impact of adverse childhood experiences such as parental substance abuse, divorce, and death during childhood on an adult's physical health. The study examined the medical history of over 17,000 participants ages 19–90 and collected data related to adverse childhood experiences (ACEs; Felitti et al. 1998). Results showed that over 64% of participants had at least one exposure, and or those 69% reported two or more incidents of childhood trauma. Further, when examining the relationship between ACEs and later health, researchers found that the presence of ACEs were associated with high-risk behaviors (e.g., smoking), chronic illness (heart disease and cancer), and early death (Dong et al., 2004). People with high ACEs scores have been found to have a reduced likelihood of high school graduation, holding a skilled job, juvenile arrests, and felony charges (Giovanelli et al., 2016). ACEs also have an impact on future violence victimization and perpetration. Figure 5.2 shows the ACE Pyramid and the framework of how ACEs impact a person across the life span.

The ACEs study is valuable in that it helps make the connection between some of the potential negative outcomes associated with adverse childhood experiences. There are some limitations and caution should be noted when interpreting and using the findings from this study. For example, the study is largely descriptive and not

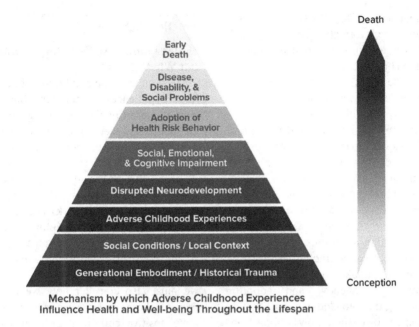

Mechanism by which Adverse Childhood Experiences
Influence Health and Well-being Throughout the Lifespan

Fig. 5.2 The ACE Pyramid shows the conceptual framework of how ACEs impact a person across the life span. (Source: CDC (2020a); Available: https://www.cdc.gov/violenceprevention/aces/about.html)

causal. Only specific traumas are included. The study does not consider factors such as resilience and protective factors. It also does not provide information about intervention. It is helpful to use the ACEs in screening, but it is equally important to focus on how screening for ACEs will be used when intervening with people who have experienced adversity. Although these experiences increase the risk of later health conditions, these factors are preventable. The Centers for Disease Control and Prevention (CDC) has outlined protective factors that have been shown to reduce ACEs and their associated harms (CDC, 2020b).

Creating and sustaining safe, stable, and nurturing relationships and environments for all children and their families can help improve health and social outcomes into adulthood. The CDC has developed a technical package that recommends six strategies to preventing ACEs that individuals, families, and communities can adopt: (1) strengthening economic supports to families through financial security and family-friendly work policies; (2) promoting social norms that protect against violence and adversity through public education campaigns and other legislative approaches; (3) ensuring a strong start for children through early childhood home visitation, high quality day care, and preschool enrichment; (4) teaching skills to children and families regarding social-emotional learning, healthy relationship building, and parenting skills; (5) connecting youth to caring adults and activities, such as mentoring and after-school programs; and (6) intervening to lessen the immediate and long-term harms through enhanced primary care, services, and treatment (CDC, 2014). (See Chap. 7 for more information about the CDC's Essentials for Childhood for information about the model.)

The effects of trauma are well-documented; however, there are a number of ways that child welfare professionals can better understand the various forms of impact and respond using a trauma-informed approach to screening and make the necessary referrals for thorough assessment and treatment. Child welfare professionals can use their skills and resources when intervening at various stages of child welfare practice, including investigation and intake; ongoing and foster care; permanency; and adoption. Having the knowledge about what are sources of trauma, how trauma manifests, and how it can have short- and long-term effects on the individual, their family, and the community helps us as professionals respond in a way that can be helpful and supportive.

Practice Highlight

Understanding ACEs Is Important, but What's Next?
Understanding one's adverse childhood experiences is important; however, it doesn't really present ways we can address prevention and treatment of these ACES. Some benefits of integrating ACEs into our practice in child welfare is that we are all "speaking the same language" across disciplines (e.g., medicine, social work), and raising awareness across disciplines and areas of practice about the impact of ACEs. However, as we are early in our understanding of the impact of ACEs, we must also consider how we can prevent these experiences and promote positive childhood experiences in their place. When we screen for ACEs, we must have a plan for how we will address the short- and long-term impact of these experiences and learn more about successful methods of prevention (Finkelhor, 2018).

Assessment Tools and Strategies for Children Who Have Experienced Trauma

Child welfare professionals are not required to provide treatment for children exposed to trauma; however, it is helpful for child welfare professionals to understand how to appropriately assess for trauma and traumatic stress responses and be aware of what treatment options are available to provide information and make referrals as necessary. There are various tools to assess for trauma (e.g., Donisch et al., 2020). (See Chap. 8 for more information about assessment.) Child welfare professionals review clinical documentation and assessments and should be aware of what they are and their implications for the child and their family. In all child welfare assessments and investigations, it is important to obtain information from multiple sources and through various methods (observation, reports, interviews, etc.), when possible. This is also true with trauma assessments. With children, it is important to observe their interactions with others; however, child welfare professionals should also interview them separately as well (as appropriate) to obtain differences in perspectives, accounts, and experiences. To begin, it is helpful to obtain details about the traumatic event or exposure and what occurred before and after. Given the varying experiences of trauma and trauma responses, this line of questioning and investigation must be approached carefully, primarily to not re-traumatize, create undue stress and discomfort, and assess immediate needs. It is quite possible the child and/or the family is not prepared during the first interview or interaction to discuss all or any of the events that have occurred; however, it is likely that with time, they will. Many agencies use standardized questionnaires or tools to ensure the necessary questions are being asked to determine whether abuse/neglect has occurred; however, when assessing for trauma exposure, these questions are used more to determine necessary services for both the child and parent/caregiver. Through assessment of trauma response, child welfare professionals can also provide additional although sometimes limited initial information about symptomology to foster or kin caregivers so that they may better respond to their needs and obtain the necessary therapeutic services promptly. Moving beyond the child welfare professional's role, clinicians will often proceed with assessing post-traumatic stress disorder (PTSD) symptomology through careful evaluation of the individual's meeting diagnostic criteria in the *Diagnostic and Statistical Manual of Mental Disorders, 5th Edition* (DSM-5). Such a diagnosis is not required in order for therapeutic services to be provided to children, youth, and their families; however, it does provide guidance in how to proceed in the clinical context. Clinicians will often assess for other psychiatric disorders alongside referrals from caregivers and child welfare professionals to primary care physicians to ensure appropriate overall development.

When assessing for trauma, it is important to note the setting where the assessment or screening occurs. For example, is the screening occurring in the home, the hospital, or at school? This will impact how the child might respond. Likewise, a child may have a different level of comfort and be impacted by who is present during an interview and what type of relationship the screener might have with the child. One should consider how the screening will benefit the child/parent. For example, it can be assumed that some kind of trauma has occurred if a child welfare professional is interviewing a child due to a report of child maltreatment; however, what other information might suggest trauma exposure and its impact. Given what child welfare professionals know now about trauma and its manifestation, child welfare professionals can use this information to guide the need for a screening or to arrange a formal assessment which includes information about trauma.

Professionals in child welfare should be aware of minimizing the need for multiple rescreening or reassessments. Protocol should include procedure for brief screenings that could lead to an assessment as needed and should be limited to that assessment to prevent re-traumatization and emotional and/or psychological damage and fatigue related to recounting the trauma events. Appropriate documentation of screenings and assessments as well as proper care coordination can be employed to avoid this. The individual conducting the screening and assessments should be adequately trained to complete the screening/or assessments and should use a client-focused, strengths-based, and culturally grounded approach.

Providers should consider when trauma screenings and assessments will be administered, and which will be used. Most child welfare agencies have an established protocol for how and when this will be done as well as by whom. The child welfare professional may document symptoms, observations, and interactions with the client that is indicative of trauma exposure; however, it is possible that they do not formally screen or assess, but make a referral for this. Timing is also important. Children and adults may not be prepared to discuss traumatic experiences immediately following the event, and the decision to screen at a specific time must be approached with care and with the client in mind. Agencies may also use different screening and assessment tools based on agency preferences, workflow systems, and culture. Assessments may be more general to capture various types of trauma exposures and behaviors, more clinical in nature, or may focus on a specific type of trauma, such as child sexual abuse. Screenings and assessments may be modified depending on the child's age or developmental stage and on the child's relationship with the caregiver or other adults. Providers using a screening tool should consider (1) factors such as the child's age, language skills, and cognitive capabilities; (2) whether the child is among the populations for which the tool has been validated and normed; and (3) if there are other factors that might affect the reliability and validity of the tool for this particular child. Tools can be completed by the provider, the child, and/or a caregiver and can be administered in a verbal or written format. Ongoing screening is also important to ensure children are safe in placements after they have been removed from their family.

Engaging Families in the Screening Process

Once it is determined that it is an appropriate time to administer the screening or assessment and how it will be administered, the provider should explain the purpose and use of the tool, why it is necessary to obtain that information, how it will be used, how it might benefit the individual/family, and potential challenges in the screening/assessment. As with all interactions, it is important to note the parameters for confidentiality. It is also good practice, as appropriate, to share the results and explain what they might mean, if possible. Consider the impact on the child of simply completing the screening or assessment and explain to the caregiver how the child may respond following the screening or assessment.

Reducing the Trauma Associated with Child Investigation, Removal, and Out-of-Home Placement

There is little doubt that children who enter the foster care system have experienced some level of trauma. However, it is important to also consider the trauma associated with the experience of the child welfare investigation process, being removed from their home, and placed in out-of-home care. These instances often involve conflict, emotions, and tension among the parties involved; however, the way that the child welfare professional and others (e.g., foster parent, law enforcement) respond can mitigate the trauma impact of these experiences. Child welfare professionals can plan investigations, assessments, and possible removals ahead as much as they can. They can slow down and explain to the family what is happening and supporting them through that process while also having identified a placement prior to removal. As much as possible, the child welfare professional should maintain a calm approach to assessment and removal, providing comfort, empathy, and support to the child and family. The child welfare professionals can help the parent in calming and caring for the child (e.g., help them to the car, gather some belongings, and explain the situation). During the process of removal, the child welfare professional can ensure the child has enough to eat and drink, has time to gather some items, and feels comfortable in their new surroundings. Child welfare professionals can ask parents about the child's needs, likes and dislikes, and routines.

It is important to be on the child's level and connect with them by attempting to understand and acknowledge their feelings. It is critical to listen and give them age-appropriate information about what is happening, assuring their safety and care, and, most importantly, that this is not their fault. Child welfare professionals should not make any promises they can't keep; however, they should make efforts to maintain relationships with family and other loved ones as much as possible. Services, such as counseling, are often helpful during these transitions, and services for the child should be assessed and implemented as soon as possible.

Reflection

Moving in the Middle of the Night

Consider for a moment that tonight you are woken up at 1am and told you have to grab some clothes in a bag and move to a stranger's house. For children being removed from their homes, this is just a small glimpse of what it would feel like in that moment. For some, they don't have many possessions, but forgetting that stuffed animal can be devastating to many. Not only are children tired, scared, and unsure of what will happen next, but also they are losing everything they know in that moment. Many children are not equipped emotionally or cognitively to understand what is happening, and all of it is out of their control. Everything about their life will change – their routine, school, friends, family, where they sleep, the soap they use, the food they eat, where they sit, activities they like, their neighborhood, house rules, and possibly their cultural traditions. As child welfare professionals, it is important to understand these elements and make every effort to recognize these changes and try to make the transition easier. Being trauma-informed means knowing the impact of having a child move and adjust to a new setting, even it is a safer, more stable home.

Overview of Treatment of Trauma

A number of individual (child and adult) and family-based interventions have been shown to be effective in treating traumatic stress and PTSD symptomology, including psychosocial interventions targeting PTSD, cognitive-based therapies, eye movement desensitization and reprocessing (EMDR), and relaxation-based psychotherapies. Various combinations of these approaches as well as pharmacological treatments have also been shown to be effective in treating PTSD and trauma symptomology. Exposure-based interventions have been shown to reduce symptoms of avoidance, fear, and anxiety that are related to a specific traumatic exposure or experience by carefully exposing the individual to the stimuli associated with the trauma in a safe, therapeutic context.

Practice Highlight

Examples of Trauma Screening and Assessment Tools

Assessment-Based Treatment for Traumatized Children: A Trauma Assessment Pathway Model (TAP) was designed for children 0 to 18 years of age who have experienced any type of trauma and who may or may not be in the child welfare system. TAP is a multifaceted assessment process that allows for screening and further assessment, if needed.

The **Brief Trauma Questionnaire (BTQ)** is a 10-item self-report trauma exposure screen that can be quickly administered and is suitable for special populations such as persons with severe mental illness as well as for general population groups.

The **Child Post-Traumatic Symptom Scale (CPSS)** assesses symptom criteria for PTSD and the corresponding impairment in functioning in children and adolescents.

Child and Adolescent Needs and Strengths (CANS): Trauma Comprehensive Version is a flexible, multipurpose tool that gathers information on a range of domains relevant to the functioning of the child and caregiving system and can organize this information to develop individualized plans of care.

Child PTSD Symptom Scale (CPSS) is a self-report measure to assess the frequency of DSM defined PTSD symptoms.

Child Report of Post-Traumatic Symptoms (CROPS) is a self-report measure for children and adolescents that assesses a range of post-traumatic symptoms and can be used to measure change in symptomology over time.

Child Trauma Screening Questionnaire (CTSQ) is a 10-item self-report screening tool that can be used to identify risk of PTSD in children. The questions assess trauma reactions following a potential traumatic event.

Life Events Checklist (LEC) is a brief 17-item self-report measure designed to screen for potentially traumatic events in a respondent's lifetime. The LEC assesses exposure to 16 events known to potentially result in PTSD or distress and includes on-item assessment any other extraordinary stressful event not captured in the other items.

PTSD Checklist (PCL) contains 17 questions that map onto the 3 DSM-IV PTSD symptom clusters: reexperiencing, avoidance, and arousal.

Post-traumatic Stress Disorder Semi-Structured Interview and Observational Record is a semi-structured caregiver report measure used to assess for PTSD symptoms for children ages 0–7 years.

Post-Traumatic Symptom Inventory for Children (PT-SIC) is a self-report measure of PTSD symptoms for children ages 4 to 8 years.

Trauma and Attachment Belief Scale (TABS) is the revised version of the TSI Belief Scale to assess individuals who have experienced traumatic events.

Trauma Symptom Checklist for Young Children (TSCYC) is a 90-item caretaker report measure to assess trauma symptomology in children ages 3 to 12.

Trauma Symptom Checklist for Children (TSCC) measures severity of post-traumatic stress and symptomology in children ages 8 to 16 who have experienced traumatic events.

The **UCLA Reaction Index** is the most commonly used measure for PTSD symptoms in children and adolescents. There are versions of this measure for children, adolescents, and parents. It assesses the respondent's trauma history and frequency of the PTSD symptoms.

The **Upsetting Events Survey** that we designed is a modification of the Traumatic Life Events Questionnaire (TLEQ). It assesses effectively for trauma history.

Evidence-Informed Interventions to Address Trauma in Children

There are a number of evidence-informed interventions used to treat trauma in children and adolescents, many of which have been tailored to address trauma in children and adolescents who have experienced maltreatment and foster care and/or who are living in out-of-home placements. Treatments used to address symptoms related to trauma often use variations of similar approaches and techniques. Although child welfare professionals working in case management with children in care will not be providing therapy or counseling for children, their parents, or caregivers, it is important to be aware of the philosophy, dynamics, and structure of commonly used interventions and therapeutic approaches. Interventions such as trauma-focused cognitive behavioral therapy (TF-CBT); attachment, self-regulation, and competency (ARC) and integrative treatment of complex trauma for children/adolescents (ITCT-C/A) use similar therapeutic techniques in their approach to treat trauma with this population. Child welfare professionals often play a role in referring clients to various community programs related to parenting education, substance abuse, and trauma-focused therapy and should be aware of evidence-informed interventions (Myers et al., 2020). A listing of evidence-based interventions can be found on the website for the California Evidence-Based Clearinghouse for Child Welfare (https://www.cebc4cw.org/). It is important to note when identifying evidence-based interventions that they have been evaluated with diverse groups by age, race/ethnicity, language, etc. to ensure fit with the client.

Children's response to maltreatment and trauma experiences differs based on age, gender, and life history. Screening, assessment, and treatment must be flexible enough to ensure individualization to meet the needs of the child and family. It is important for the treatment plan to consider the child, their caregiver, and biological family, as appropriate to develop and maintain a normal routine where a child can feel safe and cared for.

Using a Trauma-Informed Approach

Trauma experiences are common during childhood, and children respond differently to trauma. Many children recover on their own, some with support, and some struggle with managing the trauma they experienced even with treatment and support. Having the professional provider and systems in place to respond in a trauma-informed way is critical in facilitating recovery and growth among those who have experienced trauma, particularly as it relates to child welfare (Kawam & Martinez, 2016). All members of a child and family team, including the child welfare professional, their supervisor, providers (mental health, physical health, etc.), caregiver (kin, foster parent, biological parent), and other professionals (teachers, principal, staff) should use a trauma-informed approach to care. According to the Substance Abuse and Mental Health Services Administration (SAMHSA, 2014), this approach should "realize the widespread impact of trauma and understanding potential paths for recovery, recognize the signs and symptoms of trauma, fully integrate knowledge about trauma into policies, procedures, and practices, and seek to actively resist re-traumatization" (p. 9).

Practice Highlight

Common Therapeutic Approaches and Techniques to Treat Trauma

- Motivational interviewing (to engage clients)
- Risk screening (to identify high-risk clients)
- Triage to different levels and types of intervention (to match clients to the interventions that will most likely benefit them/they need)
- Systematic assessment, case conceptualization, and treatment planning (to tailor intervention to the needs, strengths, circumstances, and wishes of individual clients)
- Engagement/addressing barriers to service-seeking (to ensure clients receive an adequate dosage of treatment in order to make sufficient therapeutic gains)
- Psychoeducation about trauma reminders and loss reminders (to strengthen coping skills)
- Psychoeducation about post-traumatic stress reactions and grief reactions (to strengthen coping skills)

- Teaching emotional regulation skills (to strengthen coping skills)
- Maintaining adaptive routines (to promote positive adjustment at home and at school)
- Parenting skills and behavior management (to improve parent-child relationships and to improve child behavior)
- Constructing a trauma narrative (to reduce post-traumatic stress reactions)
- Teaching safety skills (to promote safety)
- Advocating on behalf of the client (to improve client support and functioning at school, in the juvenile justice system, and so forth)
- Teaching relapse prevention skills (to maintain treatment gains over time)
- Monitoring client progress/response during treatment (to detect and correct insufficient therapeutic gains in timely ways)
- Evaluating treatment effectiveness (to ensure that treatment produces changes that matter to clients and other stakeholders, such as the court system)

(Used with permission from the National Center for Child Traumatic Stress: National Child Traumatic Stress Network. (2016). Overview of Trauma Treatments and Practices [Web page]. Retrieved from: https://www.nctsn.org/ treatments-and-practices/trauma-treatments/overview.)

CDC's Guiding Principles to a Trauma-Informed Approach

The CDC's Office of Public Health Preparedness and Response (OPHPR), in collaboration with SAMHSA's National Center for Trauma-Informed Care (NCTIC), developed a model that outlines six principles to adopting a trauma-informed approach in various public health and child and family-serving organizations (SAMHSA, 2014). The six guiding principles include safety; trustworthiness and transparency; peer support; collaboration and mutuality; empowerment and choice; and culture, historical, and gender issues. There is no prescription or curriculum that shows how to be fully trauma-informed; however, it is critical to use a trauma-informed approach to work with clients, providers and professionals, and co-workers. It requires a high level of attention, caring awareness, and sensitivity on an individual level, and also a cultural and organizational change to reflect a trauma-informed systems approach.

Trauma-Informed Child Welfare System

Many child welfare systems have begun to consider and implement a trauma-informed approach to policies and practices. Child welfare agencies and their partners (e.g., court systems, community partners, etc.) should first use a systematic process of assessing their current system, prior to planning how to implement a system of care that is trauma-informed across the various units or departments, such as workforce development, screening and assessment, data systems, policies, funding, and interventions. It is important to focus on the workforce and take into consideration the attitudes of frontline worker (Bosk et al., 2020).

The National Child Traumatic Stress Network (NCTSN) defines a trauma-informed system as, "one in which all parties involved recognize and respond to the impact of traumatic stress on those who have contact with the system including children, caregivers, and service providers. Programs and agencies within such a system infuse and sustain trauma awareness, knowledge, and skills into their organizational cultures, practices, and policies. They act in collaboration with all those who are involved with the child, using the best available science, to facilitate and support the recovery and resiliency of the child and family." (NCTSN, n.d.) Adopting a trauma-informed approach means completing everyday tasks and conducting all interactions with the knowledge of the impact of trauma experiences of others. When all members of the system begin to incorporate these changes, it becomes a system-wide approach to practice. Using a system-wide trauma-informed approach has shown some positive changes in child and family outcomes, including a reduction in children receiving emergency or crisis services, use of psychotropic medication, fewer placement disruptions, and reduced length of stay in foster care (Child Welfare Information Gateway, 2020).

Research Brief

Promoting Positive Childhood Experiences (PCEs)

With much focus placed on adverse childhood experiences (ACEs) and the negative short- and long-term consequences to one's physical and mental health, it is often difficult to begin to consider how to prevent or intervene effectively with children, youth, and adults who have experienced such trauma. However, a new body of research has emerged that focuses on positive childhood experiences (PCEs) and how we can promote these experiences in an effort to prevent ACEs. Recent research (Bethell et al., 2019) shows adults who self-report more PCEs such as lower likelihood of depression and other mental health conditions. Positive childhood experiences (PCEs) are not simply the absence of ACEs of going to a theme park with your family every year. Examples of PCEs are being able to talk to family about feelings, having family and community traditions, having caring adults showing interest in you, and feeling safe and protected by an adult at home. Many adults as children are exposed to adverse experiences, many of which we cannot control. However, it is possible to do our best to balance these experiences with other positive experiences and promoting healthy caregiver relationships and environments for children.

Implementing a trauma-informed systems approach includes a shift in how we view the children and families we work with and how we respond and act to protect, support, and enhance well-being. Using a trauma-informed approach is one that is strengths-based, resilience-based, and culturally grounded. Instead of focusing on what someone did and what is wrong, the focus changes to what happened to that individual and how that informs what is going on now. This has been summarized by asking, "What happened to you?" rather than "What is wrong with you?" When considering a trauma-informed approach in child welfare workforce development, there has been a change in perspective of only focusing on protection, to safety, permanency, and well-being. Child welfare agencies have begun to assess and approach families more holistically and when offering services, a using family-centered approach. Trauma-informed also means prioritizing collaboration and the role of child welfare professionals. Staff and their supervisors focus more on understanding trauma, its impact, and how to move toward healing and well-being for all. There is a focus on prevention and early intervention with children and families. There is an understanding, as well, that trauma can also affect the child welfare professionals involved in cases in the form of burnout, secondary traumatic stress, and training of this issue and the role of trauma within families is critical (see Chap. 12 for information about burnout, secondary traumatic stress, self-care, and professional development.).

Training and education about trauma and its impact on children and families should also extend to caretakers, foster parents, kinship care providers, group home staff, biological parents, and providers. Education should continue as we learn more about trauma and its effects and should be infused into communication, meetings, and court hearings. Further, information and training should be available across systems in their collaboration to promote child and family well-being. (See Chap. 12 for information about trauma-informed supervision.)

Practice Highlight

Talking with Children Who Have Been Traumatized

Although this might vary by age, developmental stage, and experience of trauma, these are suggestions for talking with children who have been traumatized:

- Assess the child's readiness to talk (frequency, depth, and ability to express themselves).
- Reassure them about safety, their supports (who they can talk to), and what's going to happen next. Do not ever make promises or statements about things you don't know for sure will happen (e.g., going back to parent, visitation parameters).
- Ask what they know and how they understand the circumstances and give factual information as appropriate. This provides a better understanding of how they perceive past and current events. Ask them if they have questions they need clarification on.
- Listen closely, summarize, and use appropriate body language and facial expressions.
- Encourage and support children to show and talk about their feelings. Acknowledge their feelings about their experiences.
- Appropriately share your feelings while empathizing with the child.
- Focus on the good and the future. Discuss positive things that may or may not be related to the present circumstances.
- Give tools for the child to express emotions and process experiences.
- Make a referral for treatment as needed.

Conclusion

Child maltreatment is traumatic. Likewise, a child and family's contact with the child welfare system can be traumatic. Children and families experience a number of events that are considered traumatic, with child abuse and neglect being some of them. It is more common that they will have experienced more than one experience of trauma. Each child experiences and responds differently to trauma, and the best way to intervene is in trauma-informed ways that honor their experience. This chapter provided information about how to approach cases in a trauma-informed manner and how to promote screenings, assessments, and treatment that have been shown to address trauma appropriately that will allow for healing. There are ways for child welfare workers to respond using a trauma lens that will promote better outcomes in the case as well as with child and family well-being. Using a trauma-informed system-level approach can enhance the work that professionals and their partners are doing to improve child and family well-being.

Discussion Questions

1. What are three examples of traumatic events experienced by children?
2. Describe what trauma reminders and triggers are. What are three examples of trauma reminders or triggers for children who have experienced child maltreatment?
3. What are two ways that trauma is assessed? What tools are typically used?
4. How can child welfare professionals reduce the trauma experienced by children who are removed from their home?
5. What does it mean to use a trauma-informed approach in child welfare practice?

Suggested Activities

1. Take the ACE quiz online to reflect on the impact of your own experiences with adverse childhood experiences. https://www.npr.org/sections/health-shots/2015/03/02/387007941/take-the-ace-quiz-and-learn-what-it-does-and-doesnt-mean
2. Watch Through Our Eyes: Children, Violence, and Trauma: https://www.you-tube.com/watch?v=z8vZxDa2KPM. Consider the different types of trauma experienced by the children in the video and how it is manifested.
3. Watch How Childhood Trauma Affects Health Across a Lifetime: https://www.youtube.com/watch?v=95ovIJ3dsNk&t=1s. Explore the different ways one's health is compromised as a result of trauma.
4. Read Heleniak et al. (2016). Discuss with others how the trauma of child maltreatment can impact adolescents' behaviors and the implication for child welfare practice.
   Heleniak, C., Jenness, J. L., Vander Stoep, A., McCauley, E., & McLaughlin, K. A. (2016). Childhood maltreatment exposure and disruptions in emotion regulation: A transdiagnostic pathway to adolescent internalizing and externalizing psychopathology. *Cognitive therapy and research*, *40*(3), 394–415. (Available: https://rdcu.be/ccaW1).

Additional Resources

California Evidence-Based Clearing House for Child Welfare: https://www. cebc4cw.org/

Casey Family Programs, Why should child protection agencies become trauma-informed?: https://www.casey.org/why-become-trauma-informed/

Centers for Disease Control and Prevention, Adverse Childhood Experiences (ACEs): https://www.cdc.gov/violenceprevention/aces/index.html

National Center on Substance Abuse and Child Welfare, Child Welfare and Trauma: https://ncsacw.samhsa.gov/resources/trauma/child-welfare-and-trauma.aspx

The National Child Traumatic Stress Network: https://www.nctsn.org/

Title IV-E Prevention Services Clearinghouse: https://preventionservices. abtsites.com/

References

Bartlett, J. D., & Steber, K. (2019). *How to implement trauma-informed care to build resilience to childhood trauma*. Child Trends. Retrieved from: https://www.childtrends.org/publications/how-to-implement-trauma-informed-care-to-build-resilience-to-childhood-trauma.

Bethell, C., Jones, J., Gombojav, N., Linkenbach, J., & Sege, R. (2019). Positive childhood experiences and adult mental and relational health in a statewide sample: Associations across adverse childhood experiences levels. *JAMA pediatrics, 173*(11), e193007–e193007. https://doi.org/10.1001/jamapediatrics.2019.3007

Bosk, E. A., Williams-Butler, A., Ruisard, D., & MacKenzie, M. J. (2020). Frontline staff characteristics and capacity for trauma-informed care: Implications for the child welfare workforce. *Child Abuse & Neglect, 104536*. https://doi.org/10.1016/j.chiabu.2020.104536

Centers for Disease Control and Prevention. (2020a) *About the Kaiser-CDC ACE Study*. Retrieved from: https://www.cdc.gov/violenceprevention/aces/about.html

Centers for Disease Control and Prevention. (2020b). *Preventing adverse childhood experiences*. Retrieved from: https://www.cdc.gov/violenceprevention/acestudy/fastfact.html

Centers for Disease Control and Prevention. (2014). *Essentials for childhood: Creating safe, stable, nurturing relationships and environments for all children*. Retrieved from: https://www.cdc.gov/violenceprevention/childabuseandneglect/essentials.html

Child Welfare Information Gateway. (2020). *The Importance of a Trauma-Informed Child Welfare System*. U.S. Department of Health and Human Services, Administration for Children and Families, Children's Bureau.

Dong, M., Anda, R. F., Felitti, V. J., Dube, S. R., Williamson, D. F., Thompson, T. J., et al. (2004). The interrelatedness of multiple forms of childhood abuse, neglect, and household dysfunction. *Child Abuse & Neglect, 28*(7), 771–784. https://doi.org/10.1016/j.chiabu.2004.01.008

Donisch, K., Zhang, Y., Bray, C., Frank, S., & Gewirtz, A. H. (2020). Development and preliminary validation of the University of Minnesota's Traumatic Stress Screen for Children and Adolescents (TSSCA). *The Journal of Behavioral Health Services & Research*, 1–13. https://doi.org/10.1007/s11414-020-09725-1

Felitti, V. J., Anda, R. F., Nordenberg, D., Williamson, D. F., Spitz, A. M., Edwards, V., & Marks, J. S. (1998). Relationship of childhood abuse and household dysfunction to many of the leading causes of death in adults: The Adverse Childhood Experiences (ACE) Study. *American Journal of Preventive Medicine, 14*(4), 245–258. https://doi.org/10.1016/S0749-3797(98)00017-8

Finkelhor, D. (2018). Screening for adverse childhood experiences (ACEs): Cautions and suggestions. *Child Abuse & Neglect, 85*, 174–179. https://doi.org/10.1016/j.chiabu.2017.07.016

Giovanelli, A., Reynolds, A. J., Mondi, C. F., & Ou, S. R. (2016). Adverse childhood experiences and adult well-being in a low-income, urban cohort. *Pediatrics, 137*(4). https://doi.org/10.1542/peds.2015-4016

Heleniak, C., Jenness, J. L., Vander Stoep, A., McCauley, E., & McLaughlin, K. A. (2016). Childhood maltreatment exposure and disruptions in emotion regulation: A transdiagnostic pathway to adolescent internalizing and externalizing psychopathology. *Cognitive Therapy and Research, 40*(3), 394–415. https://doi.org/10.1007/s10608-015-9735-z

Hoffman, E. A., Clark, D. B., Orendain, N., Hudziak, J., Squeglia, L. M., & Dowling, G. J. (2019). Stress exposures, neurodevelopment and health measures in the ABCD study. *Neurobiology of Stress, 10*, 100157. https://doi.org/10.1016/j.ynstr.2019.100157

Kawam, E., & Martinez, M. J. (2016). What every social worker needs to know… trauma informed care in social work. *New Social Worker*. Retrieved from https://www.socialworker.com/feature-articles/practice/trauma-informed-care-in-social-work/.

Lambert, H. K., Meza, R., Martin, P., Fearey, E., & McLaughlin, K. A. (2017). Childhood trauma as a public health issue. In M. A. Landolt, M. Cloitre, & U. Schnder (Eds.), *Evidence-based treatments for trauma related disorders in children and adolescents* (pp. 49–66). Springer. https://doi.org/10.1007/978-3-319-46138-0_3

Myers, C., Garcia, A., Beidas, R., & Yang, Z. (2020). Factors that predict child welfare caseworker referrals to an evidence-based parenting program. *Children and Youth Services Review, 109*, 104750. https://doi.org/10.1016/j.childyouth.2020.104750

National Center for Child Traumatic Stress: National Child Traumatic Stress Network. (2016). *Overview of trauma treatments and Practices*. Retrieved from: https://www.nctsn.org/treatments-and-practices/trauma-treatments/overview.

National Child Traumatic Stress Network. (n.d.). *Creating trauma-informed systems*. Retrieved from: https://www.nctsn.org/trauma-informed-care/creating-trauma-informed-systems.

Peterson, C., Florence, C., & Klevens, J. (2018). The economic burden of child maltreatment in the United States, 2015. *Child Abuse & Neglect, 86*, 178–183. https://doi.org/10.1016/j.chiabu.2018.09.018

Substance Abuse and Mental Health Services Administration. (2014). *SAMHSA's concept of trauma and guidance for a trauma-informed approach* (HHS Publication No. (SMA) 14-4884). Rockville, MD.

U.S. Department of Health and Human Services. (2013, July 11). [Letter to State Medicaid Directors]. Retrieved from http://www.medicaid.gov/Federal-Policy-Guidance/Downloads/SMD-13-07-11.pdf

Chapter 6
Child and Family Engagement in Child Welfare Practice

Introduction

Child and family engagement is one of the most important components in child welfare practice and is key in promoting the safety, permanency, and well-being of children and families interacting with the child welfare system. In order to effectively engage parents and children in services, cooperation, and work toward positive case outcomes, it is essential for child welfare professionals to actively collaborate with all family members as well as community members, and other key partners such as mental health professionals, attorneys, child welfare staff, and extended family. Respect, patience, empathy, and collaboration are important attributes and skills to practice when engaging with families involved in the child welfare system.

Engagement

Engagement is a manner of interacting with another individual for the purpose of encouraging participation. In doing so, the child welfare professional understands the client has their own set of needs, experiences, and values (both cultural and personal) that shape their actions. Until the client believes the person they are interacting with (e.g., caseworker) understands their needs and is willing to help them meet those needs, there will be little progress made. Disregard for those needs and beliefs will often lead to estrangement and disillusionment on the part of the client.

Family engagement occurs throughout the case in child welfare. It is a family-centered and strengths-based approach that involves establishing and maintaining positive and collaborative relationships with families. Family engagement prioritizes joint efforts toward goal setting, developing case plans, making decisions, and

© Springer Nature Switzerland AG 2021
J. M. Geiger, L. Schelbe, *The Handbook on Child Welfare Practice*,
https://doi.org/10.1007/978-3-030-73912-6_6

communicating with each other to ensure safety, permanency, and well-being of the family and children involved. This collaborative process involves all members of the family (including children as appropriate depending on age), service providers, extended family, kinship caregivers, and foster/resource caregivers.

Family engagement and empowerment in child welfare practice is particularly important given the presence of a power differential. Regardless of the circumstances, child welfare professionals are in a position of great power when the child welfare system becomes involved with a family as they often have control over whether a child is removed from the home, how long a child is placed in care, whether services are offered, what types of services offered, and whether a child is returned home to their family of origin. The way that power and trust are used by child welfare professionals is an important component in parental engagement in the change process (Yatchmenoff, 2005) and may be predictive of case outcome (Damiani-Taraba et al., 2017; Graybeal, 2007). Gladstone et al. (2014) examined what casework skills contributed to parents involved in child welfare being engaged with their workers. They found three key skills: (1) workers including parents in planning, (2) workers being caring and supportive, and (3) workers praising parents for their efforts, ideas, or achievements. Other studies have found an association between engagement and workers' honesty and straightforwardness, providing information, and being able to listen and empathize (Platt, 2008), focusing on strengths and being flexible (Gockel et al., 2008), and using clear communication about agency involvement, returning calls, and being responsive (De Boer & Coady, 2007). In summary, research indicates that consistent strengths-based, family-centered, and culturally grounded practice is essential in managing potential biases and maximizing family engagement and motivation in child welfare practice (Gladstone et al., 2014).

Research has shown that family engagement in child welfare can enhance the helping relationship, promote family "buy-in," encourage parental participation in services, increase motivation to complete services and requirements, expand options for permanency and placement, improve the quality and focus of family visits, increase placement stability, improve timeliness of permanency, build family decision-making skills, and enhance the fit in family needs and services. Family engagement is relevant throughout all of child welfare. Ensuring that families believe that the services or programs are useful and relevant to them is important. Care must be taken to assess if programs and services meet the needs of families involved with the child welfare system. For example, the evidence-based parenting interventions Pathways Triple P had not been evaluated thoroughly with families in child welfare, and a recent study interviewed parents involved in the program to understand their satisfaction of the program and understanding of its appropriateness (Lewis et al., 2016). The study's main finding was parents found the program helpful and relevant. The study also highlighted barriers parents identified which can be used to help to improve interventions and better engage families.

Reflection

Initial Impressions: The Effects of Personal Bias

- What impacts someone's first impressions?
- How can initial impressions affect (negatively or positively) a purposeful helping relationship?
- When might initial impressions have positive outcomes? Negative outcomes?
- How might the client's initial impressions of the child welfare professional impact the relationship? How do these impressions impact our ability to effectively work with the client?

Strength-Based Practice in Child Welfare

A strength-based approach refers to the practice and policies that identify and cultivate the strengths of children, families, and communities. It acknowledges the individual and collective strengths and challenges and emphasizes a collaborative approach in engaging all family members in planning, implementation, and evaluation of service plan goals. Strength-based practice, in general and in child welfare, involves a number of skills and attributes, including an empowerment-focused approach in developing and maintaining a collaborative relationship between the client(s) and family that aims to create change and positive outcomes as families work toward self-sufficiency. Strengths-based practice as a philosophy is consistent with the values and ideals of social work and other helping professions and is embraced by a variety of private and public child welfare agencies used to guide practice with clients and systems. All children and families possess strengths that can be used to improve their lives. Recent research has found that strengths can improve mental health outcomes for youth with an experience of child maltreatment (e.g., Kisiel et al., 2017). By identifying children and families' strengths, we are identifying the tools that will be used to resolve many of the issues they present with. When we focus on strengths, we motivate our clients to change, give them hope, and help them view themselves in a more positive light.

Research Brief

Engaging Parents in Child Welfare System Interventions

Brittany Mihalec-Adkins, M.S.Ed.

One critical component of successful child welfare system intervention is parents' meaningful engagement with services, requirements, and helping relationships (e.g., Platt, 2012; Yatchmenoff, 2005). Briefly, parent engagement is critical because of the following: (1) parents cannot benefit from interventions unless they are sufficiently participatory, and (2) child welfare authorities cannot feel confident in parents' progress and suitability unless they observe attitudes, efforts, and commitment to remedying the conditions that led to child protection services involvement. However, cultivating and maintaining meaningful levels of parental engagement in nonvoluntary state-mandated interventions have proven challenging – particularly among parents most in need of services (e.g., Fusco, 2015; Toros et al., 2018).

Barriers to meaningful parent engagement identified include parent- or family-level factors, such as histories of intimate partner violence (Kohl et al., 2005), past and present substance misuse (Kemp et al., 2014), and poor mental health (e.g., Littell et al., 2001) – all of which are prevalent (and often comorbid; Stromwall et al., 2008) among parents in child welfare interventions (Darlington et al., 2004; Guo et al., 2006). Parents with unmet personal, social, and material needs understandably struggle to meaningfully and consistently engage; fortunately, preliminary research has found promise in interventions that provide parents with material or financial support, and that provide parents with "peer mentors" to help them navigate the intervention process (e.g., Rostad et al., 2017a, b; Summers et al., 2012).

Parent engagement can also be stifled by various factors at the caseworker- or intervention-level, including parent-caseworker relationships characterized by poor communication (e.g., unclear expectations), conflict, overt power differentials, stigma, and judgment. However, there is evidence to suggest that when services feel relevant to parents, and when parents feel "heard" and respected by caseworkers, they are more likely to persistently and meaningfully engage in services and to nourish positive helping relationships (Chapman et al., 2003; Kapp & Vela, 2004). Indeed, caseworkers' abilities to be appropriately supportive and nonjudgmental with CWS clients have shown promise for promoting parental engagement in services and positive attitudes toward CWS personnel (Kapp & Vela, 2004). Similarly, parents have been found to be more willing to earnestly engage when they felt that caseworkers were not exploiting their obvious power (Dumbrill, 2006; Gladstone et al., 2012; Maiter et al., 2006).

While initial efforts to identify paths to promoting parent engagement have been promising, more research must be done to address remaining gaps and limitations. For instance, there are vast array of definitions and assessments of parent engagement employed across practice settings and research studies. Reaching consensus on both can benefit future efforts immensely. Further, extant research on child welfare-involved parents has focused almost exclusively on mothers, leaving sizable and irresponsible blind spots in research and practice when it comes to engaging and serving fathers (Brown et al., 2009; Campbell et al., 2015; Maxwell et al., 2012).

Family-Centered Practice in Child Welfare

Family-centered practice is based upon the belief that the best way to meet a person's needs is within their families. It is also the belief that services and support can be provided to a child and their family to ensure safety, permanency, and well-being by engaging, involving, and strengthening families by considering the whole family and their communities. The key components of family-centered practice include developing a trusting, respectful, and honest relationship between family members and service providers, working closely with family members to ensure safety and well-being, strengthening families' ability to function well independently, engaging, empowering, and working collaboratively with families while making decisions and setting goals, and providing culturally grounded, individualized services and supports for each family. Child welfare professionals who are family-centered strive to preserve the family and prevent out-of-home placement while providing the necessary services and supports to ensure safety. The family-centered model views families as being capable of making decisions for their own families, prioritizes strengths, and encourages families to advocate for their own needs. When safe to do so, children should remain in their own homes to preserve the family unit. (See Chap. 7 for information about family preservation.) In situations where children must be placed in out-of-home care, the least restrictive placement is used, and families continue to be actively involved, informed, and empowered to make decisions that will lead to reunification. Community agencies can also engage in family-centered practice by providing evidence-supported interventions that cultivate individual and family strengths and empower families to keep children safe, well, and in the home with their caregivers. Family-centered practice involves meeting clients "where they are," which helps to understand that a client and their family have a unique needs, experiences, and values that shape their actions.

Despite the widespread support and promotion of these approaches in practice, the implementation of strengths-based and family-centered practice is often difficult (Lietz, 2013). Child welfare practice is challenging on an individual and systemic level and requires a collaborative approach at multiple levels. There are a number of ways that child welfare agencies can enhance family engagement on a systems level as well as an individual level. For example, agency leadership, supervisors, and staff can implement a family-focused organizational culture in practice through policies and standards, by ensuring manageable caseloads, ongoing professional development, and access to services and performance review and monitoring systems (Child Welfare Information Gateway, 2016). In casework, child welfare professionals can utilize family-centered and strengths-based skills and practices to enhance family engagement, such as being clear, honest, and respectful when communicating with families, ensure adequate time with families and check in frequently, implement shared decision-making and participatory planning, offer services that match needs, and encourage parents and children through the process.

Many agencies are implementing family engagement strategies to ensure cross-systems collaboration, shared decision-making, and family-friendly policies to engage all members of the family. One common practice is the use of Child and Family Teams (CFTs) that brings together family members and professionals involved with the case regularly to brainstorm, set, and assess goals for the children and their families in between court hearings. These meetings typically occur monthly and focus on the needs of the children and the parents to ensure they receive the social-emotional, academic, and physical health services to promote their well-being and family reunification. Similarly, some agencies use family group decision-making (FGDM) early on in the case to make decisions about placement, services, family finding, and visitation. These meetings and groups also prioritize a family's strengths and their voice in making decisions that are best for their family.

Child welfare agencies recognize the importance of fathers to the healthy development of children and how fathers have often been excluded when child welfare systems become involved. Agencies are beginning to provide resources and guidance about engaging fathers and working to enhance their positive involvement with children. Services offered vary depending on the agency; however, they often include assessment, planning, helping fathers understand the system, and strategies for obtaining custody or improving parenting skills. Recently, there have been evidence-based parent training program developed specifically for specific groups such as fathers or military families. Programs such as SafeCare Dad to Kids (Dad2K; Rostad et al., 2017b) and mDad (Mobile Device Assisted Dad; Lee & Walsh, 2015) are designed specifically for fathers. There is a need for more programs to address the needs of fathers and to target specific groups of fathers (e.g., Black fathers, fathers of adolescents) to increase engagement and ultimately child well-being (Cryer-Coupet et al., 2020). There are also programs addressing the needs of military families (e.g., Ross et al., 2020).

Another strategy is foster family – birth family meetings and increased use of shared parenting. Shared parenting refers to the practice in which foster parents cultivate positive, supportive relationships with birth parents. Shared parenting is a gradual process in which a relationship is nurtured to a point of trust and understanding. Families work together toward shared goals for the child's safety and well-being. This model helps with improving the relationship between biological parents and foster parents through communication, trust, care, and helps with modeling parenting skills, which often contribute positively to family reunification efforts. These relationships allow both sets of caregivers to establish a parenting routine and standards. Early in the case, biological

> **Practice Highlight**
>
> **Elements of Family Group Decision-Making (FGDM)**
>
> - The presence of a coordinator who acts as the group facilitator
> - Recognition and acknowledgment that the family group represents an important decision-making partner in case
> - Inclusion of private family time
> - Preference of the case plan developed by the family over other plans
> - Provision of services, resources, and supports for the case plan to be successful
> - Follow-up after the FGDM until outcomes are achieved

parents can share important information about the child necessary to their care-giving (e.g., likes and dislikes), and the foster parents can talk about the child's home environment and routine. Depending on the circumstances of the case, case investigators can discuss these issues with the biological parents at the time of removal, or this information can be exchanged during early court conferences and/or family group decision-making (FGDM) or child and family (CFT) meetings. This allows for multiple individuals who know the child well can offer their ideas to ensure the child's needs are being met.

Engaging parents as peer mentors has also been shown to improve family engagement. Peer mentoring programs enlist people who were once involved in the child welfare system as parents to help new parents navigate the system and meet case plan goals. In many states, parent partner programs or birth parent leadership groups have been successful in assisting parents faced with their children being removed from their care and child welfare system involvement. It supports parents who need the assistance and provides an opportunity for experienced parents in building skills and improving a sense of purpose and self-esteem (Rockhill et al., 2015).

Building Rapport and Developing an Alliance with the Family

Respectful and successful intervention with a family involved with the child welfare system depends heavily on the relationship between the child welfare professional and the family (Van Zyl et al., 2014). However, developing a positive relationship with families at risk for child maltreatment can be challenging for all who are involved. It is possible these families have had negative experiences in the past working with agencies and systems and therefore are distrustful, fearful, or hesitant to engage due to negative perceptions of the child protection agency. The quality of this relationship is dependent on developing a collaborative relationship with the family (DePanfilis, 2000) that begins at the first meeting and

> **Practice Highlight**
>
> **Parent Cafes: Building Protective Factors and Leadership**
>
> Parent cafes are an informal and inviting atmosphere with space for gathering that mimics a café. They typically involve a small group of four to six individuals that engage in conversations around experiences of child welfare. It is common to have a peer host who has participated in other parent cafes and who may have training to facilitate conversations that promote support and advice for other parents.

continues throughout the case. In order to develop a relationship with the client, it must be intentional, genuine, and planned. The relationship should be based on trust, care, connection, and commitment. The child welfare professional and the client must be willing to be vulnerable and understanding with one another.

The three "core conditions" of a helping relationship, according to Carl Rogers (1957), are respect, empathy, and genuineness. Other researchers highlight relationship qualities such as personal warmth, acceptance, affirmation, sincerity, and encouragement (Duncan et al., 2010). By engaging in these seemingly basic skills, the family and the worker can engage in a relationship where there is a sense of trust and security, where the core issues can be dealt with, children are safe, and families can be well together.

Respect, empathy, and genuineness are not only feelings or beliefs but also actions. These skills must also be demonstrated in daily practice with children and families. By showing respect, empathy, and genuineness, child welfare professionals can more readily make appropriate and balanced assessments, make necessary referrals, and proceed with a case as required legally and morally. Showing respect involves a child welfare professionals' ability to communicate care for the individual and family, value, and acceptance of each person in the family. Children and families experiencing child maltreatment require respect and acceptance in order for professionals to be able to understand their circumstances and provide the best care to ensure safety and well-being. Respect is communicated through words and actions.

Empathy is also a critical skill to demonstrate our ability to understand where a family is and has been, their experiences, to be able to manage our own feelings and biases, and recognize that our experiences and feelings are separate from those of the family. Empathy involves active listening, reflecting, and understanding body language, use of words, and emotions. Empathy is key in building trust with children and parents involved in child welfare and building rapport and relationships. The presence of empathy means acknowledging bias, but withholding judgment, understanding the trauma each member of the family may have experienced, and acknowledging the role of individual and collective experiences that have led the family to child welfare system involvement.

Being genuine with others may be easier than it is for others and develops and improves over time and experience. It simply means being honest, open, non-defensive, and flexible in interactions with

> **Practice Highlight**
>
> **Key Skills to Increase Family Engagement**
>
> - Provide culturally grounded services.
> - Balance discussions of problems with the identification of strengths and resources.
> - Listen to and address issues that concern the family.
> - Help families meet concrete needs (e.g., housing, food, etc.).
> - Set goals that are mutually agreed upon.
> - Focus on improving family members' skills.
> - Provide family with choices when possible.
> - Obtain commitment that the family will engage.
> - Share openly about what to expect.
> - Conduct frequent and substantive caseworker visits with parents, children, and caregivers.
> - Use effective and approved technologies to engage families.
> - Recognize and praise progress.
> - Invite all members of the support system to be a part of meetings (extended family, teachers, clergy, etc.).

children and families. People respond more openly when we present our true selves in a genuine way. Being genuine does not mean being unprofessional or overly casual in our interactions; it means balancing our knowledge of the agency's policies and procedures with a calm, engaging, open

> - Clarify goals, roles, responsibilities, and expectations.
> - Consider families' other obligations (e.g., employment) when scheduling meetings.
>
> Adapted from Child Welfare Information Gateway (2016)

response. It means using positive language that does not blame, disrespect, or show anger or disappointment. This approach reduces the likelihood of the parent or caregiver being alienated, bitter, resistant, or closed to questions. More often than not, our ability, as child welfare professionals to regulate our emotions, stay calm, and show respect helps us relate better to the individuals we are working with. Child welfare workers should focus on shared values and goals to be able to move forward.

All of these skills show others that we are there to help and empower the family to understand the need for our involvement, to explore solutions, and use strengths and resources to improve safety and promote well-being for all. Child welfare professionals should approach families with the assumption that the family has the capability of making change, and it is within their role to help them in creating change.

Connecting with Children

Engaging children is a different skill set when working with families involved in the child welfare system. Child welfare professionals must have knowledge about child development and what to expect for a specific age for a child. Additionally, in these cases, children are the victims of maltreatment and will have experienced some level of trauma from the abuse and/or neglect and possibly from being interviewed and/or removed from their caregiver and home. Skills such as empathy, warmth, and genuineness should be used, as they are with adults. Children may be suspicious and struggle to understand events and/ or consequences related to the circumstances. Child welfare professionals interviewing children should be sure to get on their level

> **Practice Highlight**
>
> **How to Show Empathy, Respect, and Genuineness**
>
> - Active listening
> - Appropriate body language
> - Understanding the other's point of view and experience
> - Using humor, appropriate self-disclosure, and warm expressions (smiles, eye contact, etc.)
> - Summarizing
> - Taking the time to understand culture and family traditions
> - Always incorporating family strengths
> - Being present, available, and honest

physically and speak to them in a way that is appropriate for their age. For example, they can sit on the floor with them and speak slowly while using words they can understand based on their age. Also, child welfare professionals can also use creative means of communicating if necessary (nonverbally, through stories, or art), be trustworthy and honest, and ensure their safety. In engaging children, child welfare professionals must be aware of trauma indicators and screen and refer for treatment as necessary.

Culturally Grounded Engagement in Child Welfare

Engagement helps to meet a family "where they are" and requires that we see a family through a culturally grounded lens. It requires that we attempt to understand the client's motivation and reasons for their actions and acknowledge that this can help us develop solutions toward planning for change. While understanding that cultures may differ in how they view discipline and corporal punishment, we must always use proper assessment tools to determine safety and risk and not excuse cultural practices that might lead to child abuse and neglect. Chapter 3 discussed appropriate discipline, and Chap. 4 presents the definition and assessment of child abuse and neglect.

Four components to consider in developing culturally "competent" or cultural "humility" include: cultural awareness, knowledge acquisition, skill development, and inductive learning (Fong, 2001). These factors allow us to better understand how others view their behaviors in relation to culture. We can learn from their beliefs and match our response in terms of services and interactions to best serve the child and family. Racial disparity and disproportionality continue to be an issue in child welfare systems. As discussed in previous chapters, in many jurisdictions, children of color are overrepresented in the child welfare system due to differential treatment by race (Fluke et al., 2010), oftentimes as a result of bias, lack of understanding, or fear. Racial bias occurs on multiple decision-making levels including reporting, investigations, and ongoing/permanency. These decisions often happen on an unconscious basis, and at the individual level, there is no intention to treat families differently; however, the bias is present, and it is often difficult to point to one individual or decision that causes overall trends in racial disparity and disproportionality.

Child Welfare Professional as Change Agent

The child welfare professional assigned to a case is not only one who manages and reports on a case – they also are a change agent, someone who takes an active role in promoting change. The intervention requiring change begins by establishing a relationship with the family so that they feel capable and motivated to make changes in their behavior, thoughts, and emotions to healthier patterns of relating to others, particularly their family members. The child welfare worker facilitates change by conducting comprehensive assessments; advocating for services; providing leadership and support for the client; assisting the family in recognizing and accessing their strengths and resources; helping the family build protective factors internally and externally; and helping to keep a strengths, solution, and family-centered focus.

Practice Tip

Strategies for Building Rapport

- Use an open mind when working with the family.
- Determine what is most important to the family.
- Use reflective strategies by taking note of the words the family uses and use similar language.
- Listen to the family's account of the situation without interrupting.
- Ask the family what their goals are.
- Use open-ended questions.
- Explain your expectations, process, and purpose in working with the family.
- Involve the family in planning throughout the process.
- Acknowledge feelings and encourage openness and honesty.
- Be consistent and follow through.
- Encourage participation in decision-making and problem-solving. (Berg & Kelly, 2000)

There are a number of skills and models that child welfare professionals can adopt to facilitate change alongside their clients, including solution-focused therapy strategies, motivational interviewing, and using a strengths-based, cognitive behavioral model for change.

In order for humans to make changes, there must be certain elements present, and they must be motivated to change. First, there must be a level of discomfort present related to something that the family wants but does not have (e.g., children removed, sense of peace and calmness, safety, stability). Second, the individual must take responsibility and see themselves not only as part of the issue but also the solution related to the discomfort. The individual must feel emotional security and vulnerability in those who are there to support them through the process of change. The individual must have a preferred alternative future, and that is how they envision the future to be. Lastly, they must have the ability and belief that they can change. These are all elements that the child welfare professional can instill, support, and promote to assist with creating change; however, there must also be buy-in on the individual's part.

Solution-Focused Approach in Child Welfare

Solution-focused brief therapy (SFBT) was developed by Steve de Shazer and Insoo Kim Berg and their team at the Milwaukee Brief Family Therapy in the early 1980s. The overall philosophy of the therapeutic intervention is to focus on solutions rather than the problems clients are facing. Main assumptions of the approach are that: (1) all clients have strengths and resources; (2) the relationship between the client and therapist has significant therapeutic value; (3) change happens all the time; (4) the focus remains on the present and future, rather than the past; (5) small change leads to bigger change; (6) clear goals are essen-

> **Practice Highlight**
>
> **Examples of Solution-Focused Questions**
>
> - Tell me what you like most about parenting.
> - Tell me about how you have been able to manage (the children/household).
> - How were you able to overcome obstacles in the past?
> - On a scale of 1 to 10, how would you rate your progress since the last time we met?

tial; and (7) it is not essential to know the cause of a problem in order to find a solution (De Jong & Berg, 2008). Using a solution-focused approach in child welfare practice helps the client consider a more positive and preferred outlook and alternate future. The approach is accepting of all individuals, no matter their pasts, actions, or experiences. Several strategies within SFBT are helpful in developing positive rapport and change with clients. When using a solution-focused approach, child welfare professionals use questions about past successes, exception questions (when the issue/problem does not occur), the miracle question, scaling questions, and coping questions. The purpose of asking questions about past successes allows us to discover instances when the family was functioning well. Exception questions allow us to learn more about the times when the problem was not occurring but could have (e.g., where, when, how, who, etc.). The miracle question asks the family to describe how things would look if the problem no longer existed as if a miracle had occurred overnight. Scaling questions involve clients rating the severity of the problem (on a scale of 1–10), from their perspective, and relationship questions ask how other individuals (typically other family members) would view the problem/issue. Finally, coping questions help clients discover their own resources and strengths by asking them how they managed to cope given the challenging circumstances.

When applying this model to child welfare, practitioners should focus on capitalizing on family strengths and setting goals that use a family's specific language and support "family ownership" and track progress while celebrating successes. Solution-focused casework has been shown to be effective in increasing families' involvement in their case plan, follow-through on referrals to service, and less recidivism in terms of reports for repeat maltreatment.

Motivational Interviewing in Child Welfare Practice

Motivational interviewing, developed by William Miller and Steven Rollnick (2002), is a directive, client-centered approach of eliciting behavior change by helping clients to explore and resolve ambivalence. Compared with nondirective counseling, it is more focused and goal-directed. The examination and resolution of ambivalence are its central purpose, and the interviewer is intentionally directive in pursuing this goal. Motivational interviewing is also a common method to support families that may be ambivalent or resistant to engage in change with the child welfare agency. There are four core techniques that allow individuals in families to explore this ambivalence and motivate them to make changes at various stages of the case, including the first interaction. The acronym used to describe these techniques is OARS (**O**pen-ended questions, **A**ffirmations, **R**eflections, **S**ummary).

Practice Tip

Motivational Interviewing Techniques

O – Open Questions: These encourage family members to use their own words and elaborate on a topic.

"What do you know about why I am here today?"
"What is a typical day like for your family?"
"What has been challenging in your ability to parent lately?"

A – Affirm Client: This builds productive and cooperative working relationships with families by engaging their positive intents, characteristics, or traits.

"Sounds like you've had a lot of challenges lately, but you have really worked hard to make things better."
"I've really noticed how positive you've been and open to making changes. Thank you."
"I know it's not easy to parent a child with special needs, but I admire how organized you are and what great care you've taken."

R – Reflect: This engages others in the relationship, builds trust, and fosters motivation to change by ensuring breakdowns in communication don't occur.

"You were angry with Bart for soiling his pants."
"It sounds like this was a very frustrating situation."
"You're worried that LeeAnn will have a temper tantrum at the store next time."

S – Summarize: This ensures there is clear communication between the speaker and listener.

"Here's what I heard you say…"
"Tell me if I understand this correctly…"

Open-ended questions are important to gather information from the client's perspective. By asking open-ended questions, we avoid making any assumptions and allow the client to offer information in their own words and experience. Affirmations are used to recognize individual and family strengths and to use those to encourage and motivate the client toward making a change. It also shows them that they have the tools to make changes and helps them to build confidence. Statements about progress and positive actions can also motivate a client toward change. Clients respond to statements that show empathy and how we relate. This also allows for open-ended questions to elicit more information about their abilities, motives, and strengths.

Active listening is a critical skill in the helping profession when interviewing and engaging clients. The key part of active listening is being able to reflect back what the individual is saying in a way that shows understanding. It involves more listening and less talking to avoid giving advice or offering solutions, which is challenging for many to do. Reflecting involves statements of the client's words to "check" what the client is saying. For example, reflective statements use language that shows understanding of their thoughts, feelings, and emotions based on what they have said. Miller and Rollnick (2002) describe various types of reflections, including simple, complex, double-sided, and amplified reflections.

Finally, summarizing is a key technique in motivational interviewing that allows the listener to pull together important aspects of the conversation that summarize what was said, getting agreement on issues, and going forward, what next steps are. It involves obtaining a commitment to actions (from all involved) and addressing some of the ambivalence that families may have.

A *change agent* is often the source of support that helps motivate the client through the process. This process can start in the first meeting and in as little as 5–30 min and best used in subsequent meetings with the client. The child welfare professional can adopt the following several principles when motivating change. First, they should *express empathy*. They can highlight apparent conflicts between stated goals and current behaviors by *developing discrepancies*. It is important to *avoid argumentation* and *roll with resistance*. Acknowledging and accepting resistances as normal while *supporting self-efficacy* encourages even small attempts with change.

> **Practice Highlight**
>
> **Types of Reflective Statements**
>
> **Client statement**: "I don't think this is fair."
>
> **Simple:** "This doesn't seem fair to you."
>
> **Complex:** "This feels unfair to you when nobody will listen."
>
> **Double-sided:** "While you don't think this is fair, you are willing to participate in the classes."
>
> **Amplified:** "Even with all of your efforts, none of this seems fair to you."

Other motivational interviewing strategies include asking for permission, eliciting change talk, exploring importance and confidence, normalizing, decisional balancing, using a supporting self-efficacy, and gauging readiness to change. Practitioners also use what is referred to as the "Columbo" approach, which involves presenting the facts that appear to conflict, giving the person an opportunity to respond, and then asking questions to clarify the issues. Eliciting change talk can be challenging when clients view themselves as being unable to change or unwilling to change. The more we encourage them to talk about change, the more likely they begin to think about change and take action to change. Some strategies for eliciting change talk include asking them to scale the importance of an issue and their confidence level. This allows them to think about where they are in the change process and establish a reference point for measuring change. Second, asking clients to verbalize extremes, using terms such as worst, best, biggest, and lowest, also gets clients to think about moving toward change. Assessing progress with clients by asking them to look back (to the beginning) and looking forward toward what change looks like can be effective. Another strategy elicits the exploration of pros and cons of change for the individual and their family. For example, "what are the positives of not changing?" or "what are the downsides to not changing?"

Managing Difficult Encounters with the Family

Working with individuals and families who did not seek help can be challenging and can often present with difficult circumstances. As a child welfare professional, we have the authority and responsibility to investigate and monitor situations where child safety is involved. Oftentimes in those circumstances, the adult caregivers or biological parents are the individuals who are responsible or suspected of abuse or neglect of the child. As a result, they will be hostile, resistant, and possibly reactive. The child welfare professional's approach in these situations can often predict how the encounter will go; in other situations, they may have little control in what occurs. There are a range of challenging encounters with families, from adults who do not want to open the door and allow entry to those who are threatening violence. Verbal and physical threats are all too common in situations that are as volatile as the threat of removing a child from their parent. When dealing with resistance, denial, or hostility, it is possible to still navigate a productive meeting or interview with another adult without law enforcement involvement. By staying calm, in control, and non-defensive, child welfare professionals can work toward small steps in engaging in discussion with the adult(s). Child welfare professionals can normalize the circumstances, avoid blaming or labeling, and acknowledge the difficult situation both the child welfare professional and the parents placed in. It is important to note any behaviors that are escalating or if feeling unsafe. In those situations, child welfare professionals should prioritize their safety and leave and request support from a supervisor or law enforcement. Be aware, use active listening, stay focused, and keep an appropriate distance. Use discretion, be strategic, and know how to remain safe. See Chap. 12 for more information about safety in child welfare practice.

Working with Families Experiencing Mental Health Challenges, Substance Abuse, and Intimate Partner Violence

When working with families, it is important to note various underlying conditions that play a role in how a parent is able to care for a child. There may be issues that are preventing a parent from providing the care a child needs, such as the presence of mental health symptoms, developmental disabilities, substance abuse, and/or domestic violence. These experiences vary and can change over time; however, the presence of these underlying conditions may negatively impact a parent's ability to meet the child's needs and may increase the risk of abuse or neglect. This does not mean that abuse and neglect are present if a family is experiencing one of the underlying conditions. Once one of the underlying conditions has been identified with the child or the parent, it must be assessed for a regular basis. Treatment or attention to the condition may also be a part of the case plan goals and therefore must be monitored throughout the case.

Practice Highlight

Motivational Interviewing: Sample Questions and Statements

Open-Ended Questions

"Tell me about your parenting experiences."
"What concerns do you have about your parenting?"
"How can I help you with your parenting?"

Reflective Listening (Ambivalence)

"I hear you."
"I'm accepting, not judging you."
"Please say more."

Affirmative Statements (Building Trust and Confidence)

"You are very courageous to be so honest about this."
"You've accomplished a lot in a short time."
"I can understand why this has been so hard for you."

Summary Statements

"What you said is important. I value what you say. Here are the salient points."
"Did I hear you correctly?"
"We covered that well. Let's talk about ..."

Elicit Self-Motivational Statements

Problem recognition: *"I never realized how this has been a problem." "Maybe I have been doing something wrong."*
Expression of concern: *"I am really worried about parenting and how my kids are being affected."*
Intention to change: *"I don't know how but I want to try."*
Theme about optimism: *"I think I can do it. I am going to overcome this problem."*

Substance Abuse

It is estimated that more than a third of child welfare cases involve alcohol or other drugs as a contributing factor for removal (U.S. DHHS, 2020). With cases that involve alcohol and other drugs, it's important to consider timeframes. Policies regarding permanency have certain timeframes for reunification or another plan for children. (See Chap. 10 for more details about required timeframes.) In these cases, we must consider time for treatment and recovery and the child's sense of time based on their age, attachment, and relationships with biological parents and foster or kinship providers. As a child welfare professional, it is not our responsibility to provide substance abuse treatment; however, it is our responsibility to assess for the need for treatment by conducting a screening and assess the impact of the substance abuse condition that impacts the child's need for safety and well-being, and work alongside the parent to obtain treatment and support success through child-parent visits, providing tangible supports, and monitoring the use of the following treatment. To facilitate success for parents experiencing substance abuse issues, a child welfare professional can provide transportation for drug screenings, treatment, groups, therapy, and visitation. It is important to work closely with the parent to ensure they understand what is required of them and how they can work toward reunification. Being aware of what substance abuse treatment typically entails is also helpful. No one treatment approach is appropriate for everyone, and treatment may be lengthy. Recovery often includes relapse; therefore, treatment should include planning and supports to prevent relapse and promote long-term recovery.

Parents may deny the need for treatment, particularly inpatient treatment, and they may be resistant to change. This does not mean they do not want to parent or do not love their child. They may be without support, or may have legal or financial barriers to treatment, which should be addressed to promote family reunification.

Note from the Field

A Family's Struggle with Substance Abuse

Carol Taylor, MSW, LCSW

Maya[1] was an African-American woman in her late 30s when she came to the attention of DCFS for a second time. Maya had given birth to a baby girl that tested positive for cocaine. When DCFS was alerted of the case, they realized that mom had two adolescent boys age 13 and 16 already in foster care. The boys had come into care over 10 years earlier due to Maya's substance abuse. Maya's two sons had spent the majority of their lives in the DCFS system and bounced around to several homes but had been in the current home for the last 3 years. Maya was in and out of their lives over the 10 years but never actively working toward their reunification, and at the same time, no home until now had been willing to do permanency. The current foster parent was also vacillating in her commitment to move forward with adoption.

When the private agency was notified of Maya's new baby, investigations unit was making a decision on whether to remove the baby from her care. The current situation was that Maya was now in a long-term relationship with the baby's father, John. John had a history of substance abuse and domestic violence but had been clean for the last couple of years. Maya agreed to go to inpatient substance abuse treatment, and John was willing to take the baby home. DCP made the decision to allow for John to be the primary caregiver with a safety plan for Maya to complete treatment and be monitored by the family case worker at the private agency.

The family case worker monitored Maya as she successfully completed drug treatment; both Maya and John completed domestic violence classes and continued to both drop clean. Since the new baby arrived, the family case worker started visitation between both older boys, Maya, the baby, and John. Since Maya and John continued to do well, the child and family team decided to staff the case and discuss the possibility of changing the goal to return home for the older boys. The boys wanted to go home, and Maya and John desired them to be reunified.

At the next court date, the goal was changed to Return Home within 12 months. The case moved quickly since the risks that were in place years ago were less due to Maya's stability but also do to the boys being older and able to protect themselves. Within several months, the youngest of the two boys was returned home. Maya relapsed once but immediately went back to treatment for the family to remain intact.

The oldest son did not return home. He had stopped attending school and struggled with his own substance use. The child and family team decided that a goal of Independence was best for him and the family in order to allow him to focus on his own needs while Maya focused on raising her youngest two children and remaining sober.

[1]All names and other personal identifiers in cases and examples throughout this book have been changed to protect privacy and confidentiality.

Intimate Partner Violence (IPV)

Intimate partner violence (IPV) is also common among families reported for child maltreatment. The National Coalition Against Domestic Violence (n.d.) defines domestic violence/intimate partner violence as the "willful intimidation, physical assault, battery, sexual assault, and/or other abuse behavior as a part of a systematic pattern of power and control perpetrated by one intimate partner against another." Violence includes physical violence, sexual violence, psychological violence, and emotional abuse directed at one's partner. When interviewing a client who presents with an intimate relationship, whether it is a spouse or paramour/significant other, we should assess for any violence and how the violence may affect the child and caretaker.

Child maltreatment is more likely to occur in cases where there is intimate partner violence (e.g., Hartley, 2002; Herrenkohl et al., 2008). It is also often linked to severe and fatal cases of child abuse. Perpetrators of intimate partner violence may use children to establish or maintain control over the victim by physically, emotionally, or sexually attacking the children. Further, research has begun to document the impact on children living in homes where intimate partner violence is present. Proper assessment is critical in the early stages and throughout the case. Child welfare professionals can assist with treatment – therapy, shelter services, financial services, and housing to assist in preventing intimate partner violence and preventing out-of-home care for the child.

> **Practice Tip**
>
> **Assessing for Intimate Partner Violence**
>
> - Tell me about your relationship.
> - How are decisions made in your relationship? How are disagreements resolved?
> - Do you feel free to do, think, or believe what you want?
> - Does your partner ever act jealous or possessive?
> - Have you ever felt afraid of your partner? In what ways?
> - Have you ever been afraid for the safety of your children?

Collaboration between child welfare professionals and advocates providing services and supports to families who have experienced intimate partner violence is important in working toward family reunification, family safety, and well-being. Advocates can work with child welfare professionals to develop safety plans, enhance family resilience, and provide necessary services and supports to families in need of housing, counseling, etc. Child welfare professionals can offer expertise around issues of child maltreatment, share information about the dependency case (as appropriate), and collaborate on accessing services for children and families exposed to intimate partner violence.

Mental Illness

One in 5 adults experiences a mental illness any given year, and 1 in 25 lives with a serious mental illness (NAMI, 2019). A mental illness is a condition that impacts a person's thinking, feeling, or mood and may affect their ability to relate to others and function on a daily basis. A diagnosis of mental illness according to the *Diagnostic and Statistical Manual of Mental Disorders* (DSM), one must experience clinically significant impairment or distress in one's personal, social, or occupational life. National data are not collected regarding mental illness being the primary reason for child removal; however, in a study of birth records in California, it was estimated that more than a third (34.6%) of infants born to mothers with a mental health disorder were reported by Child Protective Services within 1 year (Hammond et al., 2017). Research also shows that approximately two-thirds of women with mental illness are mothers (Nicholson et al., 2002), which may increase the risk for child maltreatment (Chaffin et al., 1996; Kohl et al., 2011; Moore et al., 2004) and foster care entry (Park et al., 2006). It is also documented that parental mental health can impact children's well-being (e.g., Marçal, 2020). This has implications for child welfare professionals. Although as a child welfare professional, we do not diagnose clients; it is helpful to be aware and become familiar with signs and symptoms of mental illness that may warrant referral for further assessment or treatment. Some common types of mental illnesses encountered in child welfare work include major depressive disorder, anxiety disorders, bipolar or mood disorders, and schizophrenia.

The most important issue to consider when working with families faced with mental health challenges is the impact of the mental illness on parenting ability. If a parent or caretaker has been diagnosed with a mental illness, it does not mean they are incapable of parenting. However, children whose parents have mental illness are at increased risk for mental health problems, which have implications for the child's needs and possible treatment. Maternal depression (and schizophrenia) is associated with other risk factors (e.g., psychosocial stress, poverty, or marital difficulty), and mothers who experience depression, particularly new mothers or mothers who have recently given birth, may be more negative when interacting with their infant. It has been shown that insecure attachment is more common in children of mentally ill parents, and conflict between parents and children is more prevalent in families where a parent is mentally ill. Child welfare professionals should be able to recognize when a parent's mental illness might be a concern, determine when a mental health assessment is needed, and be able to refer the parent to a mental health provider. Close collaboration with the parent and the provider is important, as well as including appropriate mental health interventions in the case plan and monitoring mental health throughout the case.

Practice Highlight

Mental Illness and Symptomology

Major Depressive Disorder

- Depressed mood
- Diminished interest or pleasure
- Significant weight loss
- Insomnia
- Chronic fatigue
- Feelings of worthlessness
- Lack of concentration or decisiveness
- Recurrent thoughts of death

Bipolar Disorder

- Significant mood swings
- Inflated self-esteem
- Racing thoughts
- Distractibility
- Decreased need for sleep
- Irritability

Schizophrenia

- Delusions
- Hallucinations
- Disorganized speech
- Grossly disorganized behavior
- Magical thinking

Promoting Collaborative Practice in Child Welfare

There are many different professionals and individuals who serve various roles in the child welfare system. Further, as child welfare professionals, we interact with individuals who are a part of other systems as well, such as the judicial system, health, mental, and behavioral health system, and educational system. To promote positive family and child outcomes, it is necessary to collaborate with various individuals who play a role in the life of the child and family and the case process. These individuals may be providing care for the child (e.g., foster and kinship caregivers, group home, or residential staff), be involved with the legal aspects of the case (e.g., law enforcement, dependency court staff, attorneys, etc.), serve as a mentor or advocate for the child or parent (e.g., CASA, guardian ad litem), provide necessary services for the child or parent (e.g., therapist, medical provider, specialist, home visitor), or may be a part of the immediate or extended family.

Child protection requires people working together. It may not always be easy due to differences in professional training and personalities. While we all have the overarching goal of child safety, sometimes there are different views of how best to accomplish this. Sometimes there are certain protocols within an agency that may seemingly conflict with the protocols of another agency or views of a professional. There may be "turf" issues where different professionals do not readily share information and work together when possible. Sometimes there are communication issues stemming from differences in professional training. Professional skills and practice are generally necessary in all of these relationships; however, there are some differences in interactions, requirements, and considerations, as the child welfare professional that may show to improve collaboration with these individuals and groups.

Working with Substitute Caregivers

When children are in out-of-home placements, they are placed in a variety of settings, and often multiple settings during their time in care. (See Chapter 9 for details about out-of-home placements.) Children are most often placed in family-like settings, with relatives or not relatives or in residential homes and facilities or group homes, depending on the child's needs. As discussed in earlier chapters, many factors play into the child's initial and ongoing placements, including preferences, availability, safety, and the child's needs. Those residing or working in those placements play a critical role in the care, safety, and well-being of the child and spend a considerable amount of time with them. They are charged with ensuring the medical, educational, and social-emotional needs of the child is being met on a daily basis. They must also stay apprised on case processes and promote or facilitate parent or sibling visitation, court attendance (for older youth), and therapy or other appointments the child requires. Given the nature of a child being in care and the trauma associated with child maltreatment and removal from their parents' care, a child may need therapy or additional medical attention. Caregivers also need to be available for home visits from case managers, attorneys (e.g., guardians ad litem) or family or service providers. They are the ones who spend a considerable amount of time with the child and are responsible for their care and well-being; therefore, it is critical to have open and regular communication with them as a child welfare professional, as well as fair expectations, while also allowing for decision-making skills and autonomy in care, as appropriate.

In a recent study, researchers asked foster care providers for their suggestions to improve relationships with child welfare workers and found that foster care providers wanted caseworkers who were responsive to their needs, provided concrete and emotional support, and improved communication and teamwork (Geiger et al., 2017). They also recognized that many child welfare professionals were often overwhelmed with system challenges. Foster parents' decisions to continue fostering are influenced by the level of respect and recognition as integral members of the team (Geiger et al., 2013). Many discontinue fostering early due to issues with the child welfare system or navigating the system, concerns about the child's behavior, stressful interactions with the biological parents, or being named in allegations of abuse (Rhodes et al., 2001). All of these reasons can be mitigated through positive support and relationships with the child welfare agency and staff. For example, the case manager can provide social-emotional and behavioral services or therapy for the child; promote shared parenting as appropriate and make sound decisions about biological parent-foster parent interactions; reduce the impact of abuse allegations through support; system response; and service provision. Further, studies show several important interpersonal and professional skills that promote positive relationships between child welfare professionals and foster parents, including

---

Practice Tips

Supporting Caregivers in Promoting Mutual Attachments with Children

Children in care have extensive needs.
- *Support the foster family to be accepting of the child's needs.*
- *Help caregivers prioritize needs and understand they do not have full responsibility for meeting all the child's need.*
- *Encourage them to not neglect their own needs.*

Child's emotional energy is devoted to the grieving process.
Give children "permission" and space to express their feelings.
- *Work with families in providing the child with consistent/accurate information about his/her family, placement, and visitation.*
- *Secure appropriate therapeutic services as needed.*

Child may not have a foundation for healthy attachment.
Encourage the caregivers' consistent efforts to protect, nurture, and meet the child's needs.
- *Help them to not expect "too much, too fast."*
- *Assist foster families in finding additional support (e.g., agency resources, caregiver support groups).*

having a physical presence and open communication (MacGregor et al., 2006), trust (Chipungu & Bent-Goodley, 2004), and establishing and maintaining a positive rapport (Rhodes et al., 2003).

The relationships between foster care providers and child welfare professionals are critical in recruiting and retention efforts in child welfare. Improved relationships often can prevent placement disruption and enhance the over well-being of the child, their caregiver, and family. Positive relationships can improve overall satisfaction and feelings of inclusion and respect. Child welfare professionals will interact the most with foster care providers and are the ones who are able to provide services to the child and the family, highlighting the importance of this relationship in promoting safety, permanency, and well-being. Retaining quality foster care providers has implications for child well-being by promoting placement stability, the development of secure attachments, and pro-social behaviors (Ramsay-Irving, 2015). Increased stability and support from their caregivers can improve a child's mental and emotional health and reduced risk of re-traumatization (Rubin et al., 2007).

Child welfare workers can also learn more about the licensing requirements for foster parents, stay attuned to available trainings to take part in and recommend to foster parents, and include foster parents as team members in case management, promoting permanency, and making decisions. Foster parents should be kept apprised about the case, its status, any changes, and should be consulted about the child's needs and desires.

Licensed foster care providers receive hours of pre-service and ongoing training and have to complete a number of assessments and evaluations to become licensed. Many have experience working with children and the child welfare system and often know how to advocate for services and the needs of the children. However, many kinship care providers have not interacted with the child welfare system as caregivers or professionals or may possibly have a negative impression, or experience with the system may present with challenges in understanding and navigating the system.

Working with Kinship Placements

There are many similarities in terms of what kinship caregivers need when caring for children in out-of-home placement. Children placed with kin still need the stability, services, and support as licensed foster caregivers. Caseworkers should identify the child and family's needs and tailor them to support kinship placements, while also helping children in foster care maintain positive family connections. In all cases, child welfare professionals should work with kinship caregivers and provide full disclosure throughout the case, including prior to placement. They should provide information about the child welfare system, what one can typically expect in the course of a case (e.g., court hearings), their roles and responsibilities as a kinship caregiver, and sources of support (e.g., financial support, social support, tangible support) within the agency and in the community. Discussions should include options about permanency and their thoughts, beliefs, and feelings about those options.

Working with Residential and Group Home Placement Staff

Child welfare collaboration with residential or group home staff is very similar to working with other care providers; however, some differences exist in terms of the environment, communication, and involvement. Due to the nature of a staffed facility as a placement, there will be more than one or two caregivers in the home or placement, and these staff work in shifts and may also not be long term. Relationships between the youth and staff vary, with some establishing strong relationships, similar to a mentoring role that is built on trust and understanding, while others are based on meeting basic needs within the setting. Again, many of the staff and management may spend a great deal of time with the youth, getting to know them and can offer support and guidance throughout their case. The home leader or manager may participate in child and family teams, educational meetings (e.g., IEP, caregiver conferences), and facilitate visitation, recreation, etc. They also are a key member of the team to assist with implementing the case plan in the home with the youth and providing important feedback to the child and family team and the case manager.

Note from the Field

Child Removals Are Never Easy

Carol Taylor, MSW, LCSW

Lia is a 14-year-old African-American girl who had been living with her grandmother for most of her life in kinship care within the child welfare system. Grandma was struggling with the normal ups and downs of adolescence. The permanency plan for Lia was to have Grandma to adopt her. On a Friday afternoon, I, who had been working with the family for over a year received a call that the Grandma could no longer care for Lia and requested her removal immediately. I attempted to deescalate the situation and offered support, but Grandma was unwilling to give it any more time.

I arrived at the home to find the tension very high. Grandma reported that Lia was being disrespectful toward her and that she could not have her live there any longer. I talked with Lia who was unusually quiet and visibly sad. Lia had the perspective that Grandma was too strict and would not allow her to do anything.

I attempted to offer support and see if there was anything that would help Grandma to allow her to stay, but she was tired and needed the break. I talked with Grandma alone to see if there were any family that she was aware of that may take Lia at this time to allow for Lia to stay with family. Grandma did not have any suggestions.

Lia and I left the home with Lia's belongings in a combination of bags and garbage bags. The protocol was to rule out kinship care, then consider foster care, and as a last resort contact a shelter. Since this was a Friday afternoon, there was an additional challenge of not being able to quickly be in contact with anyone, and additionally, the child welfare office was closing and would not be an option.

Once Lia was out of the house, she asked about her Aunt as an option for placement. We attempted to reach her Aunt with no avail. At the same time, I continued to leave messages for foster parents and as a last resort start the process of having Lia go to the shelter. The foster parents that were reached were hesitant to take on a soon-to-be freshman in high school despite that she received good grades and had no behavior concerns outside of the normal desires for more independence that adolescence brings. The shelter process required proof of contact with multiple caregivers prior to consideration for Lia to be placed at the shelter; since I was not hearing back from several caregivers, we were at a standstill.

During this time, Lia remained quietly distraught with her current situation. I continued to talk and encourage Lia despite the difficult situation. I eventually was able to reach her Aunt to discover she would be willing to have her come to the home but would not be home until 10:00 pm that evening. After a trip to McDonald's and hours of time together, we arrived to the Aunt's home around 10:00 pm. Lia visibly showed signs of relief when she was welcomed by her Aunt to the home.

Working with Law Enforcement

Law enforcement officers can be important allies in keeping children safe. Child welfare professionals and systems can enhance partnerships with law enforcement by educating them about the nature of their work and the laws governing child protection. They can also help law enforcement systems and officers about child welfare's focus on strengths-based, family-centered practice with children and families and can help them to understand the similar and different approaches professionals within each sector respond to and address the needs of children and families. Law enforcement officers may be the first responder in a situation where a child welfare professional is needed to assess and provide a safe and stable placement for the child. Likewise, child welfare professionals may require the support of law enforcement in cases where the safety of the child, caseworker, or other household member might be at risk in the home, court, or meeting place. Law enforcement may accompany the child welfare worker in situations where there is potential danger or if a family member has a history of being violent. It is important to understand the roles, responsibilities, and skill sets of each of the professionals, given the circumstances.

Both professionals work together by sharing information, communicating effectively, and collaborating to ensure the safety of all involved. Both units should be cross-trained on issues where child welfare professionals and law enforcement officers might interact. Both should be trained in using a trauma-informed approach when working with families, which means minimizing trauma to all parties involved, and understanding that trauma may play a role in the family's circumstances.

Working with Attorneys and Court Personnel

As with practice with other professionals, child welfare workers must be aware of the roles, responsibilities, and common practice of those they work with and, likewise, help them to be aware of the roles, responsibilities, and common practice of child welfare professionals. By delineating these roles, we can promote a healthier, more productive collaboration with shared goals. As discussed in Chap. 2, attorneys and court personnel serve different roles based on the practice jurisdiction; however, getting to know these roles and what the child welfare professionals' relationships are to them and within the case is helpful in collaboration. The parents' attorneys, child's attorney, guardian ad litem (typically an attorney), and state's attorney (agency attorney) all represent different members involved in the case. In other words, their responsibility is to represent the wishes and best interest of that individual or group. In most cases, all or many parties to the case can come to an agreement about decisions and/ or recommendations made to the court, and sometimes they may not. As child welfare professionals, it is our responsibility to provide reports and information (as appropriate and required) to each party within a reasonable amount of time. Attorneys will often be invited to agency and family meetings and may or may not attend or send a representative but should always be informed of meetings involving their client. With regard to legal matters, attorneys should always talk to other attorneys (instead of the clients of other attorneys); however, it is often common practice for the attorneys to approach the child welfare professional about specifics of the case (e.g., progress, case plan, visitation) when appropriate. By using effective communication, members involved with the case can create more efficient case processes and ensure safety, permanency, and well-being for the child and family.

Court personnel (e.g., bailiff, judicial assistant, court reporter) are also integral parts to the team. They may not be actively involved in the case processes or be aware of case details; however, they serve an important role in facilitating information sharing with the judicial officer (e.g., judge, commissioner) on the case, who also requires all court reports and information shared with all parties. This individual also serves as a liaison with the judge in terms of motions and other court documents being filed, reviewed, and approved and often manages the court calendar. The bailiff helps maintain security and safety and may coordinate court proceedings at times. Maintaining positive relationships with the court personnel can facilitate efficient and productive court proceedings.

Practice Highlight

The Importance of Understanding the Needs of the Children Entering Foster Care

Barbara H. Chaiyachati, MD, PhD

Entrance into the child welfare system may represent a vulnerable transition for children with regard to medical care. Medical history may be lost amidst the many simultaneous priorities of information gathering. Caregivers may not provide complete information, intentionally or unintentionally. For example, caregivers may not have immediate recall of complete information at this high stress point. Caregivers may wish to obfuscate for any number of reasons including insight to inadequate utilization of health care. Transmission of health information between responsible caregivers – from biological parents to foster parents and hopefully back to biological parents – is typically completed via child welfare professionals. This game of telephone can be fraught with errors and omissions.

Removing a child from a home without having adequate information may result in loss of access to life-saving medications or vital equipment for daily success, such as eyeglasses. It may also impede children's ability to continue in established medical homes depending on location of foster care placement as well as perceived or actual impacts on insurance. After entrance to foster care, unstable placements may further disrupt normal access to health care. Even if outreach is initiated by healthcare providers, the medical records may not contain appropriate contact information for current foster care providers. Additionally, issues of who can consent for medical care of a minor can create real and perceived barriers to receiving appropriate medical care. There is a need to prioritize communication and continuity to ensure children receive the necessary medical care while in the child welfare system.

Working with Medical and Behavioral Health Providers

Pediatric professionals, emergency staff and personnel, nurses, counselors, family medicine professionals, and others who help to promote physical and mental health are key members of the child welfare team. Not only do they provide services and supports for children and families already involved in the child welfare system, but also they are responsible for identifying and reporting suspected abuse and neglect. It is well documented that children with a history of child maltreatment and those who enter the foster care system often have greater physical and mental health needs when compared to their same-aged peers who have not had those experiences (e.g., Minnis et al., 2006). As a result, it is critical that child welfare professionals work alongside healthcare and mental health professionals by providing the information and support needed for them to best treat the child, meet with and discuss progress and/or concerns to facilitate a joint decision-making process, work together to facilitate improved access and service delivery and coordination of care, and make the necessary referrals and recommendations for needed care. Coordinating physical and mental health care requires good communication, obtaining, maintaining, and consolidating records to ensure proper care, enrolling, and ensuring appropriate coordination when coverage or services change (e.g., aging out, family reunification). These professionals share common philosophies of care with child welfare professionals in that they take responsibility to prevent child maltreatment, uphold confidentiality and privacy of children and families, use trauma-informed care and practice, and serve as a resource to children, families, and those who manage cases in child welfare.

Note from the Field

Advocating for Therapy and Academic Supports

Libby Fakier, MBA

Most of the children who have been placed in our care struggle academically, either because of the circumstances in their birth home or due to changes in school placement as a result of moves from placement to placement. Exacerbating the issue is that many children in care have learning disabilities, psychosocial challenges, and generalized anxiety that inhibit their ability to learn.

When a child comes into our home, we meet with the case management team to assess grades, individualized educational programs (IEPs), learning disabilities, psychological evaluations, and supports that are currently in place. Often, we find that the child has not been evaluated for services or that evaluations were not followed up with approvals and implementation of therapeutic services. We see that children go years without services and suffer academically, psychologically, and physically because by the time they are evaluated at one placement, they are moved again before services are implemented. At the outset of receiving a new placement in our home, I advocate for my children to immediately receive psychological counseling with a professional that I have worked with for years. This creates the foundation of care for my kids on which we can build supports for all the other areas where the child needs help.

Wading through the bureaucracy is not for the faint of heart and requires a determined and unrelenting mindset to ensure that children in care get the services and support they need and deserve. Foster parents must be vigilant about advocating for their children's needs and not give up when the case management team or public school system either denies services or drags their feet about getting evaluations completed and services implemented. Daily calls, weekly emails, and constant follow-up with everyone on the case management team are essential to securing services in a timely manner.

There's a very small window to address children's psychological or thera-peutic (physical therapy, occupational therapy, and speech therapy) needs to get them back on track. Medication evaluation and management must be streamlined so children have continuity of care and mental health issues are addressed before the child decompensates. Time is of the essence. Foster par-ents have the moral obligation and responsibility to ensure that their chil-dren's needs are met as quickly as possible. They must remain unconquered in their fight to advocate for the support services their children need to grow, heal, and succeed.

Working with Educators and the School System

Educators (especially elementary, secondary, and early childhood) play an impor-tant role in the well-being of children in general, and in particular children involved with the child welfare system. They spend a great deal of time with children and their families, build strong relationships with them and the community, and can be a great resource to them. They are also the most common professional to report child maltreatment and are critical in the prevention of child maltreatment. Educators can provide critical information to child welfare professionals who are investigating an allegation of child maltreatment and can also offer knowledge about child and family strengths, sources of supports, as well as needs. They have insight into the community and its resources, as well. When a child is in out-of-home placement, educators and other school professionals (e.g., school social workers) can assist with obtaining school records, making referrals, conducting, and evaluating educa-tional and behavioral assessments as needed. Educators and school professionals can help with ensuring stability and normalcy by offering extracurricular activities, remedial support, tutoring, and promote social-emotional well-being. Child welfare professionals rely on educators and other school-level professionals to support chil-dren and their families in learning and improving overall family functioning.

Child welfare professionals can partner with educators and school staff to ensure children are ready to learn and are offered the resources and supports for an optimal learning environment. Children who have been maltreated and/or who enter the child welfare system are often behind academically. Specifically, children entering foster care may not be at grade level for their age, may require special education, or other supportive services (speech, occupational therapy, etc.), and may not have all of the necessary paperwork and documentation required to enroll. Child welfare professionals can work with schools and districts to make efforts to keep children in their school of origin to reduce the emotional and academic impact of moving schools and peer groups. The Fostering Connections Act provides guidance regard-ing keeping children in their home schools by providing transportation and sup-ports. When this is not possible, child welfare professionals and schools should work together to ease the transition. The Uninterrupted Scholars Act of 2013 also assists with records access and sharing with appropriate personnel and systems. Similarly, Every Student Succeeds Act (ESSA) of 2015 promotes collaboration among education and child welfare professionals to ensure stability and decision-making. Child welfare professionals can also ensure that educators and other school professionals are aware of the child's situation regarding child welfare system involvement and invite them to be a part of the child and family team.

Research Brief

Engaging Fathers in Child Welfare Practice

Justin S. Harty, MSW, LCSW and Tova B. Walsh, PhD, MSW

Father involvement in children's lives and in child and family services has important consequences for child well-being. Father involvement in children's lives is associated with positive social, emotional, and cognitive outcomes for children from infancy to adolescence and into adulthood. Father engagement in child and family services including parent training, family therapy, and permanency planning is associated with improved child outcomes. A growing body of research demonstrates that fathers provide a unique contribution to their children's development and suggests that outreach, engagement, and inclusion of fathers are an important strategy for improving well-being, permanency, and safety of children and families involved with the child welfare system.

Yet father involvement in child welfare services is generally low. It is widely recognized that fathers face numerous obstacles and barriers to engagement in child welfare services. Trauma, mental health issues, substance use disorders, incarceration, or other challenges may limit their capacity to be fully engaged. Competing demands, time constraints, intermittent employment, and housing instability may present additional barriers. Fathers may have a decreased willingness to engage when they have adversarial relationships with their child's mother; the mother holds negative views of their parenting; or the mother acts as a gatekeeper. Child welfare practitioners who believe fathers cannot be trusted are reluctant to participate in services, or present risk to children and families also creates conditions in which fathers are less likely to engage in services. It may be challenging to engage some fathers in child welfare practice. However, there are things that child welfare practitioners can do to more effectively engage fathers. Strategies include:

- Engage with fathers as early and equally as mothers, including engaging fathers in case planning, meetings, and court dates, and other important case-related tasks.
- Engage fathers whenever possible, even when fathers have not engaged in the past.
- View every decision point, case event, and exchange as an opportunity for father engagement.
- Use a father-focused, strengths-based approach that emphasizes fathers' self-determination and strengths.
- View fathers as an asset and not a risk. Recognize that fathers generally want what is best for their child and address obstacles or barriers preventing them from engaging in services or from meeting the needs of their child.
- In cases where fathers have presented risk to children or mothers, continue to assess if, when, and how fathers may be safely engaged in the future.
- Explore fathers as viable placement options and paternal family members as resources for support and permanency planning.

Engaging fathers in child welfare practice is not limited to fathers with children involved in the child welfare system. Child welfare practitioners need to be prepared to engage men as foster fathers, including single and same-sex fathers, as well as young fathers in foster care. Practitioners must also recognize that fathers are not a homogenous group, and child welfare practice must be tailored to meet the needs of diverse fathers and families.

Child and Family Teams

A child and family team are a group of individuals identified by the child and family, as well as the professionals familiar with the case to brainstorm strategies around strengths, resources, and needs of the child and the family. The goal of the child and family team is to establish shared goals that will meet the needs of the family and keep all team members apprised so that they may contribute resources and supports in attaining the family's goals. Teams can consist of children/youth, substitute caregivers, biological parents, extended family, educators and school personnel, natural supports (e.g., clergy, neighbor, mentor, friend), mental health providers, Court Appointed Special Advocate (CASA), or legal/law enforcement staff (e.g., attorneys, probation).

Child and family teams are intentional and critical to strengthening and supporting a family involved with the child welfare system. They involve planning, creating a mission statement, documenting strengths and needs, and developing and monitoring of a plan of care. The planning stage involves developing a team through outreach and engagement, developing a family mission, and helping to orient the family to the child and family process. After exploring and noting all family strengths, a family will develop a needs statement, which addresses the "what" of the circumstances. For example, there may be specific reasons a child came to the attention of the child welfare system; however, there may also be some underlying reasons that have led the family to require additional services or resources. However, needs are not services.

> **Practice Tip**
>
> **Facilitating a Child and Family Team**
>
> Encourage participation and collaboration.
>
> Address any conflict that occurs through discussion.
>
> Be aware and promote child and family voice.
>
> Be cognizant of agency and policy requirements for meetings (e.g., frequency, duration, membership).
>
> Acknowledge successes, strengths, and effort of all team members.

Child welfare professionals may be asked to facilitate child and family teams. Other times, this is the responsibility of a mental health team leader or another team member. Some ideas to facilitate the process of the meeting and team are to allow for introductions, establish ground rules, develop a family vision and/or mission, and review any safety or crisis plans to begin. The team will identify needs in early meetings and develop goals accordingly. The team will brainstorm ideas about services that will address the needs identified, followed by who will complete specific tasks related to the goals and objectives. During the facilitation of child and family teams, it is important to establish and follow the group rules set forth by the team and to be aware of the time and manage it well. It helps to have an agenda to follow to ensure time management. It is important to be flexible, in control, creative, and think beyond traditional services offered. Keep the family central to the team and the meetings and focus on solutions rather than the problems that are creating barriers.

Conclusion

Family engagement is the core of child welfare casework and helps us work toward child safety, permanency, and well-being. Effective engagement with the child and the family requires individual skills and collaboration among providers, extended family, and must be infused into the child welfare systems. Despite the challenges often encountered when engaging families in a difficult process, child welfare professionals acknowledge the benefits of including all family members in a family-centered, strengths-based approach to making decisions, setting goals, and working alongside to achieve those goals to strengthen the family.

Acknowledgments The authors thank Brittany Mihalec-Adkins, M.S.Ed; Carol Taylor, MSW, LCSW; Barbara H. Chaiyachati, MD, PhD; Libby Fakier, MBA; Justin S. Harty, MSW, LCSW; and Tova B. Walsh, PhD, MSW, for their contributions to Chap. 6.

Discussion Questions

1. Why is engagement so important in child welfare practice?
2. What are three ways child welfare professionals can increase family engagement with child welfare services?
3. What are three ways to build rapport with children and families?
4. How are cases involving substance abuse, intimate partner violence, and mental illness different from other cases in child welfare?
5. What are three strategies for healthy collaboration with other key partners in child welfare (e.g., foster parents, residential staff, educators, etc.)?

Suggested Activities

1. Listen to the "Engaging Fathers" Podcast series with Child Welfare Information Gateway. Consider ways to engage fathers throughout the life of a case. https://www.childwelfare.gov/more-tools-resources/podcast/episode-6/
2. Watch: "Building Partnerships in Child Welfare" and think about ways to work collaboratively among multiple team members: https://www.youtube.com/watch?v=ES8Vij2CNBA
3. Watch: "Interviewing the Child Client" to better understand how attorneys and other professionals can interact appropriately with children in cases of child welfare investigations: https://www.youtube.com/watch?v=OYLWkVHvgOM&t=45s
4. Read Kisiel et al. (2017) and write a reflection paper on the value of using strength-based practice in child welfare in interventions with children.
Kisiel, C., Summersett-Ringgold, F., Weil, L. E., & McClelland, G. (2017). Understanding strengths in relation to complex trauma and mental health symptoms within child welfare. *Journal of child and family studies*, 26(2), 437-451. (Available: https://rdcu.be/ccbwI).

Additional Resources

Child Welfare Capacity Building Collaborative: https://capacity.childwelfare.gov/

Child Welfare Information Gateway, Family Engagement: https://www.childwelfare.gov/pubs/f-fam-engagement/

Child Welfare Information Gateway, Partnering with Birth Parents to Promote Reunification: https://www.childwelfare.gov/pubs/factsheets-families-partnerships/

Child Welfare Information Gateway, The Importance of Fathers in the Health Development in Children: https://www.childwelfare.gov/pubs/usermanuals/ fatherhood/

National Responsible Fatherhood Clearinghouse: https://www.fatherhood.gov/

Youth.gov, Family Engagement: https://youth.gov/youth-topics/family-engagement

References

Berg, I. K., & Kelly, S. (2000). *Building solutions in child protective services*. W. W. Norton & Company.

Brown, L., Callahan, M., Strega, S., Walmsley, C., & Dominelli, L. (2009). Manufacturing ghost fathers: The paradox of father presence and absence in child welfare. *Child and Family Social Work, 14*(1), 25–34. https://doi.org/10.1111/j.1365-2206.2008.00578.x

Campbell, C. A., Howard, D., Rayford, B. S., & Fordon, D. M. (2015). Fathers matter: Involving and engaging fathers in the child welfare system process. *Children and Youth Services Review, 53*, 84–91. https://doi.org/10.1016/j.childyouth.2015.03.020

Chapman, M. V., Gibbons, C. B., Barth, R. P., & McCrae, J. S. (2003). Parental views of in-home services: What predicts satisfaction with child welfare workers? *Child Welfare, 82*, 571–596.

Child Welfare Information Gateway. (2016). *Family engagement: Partnering with families to improve child welfare outcomes*. U.S. Department of Health and Human Services, Children's Bureau.

Chipungu, S. S., & Bent-Goodley, T. B. (2004). Meeting the challenges of contemporary foster care. *The Future of Children*, 75–93. https://doi.org/10.2307/1602755

Chaffin, M., Kelleher, K., & Hollenberg, J. (1996). Onset of physical abuse and neglect: Psychiatric, substance abuse, and social risk factors from prospective community data. *Child Abuse & Neglect, 20*(3), 191–203. https://doi.org/10.1016/S0145-2134(95)00144-1

Cryer-Coupet, Q. R., Dorsey, M. S., Lemmons, B. P., & Hope, E. C. (2020). Examining multiple dimensions of father involvement as predictors of risk-taking intentions among black adolescent females. *Children and Youth Services Review, 108*, 104604. https://doi.org/10.1016/j.childyouth.2019.104604

Damiani-Taraba, G., Dumbrill, G., Gladstone, J., Koster, A., Leslie, B., & Charles, M. (2017). The evolving relationship between casework skills, engagement, and positive case outcomes in child protection: A structural equation model. *Children and Youth Services Review, 79*, 456–462. https://doi.org/10.1016/j.childyouth.2017.05.033

Darlington, Y., Feeney, J. A., & Rixon, K. (2004). Complexity, conflict and uncertainty: Issues in collaboration between child protection and mental health services. *Children and Youth Services Review, 26*(12), 1175–1192. https://doi.org/10.1016/j.childyouth.2004.08.009

De Boer, C., & Coady, N. (2007). Good helping relationships in child welfare: Learning from stories of success. *Child & Family Social Work, 12*(1), 32–42. https://doi.org/10.1111/j.1365-2206.2006.00438.x

DePanfilis, D. (2000). How do I develop a helping alliance with the family. *Handbook for Child Protection Practice*, 36–40. https://doi.org/10.4135/9781452205489.n8

Dumbrill, G. C. (2006). Parental experience of child protection intervention: A qualitative study. *Child Abuse & Neglect, 30*(1), 27–37. https://doi.org/10.1016/j.chiabu.2005.08.012

Duncan, B. L., Miller, S. D., Wampold, B. E., & Hubble, M. A. (2010). The heart and soul of change: Delivering what works in therapy. *American Psychological Association*. https://doi.org/10.1037/12075-000

Fluke, J. D., Chabot, M., Fallon, B., MacLaurin, B., & Blackstock, C. (2010). Placement decisions and disparities among aboriginal groups: An application of the decision making ecology through multi-level analysis. *Child Abuse & Neglect, 34*(1), 57–69. https://doi.org/10.1016/j.chiabu.2009.08.009

Fong, R. (2001). *Culturally competent social work practice: Past and present* (pp. 1–9). *Skills, Interventions, and Evaluations.*

Fusco, R. A. (2015). Second generation mothers in the child welfare system: Factors that predict engagement. *Child and Adolescent Social Work Journal, 32*(6), 545–554. https://doi.org/10.1007/s10560-015-0394-4

Geiger, J. M., Hayes, M. J., & Lietz, C. A. (2013). Should I stay or should I go? A mixed methods study examining the factors influencing foster parents' decisions to continue or discontinue providing foster care. *Children and Youth Services Review, 35*(9), 1356–1365. https://doi.org/10.1016/j.childyouth.2013.05.003

Geiger, J. M., Piel, M. H., & Julien-Chinn, F. J. (2017). Improving relationships in child welfare practice: Perspectives of foster care providers. *Child and Adolescent Social Work Journal, 34*(1), 23–33. https://doi.org/10.1007/s10560-016-0471-3

Gladstone, J., Dumbrill, G., Leslie, B., Koster, A., Young, M., & Ismaila, A. (2014). Understanding worker-parent engagement in child protection casework. *Children and Youth Services Review, 44*, 56–64. https://doi.org/10.1016/j.childyouth.2014.06.002

Gockel, A., Russell, M., & Harris, B. (2008). Recreating family: parents identify worker-client relationships as paramount in family preservation programs. *Child Welfare, 87*(6).

Graybeal, C. T. (2007). Evidence for the art of social work. *Families in Society, 88*(4), 513–523. https://doi.org/10.1606/1044-3894.3673

Guo, S., Barth, R. P., & Gibbons, C. (2006). Propensity score matching strategies for evaluating substance abuse services for child welfare clients. *Children and Youth Services Review, 28*(4), 357–383. https://doi.org/10.1016/j.childyouth.2005.04.012

Hartley, C. C. (2002). The co-occurrence of child maltreatment and domestic violence: examining both neglect and child physical abuse. *Child Maltreatment, 7*(4), 349–358. https://doi.org/10.1177/107755902237264

Herrenkohl, T. I., Sousa, C., Tajima, E. A., Herrenkohl, R. C., & Moylan, C. A. (2008). Intersection of child abuse and children's exposure to domestic violence. *Trauma, Violence & Abuse, 9*(2), 84–99. https://doi.org/10.1177/1524838008314797

Hammond, I., Eastman, A. L., Leventhal, J. M., & Putnam-Hornstein, E. (2017). Maternal mental health disorders and reports to child protective services: a birth cohort study. *International Journal of Environmental Research and Public Health, 14*(11), 1320. https://doi.org/10.3390/ijerph14111320

Kapp, S. A., & Vela, R. H. (2004). The unheard client: Assessing the satisfaction of parents of children in foster care. *Child and Family Social Work, 9*(2), 197–206. https://doi.org/10.1111/j.1365-2206.2004.00323.x

Kemp, S. P., Marcenko, M. O., Lyons, S. J., & Kruzich, J. M. (2014). Strength-based practice and parental engagement in child welfare services: An empirical examination. *Children and Youth Services Review, 47*, 27–35. https://doi.org/10.1016/j.childyouth.2013.11.001

Kisiel, C., Summersett-Ringgold, F., Weil, L. E., & McClelland, G. (2017). Understanding strengths in relation to complex trauma and mental health symptoms within child welfare. *Journal of Child and Family Studies, 26*(2), 437–451. https://doi.org/10.1007/s10826-016-0569-4

Kohl, P. L., Edleson, J. L., English, D. J., & Barth, R. P. (2005). Domestic violence and pathways into child welfare services: Findings from the National Survey of Child and Adolescent Well-Being. *Children and Youth Services Review, 27*(11), 1167–1182. https://doi.org/10.1016/j.childyouth.2005.04.003

Kohl, P. L., Jonson-Reid, M., & Drake, B. (2011). Maternal mental illness and the safety and stability of maltreated children. *Child Abuse & Neglect, 35*(5), 309–318. https://doi.org/10.1016/j.chiabu.2011.01.006

Lee, S. J., & Walsh, T. B. (2015). Using technology in social work practice: the mDad (Mobile Device Assisted Dad) case study. *Advances in Social Work, 16*(1), 107–124. https://doi.org/10.18060/18134

Lewis, E. M., Feely, M., Seay, K. D., Fedoravicis, N., & Kohl, P. L. (2016). Child welfare involved parents and Pathways Triple P: perceptions of program acceptability and appropriateness. *Journal of Child and Family Studies, 25*(12), 3760–3770. https://doi.org/10.1007/s10826-016-0526-2

Lietz, C. A. (2013). Strengths-based supervision: Supporting implementation of family-centered practice through supervisory processes. *Journal of Family Strengths, 13*(1), 6.

Littell, J. H., Alexander, L. B., & Reynolds, W. W. (2001). Client participation: Central and under-investigated elements of intervention. *Social Service Review, 75*(1), 1–28. https://doi.org/10.1086/591880

MacGregor, T. E., Rodger, S., Cummings, A. L., & Leschied, A. W. (2006). The needs of foster parents: A qualitative study of motivation, support, and retention. *Qualitative Social Work, 5*(3), 351–368. https://doi.org/10.1177/1473325006067365

Maiter, S., Palmer, S., & Manaji, S. (2006). Strengthening social worker-client relationships in child protection services: Addressing power relationships and ruptured relationships. *Qualitative Social Work, 5*(2), 161–186. https://doi.org/10.1177/1473325006064255

Marçal, K. (2020). Caregiver depression and child behaviour problems: A longitudinal mixed effects approach. *Child & Family Social Work.* https://doi.org/10.1111/cfs.12786

Maxwell, N., Scourfield, J., Featherstone, B., Holland, S., & Tolman, R. (2012). Engaging fathers in child welfare services: A narrative review of recent research evidence. *Child and Family Social Work, 17*(2), 160–169. https://doi.org/10.1111/j.1365-2206.2012.00827.x

Miller, W. R., & Rollnick, S. (2002). *Motivational interviewing: Preparing people for change. 2002.* Guilford Press.

Minnis, H., Everett, K., Pelosi, A. J., Dunn, J., & Knapp, M. (2006). Children in foster care: Mental health, service use and costs. *European Child & Adolescent Psychiatry, 15*(2), 63–70. https://doi.org/10.1007/s00787-006-0452-8

Moore, P. S., Whaley, S. E., & Sigman, M. (2004). Interactions between mothers and children: impacts of maternal and child anxiety. *Journal of Abnormal Psychology, 113*(3), 471. https://doi.org/10.1037/0021-843X.113.3.471

National Alliance on Mental Illness. (2019). *Mental health by the numbers.* Retrieved from: https://www.\.org/mhstats

National Coalition Against Domestic Violence. (n.d.). *Learn more.* Retrieved from: https://ncadv.org/learn-more

Nicholson, J., Biebel, K., Katz-Leavy, J., & Williams, V. (2002). The prevalence of parenthood in adults with mental illness: Implications for state and federal policymakers, programs, and providers.

Park, J. M., Solomon, P., & Mandell, D. S. (2006). Involvement in the child welfare system among mothers with serious mental illness. *Psychiatric Services, 57*(4), 493–497. https://doi.org/10.1176/ps.2006.57.4.493

Platt, D. (2012). Understanding parental engagement with child welfare services: An integrated model. *Child and Family Social Work, 17*(2), 138–148. https://doi.org/10.1111/j.1365-2206.2012.00828.x

Platt, D. (2008). Care or control? The effects of investigations and initial assessments on the social worker-parent relationship. *Journal of Social Work Practice, 22*(3), 301–315. https://doi.org/10.1080/02650530802396643

Ramsay-Irving, M. (2015). The foster care systems are failing foster children: The implications and practical solutions for better outcomes of youth in care. *Canadian Journal of Family and Youth/Le Journal Canadien de Famille et de la Jeunesse, 7*(1), 55–86. https://doi.org/10.29173/cjfy24298

Rhodes, K. W., Orme, J. G., & Buehler, C. (2001). A comparison of family foster parents who quit, consider quitting, and plan to continue fostering. *Social Service Review, 75*(1), 84–114. https://doi.org/10.1086/591883

Rhodes, K. W., Orme, J. G., Cox, M. E., & Buehler, C. (2003). Foster family resources, psychosocial functioning, and retention. *Social Work Research, 27*(3), 135–150. https://doi.org/10.1093/swr/27.3.135

Rockhill, A., Furrer, C. J., & Duong, T. M. (2015). Peer mentoring in child welfare: A motivational framework. *Child Welfare, 94*(5), 125.

Rogers, C. R. (1957). The necessary and sufficient conditions of therapeutic personality change. *Journal of Consulting Psychology, 21*(2), 95. https://doi.org/10.1037/h0045357

Ross, A. M., DeVoe, E. R., Steketee, G., Emmert-Aronson, B. O., Brown, T., & Muroff, J. (2020). Outcomes of a reflective parenting program among military spouses: The moderating role of social support. *Journal of Family Psychology, 34*(4), 402–413. https://doi.org/10.1037/fam0000637

Rostad, W. L., Rogers, T. M., & Chaffin, M. J. (2017a). The influence of concrete support on child welfare program engagement, progress, and recurrence. *Children and Youth Services Review, 72*, 26–33. https://doi.org/10.1016/j.childyouth.2016.10.014

Rostad, W. L., Self-Brown, S., Boyd, C., Jr., Osborne, M., & Patterson, A. (2017b). Exploration of factors predictive of at-risk fathers' participation in a pilot study of an augmented evidence-based parent training program: A mixed methods approach. *Children and Youth Services Review, 79*, 485–494. https://doi.org/10.1016/j.childyouth.2017.07.001

Rubin, D. M., O'Reilly, A. L., Luan, X., & Localio, A. R. (2007). The impact of placement stability on behavioral well-being for children in foster care. *Pediatrics, 119*(2), 336–344. https://doi.org/10.1542/peds.2006-1995

Stromwall, L. K., Larson, N. C., Nieri, T., Holley, L. C., Topping, D., Castillo, J., & Ashford, J. B. (2008). Parents with co-occurring mental health and substance abuse conditions involved in child protection services: Clinical profile and treatment needs. *Child Welfare, 87*(3), 95–113.

Summers, A., Wood, S. M., Russell, J. R., & Macgill, S. O. (2012). An evaluation of the effectiveness of a parent-to-parent program in changing attitudes and increasing parental engagement in the juvenile dependency system. *Children and Youth Services Review, 34*(10), 2036–2041. https://doi.org/10.1016/j.childyouth.2012.06.016

Toros, K., DiNitto, D., & Tiko, A. (2018). Family engagement in the child welfare system: A scoping review. *Children and Youth Services Review, 88*, 598–607. https://doi.org/10.1016/j.childyouth.2018.03.011

US Department of Health and Human Services. (2020). *Administration for Children and Families, Administration on Children, Youth, and Families, Children's Bureau*. The AFCARS report. Preliminary FY 2017 estimates as of August 10, 2018. 2018.

van Zyl, M. A., Barbee, A. P., Cunningham, M. R., Antle, B. F., Christensen, D. N., & Boamah, D. (2014). Components of the solution-based casework child welfare practice model that predict positive child outcomes. *Journal of Public Child Welfare, 8*(4), 433–465. https://doi.org/10.1080/15548732.2014.939252

Yatchmenoff, D. K. (2005). Measuring client engagement from the client's perspective in nonvoluntary child protective services. *Research on Social Work Practice, 15*(2), 84–96. https://doi.org/10.1177/1049731504271605

Chapter 7
Child Maltreatment Prevention and Family Preservation

Introduction

Child maltreatment prevention efforts have improved in the last several decades as we learn more about the etiology of child maltreatment and better understand ways to support families before child maltreatment occurs. One major challenge in child abuse prevention is that it is so varied in its manifestation, etiology, and how it can be managed. Instead of managing a biological public health threat, we are instead having to account for human behavior, which is more complicated, less predictable, and difficult to manage. It is also challenging to reach all those who are in need of support and services.

Child Maltreatment Prevention

Child maltreatment prevention can be conceptualized within three levels in terms of its approach: primary, secondary, and tertiary. This conceptualization delineates different types of activities used to address public health threats, such as child maltreatment at different time points (Caplan, 1964). The types of prevention as a framework in child welfare are outlined in Fig. 7.1. Primary prevention activities target the general population in an effort to prevent maltreatment before it occurs. Primary prevention is a universal approach where everyone in the community has access to services. Primary prevention approaches also focus on addressing systemic factors that may place children and families at risk of maltreatment.

© Springer Nature Switzerland AG 2021
J. M. Geiger, L. Schelbe, *The Handbook on Child Welfare Practice*,
https://doi.org/10.1007/978-3-030-73912-6_7

Practice Highlight

Examples of Primary Prevention of Child Maltreatment Activities

- Public service announcements regarding positive parenting
- Parent education programs and groups with information and support related to child development and parenting
- Family support and family strengthening programs designed to improve access to services, resources, and support
- Public awareness campaigns with information on reporting suspected child maltreatment

Secondary prevention activities focus on populations that are at a greater risk for child maltreatment and are exposed to one or more risk factors associated with child maltreatment (e.g., poverty, parental substance abuse, parental mental health concerns, and young parental age). Programs and approaches may include parent education programs focused on specific groups such as teen parents and parents with substance abuse issues; parent support groups that help parents manage stress and parenting challenges; home visitation programs with expecting and new mothers; and respite care services for parents with children who have special needs.

Tertiary prevention activities target children and families who have experienced maltreatment and are focused on treatment and reducing the risk of recurrence of maltreatment. Tertiary prevention aims to reduce the impact of child maltreatment. Some activities include intensive family preservation services, parent mentoring and support groups for parents whose children are in care, and mental health services for children and families who have experienced child maltreatment.

Many child welfare agencies as well as the federal government use a comprehensive approach to child maltreatment prevention that includes all levels of prevention, where individuals, systems, and communities are involved in efforts. Each child welfare agency is required to develop plans that outline primary, secondary, and tertiary prevention activities

Practice Highlight

Examples of Child Maltreatment Prevention Programs

Primary Prevention

- Nurse-Family Partnership
- Safe Environment for Every Kid (SEEK)
- Body Safety Training Workbook
- Period of Purple Crying

Secondary Prevention

- Incredible Years
- Coordination, Advocacy, Resources, Education, and Support (C.A.R.E.S.)
- CICC Effective Black Parenting Program
- Nurturing Parenting Program

in order to receive funds from the state and federal government. More recently a greater emphasis has been placed on primary prevention efforts to curb the significant social and economic impact of child maltreatment.

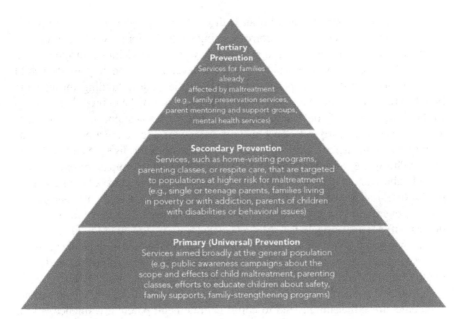

Fig. 7.1 Levels of prevention services. (Source: Child Welfare Information Gateway. (n.d.). Framework for prevention of child maltreatment.
https://www.childwelfare.gov/topics/preventing/overview/framework/)

The Children's Bureau highlights the importance of proactively preventing child maltreatment and investing in the capacity of parents to keep their children safe early on through collaboration with the legal, judicial, educational, and child welfare systems through an increased focus on primary prevention and by strengthening the capacity of communities to support the children and families who live there and provide the critical services they need before (and after) child welfare system involvement (Child Welfare Information Gateway, 2018). Part of child maltreatment prevention is increasing awareness, which can be delivered through public awareness campaigns (e.g., Drazen et al., 2009).

History of Child Maltreatment Prevention

Child maltreatment has been a growing concern in the United States with the recognition of the impact of child neglect and physical abuse. Henry Kempe et al.'s (1962) work in the 1960s led to the implementation of federal and state policy directed at forming a reporting system, laws against child abuse and neglect, followed by the Child Abuse Prevention and Treatment Act (CAPTA) of 1974, which mandated reporting of child abuse and neglect cases. A greater awareness of the issue led to an increase in education directed at the general public about identifying child abuse and neglect and its consequences.

The shift towards prevention began with funding to projects that examined the causes of child maltreatment and corresponding strategies for preventing child maltreatment. Some of the earliest projects funded were home visitation programs that promoted education on pregnancy and child development, healthy mother-child bonding, and a positive home environment. In the 1990s, funding through the Family Preservation and Support Services Program Act of 1993 provided services for families in need of counseling, in-home services, parent support, and childcare. The importance of early relationships with caregivers and connection to the community was emphasized with new research from the Neurons to Neighborhoods Study (Phillips, & Shonkoff, 2000). It further discussed the impact of experiences of child abuse and neglect on the growing child within the context of their environment. Research began to focus on protective factors, those elements that helped families overcome risks and promoted improved outcomes. Protective factors function as buffers and mitigate the risks associated with maltreatment while also promoting resilience (Walsh et al., 2015). These protective factors became the basis for programs and policies that invested in family strengths, early education, and community building and supports. The Center for the Study of Social Policy (CSSP) described five overarching protective factors that when promoted could help parents overcome stress that might lead to child maltreatment: parental resilience, social connections, concrete support in times of need, knowledge of parenting and child development, and development of social and emotional competence in children.

CAPTA has been amended numerous times over the last several decades and continues to fund programs that focus on preventing child maltreatment through programs that infuse protective factors targeting children and families and those that address issues related to child maltreatment risk. The Administration Children and Families (ACF) identified 10 protective factors from the research that help guide programming and policy that promote child and family well-being: self-regulation, relational skills, problem-solving skills, involvement in positive activities, parenting competencies, caring adults, positive peers, positive community, positive school environments, and economic opportunities (Child Welfare Information Gateway, 2014).

Reflection

Moving Upstream

There is a commonly used story that people often use to describe the concept of "going upstream" address certain problems. It tells the story about a group of campers on a riverbank who are gathering when one of them sees a baby in the water. Of course, he immediately jumps in and rescues the infant. But as he climbs out of the water, one of the other campers spots another baby in the river headed their way, followed by another. And another. Overwhelmed by the number of babies, the campers grab anybody around them so that they can help them get babies from the water.

Before they know it, the river is filled with babies, and more and more rescuers are needed to help the campers. But not all the babies can be saved. Also, some of the brave rescuers occasionally drown. But they somehow continue to work together to create a complex system that involves multiple supports to be able to keep pulling babies from the river.

At one point, one of the rescuers starts walking upstream. The others ask them, "Where are you going? We need your help to pull the babies out." The rescuer replies: "You carry on here ... I'm going upstream to find the bugger who keeps chucking all these babies in the river."

Prevention Strategies

Given what is known about the individual, family, and community risk and protective factors associated with child maltreatment, several national organizations have established approaches to prevent child maltreatment and provide guidance to child welfare agencies and practitioners, as well as policy-makers, to further implement priorities in practice as it fits with their population and needs. Many of these approaches have adopted a public health perspective. Experts have argued that to address child maltreatment it is necessary to have a universal system that seeks to help all children and families (Daro, 2016). Various communities are attempting to address child maltreatment systematically, as is the case in South Carolina and Colorado (Daro et al., n.d.). South Carolina has embraced public health policies and the Positive Parenting Program (Triple P), a population parenting program working with experts in communities across the state to ensure its implementation (Strompolis et al., 2020). To assist communities, the Centers for Disease Control and Prevention (CDC) Essentials for Childhood Framework and the Center for the Study of Social Policy Strengthening Families Framework provide direction on how to address and prevent child maltreatment.

Center for the Study of Social Policy (CSSP)
Strengthening Families

The CSSP Strengthening Families is a research-informed approach to "increase family strengths, enhance child development, and reduce the likelihood of child abuse and neglect." (CSSP, n.d.). It is family-centered, rooted in communities, and focused on building five key protective factors. The Strengthening Families framework is based on the idea that all families possess strengths and that it is possible to cultivate existing and new characteristics to promote child and family well-being. They draw on the above protective factors at multiple levels to guide programs, practice, and policies. The framework's logic model outlines core functions of state and system alongside program and community leaders to build parent partnerships; deepen knowledge and understanding; shift practice, policy, and systems; and ensure accountability. It further outlines worker and program practice serving children and families that support families to build and cultivate the five protective factors to strengthen families, achieve optimal child development, and reduce child maltreatment (CSSP, n.d.) See Table 7.1 for details about the Strengthening Families approach.

Across multiple frameworks and strategies to prevent child maltreatment, there is general consensus that in order to achieve positive child and family outcomes, providers should work alongside parents as partners, providing the necessary support and resources in order for them to be successful. Most would agree that changing the circumstances so that parents can enhance relationships with their children and provide nurturing environments for their families can mitigate some of the risks associated with child maltreatment. Overall, we should focus on promoting family strengths and protective factors on an individual level and changing systems that create circumstances that lead to child maltreatment. Child maltreatment prevention must be a multisystemic, collaborative effort in order for it to be effective. Children and families interact with a number of systems that can collectively provide the support, guidance, and resources needed for well-being. Strategies to prevent child maltreatment must incorporate data-driven methods and rely on evidence-informed programs when available. Funding is also essential to establish a strong research base and to pilot prevention programs targeting the families who need them.

Table 7.1 Components and description of the Strengthening Families approach

Parental resilience	• Honor family's, language, culture, history, and approach to parenting • Support parents as decision-makers • Help parents to intervene and support their children during challenging times
Social connections	• Help families to value, build, and sustain social networks • Create an inclusive environment • Promote community engagement and participation
Knowledge of parenting and child development	• Provide information and resources on parenting and child development • Provide opportunities to practice new parenting skills • Model and teach developmentally appropriate interactions with children
Concrete support in times of need	• Provide connections to services in the community • Respond immediately to families in crisis • Support families in developing skills and strengths to identify needs and access supports
Social and emotional competence of children	• Help parents to foster child's social-emotional development • Help children develop a positive cultural identity and interact in a diverse society • Model nurturing support to children

Source: Used with permission from the Center for the Study of Social Policy. (n.d.). Strengthening Families

CDC Essentials for Childhood

The CDC's Division of Violence Prevention (2014) developed a technical package that outlines four overarching areas of focus that lead to safe, stable, and nurturing relationships (SSNRs) and promote primary prevention of child maltreatment. Strategies related to these areas involve targeting child maltreatment at multiple levels, including individual, familial, societal, and community levels. In order to prevent child maltreatment and reduce risk for child maltreatment, they recommend policies, programs, and supports (Fortson et al., 2016): (1) Strengthen economic supports for families, (2) change social norms to support parents and positive parenting practices, (3) provide quality care and education in infancy and early childhood, (4) enhance parenting skills to promote healthy child development, and (5) intervene when necessary to lessen the potential for harm and prevent future risk.

Research shows that policies that improve an individual and family's financial stability can have an impact on health outcomes (Frieden, 2010) and reduce child abuse and neglect (Stith et al., 2009); however, little is known about the effectiveness and economic efficiency of policies and practices that provide economic supports to families to prevent child abuse and neglect. By supporting family financial security, parents are able to better meet their children's basic needs, such as shelter, food, and health care. Improved health can have positive effects on child

> **Practice Highlight**
>
> **Contributors to Safe, Stable, and Nurturing Relationships (SSNRs)**
>
> - Greater awareness of child maltreatment and a commitment to prevent it
> - Use of data to inform actions
> - Programs to create the context for healthy children and families
> - Policy that develops such a context

development and educational and social outcomes. In order to strengthen household financial security, policies can address family needs related to tax credits; nutrition assistance programs; child support payments and financial assistance; safe, stable, and affordable housing; and childcare. In addition, the Fortson et al. (2016) highlights the need for livable wages, paid leave for family members, and flexible and consistent schedules as a means of improving financial security for families. It is also critical to identify community conditions that increase or reduce the incidence of child maltreatment to promote the development of SSNRs. Finally, research is needed to evaluate the economic effectiveness of programs that reduce multiple forms of child maltreatment and their relationship with other forms of violence, such as youth violence, intimate partner violence (IPV), and suicide.

Note from the Field

Home Visitation as a Game Changer

I worked with Jada,[1] a 19-year-old new mom of a beautiful baby girl. Jada has been in foster care since she was 11 and lived in a series of group homes and shelters, until 3 months ago, when she received notice that she had was able to use Section 8 housing. She moved into a one-bedroom apartment with her baby. She didn't have much work experience and hoped she could get a job soon. While she was in the hospital, a social worker referred her to the Healthy Families program offered in the county she lived. The social worker told her that she would have someone come visit her, teach her about parenting, help her to access benefits and training, and offer support in her parenting journey. Jada wasn't sure she needed the help, but after being in foster care, she didn't have much of a role model for good parenting and didn't want her daughter to be taken from her. She was worried they would judge her parenting and report her to the child welfare authorities. She took a chance, and Tracy was assigned her case. Tracy came to her home almost every day to begin. She first focused on helping her access things for the baby: diapers, a breast pump, and identifying a pediatrician for the baby. She sat down and showed her how to hold her, soothe her when she was upset or fussy, and helped her set up a safe sleeping environment for her. When the baby was sleeping during their visits, she talked to her about her boyfriend who doesn't come around anymore, her fragmented relationship with her mom, and her friends who don't call as much because the baby cries a lot. Tracy helped her to map out some plans and goals for her future with school and work and encouraged her to apply for government assistance to help her spend more time with her baby before going back to work. Jada called Tracy when she was struggling with her baby refusing to nap or crying when she was teething. When Jada was ready to start going to school part-time, Tracy helped her organize her applications and scholarships. She helped her find childcare so she could complete her prerequisite courses to apply to business school to study accounting. Jada didn't have many positive adults in her life when she had her baby and relied on Tracy to help her to learn how to do the things most new parents learn from their parents. She helped her establish a social support network and how to navigate the various systems. Without home visitation, Jada would have struggled to keep her baby in her care.

[1]All names and other personal identifiers in cases and examples throughout this book have been changed to protect privacy and confidentiality.

Evidence suggests that providing quality care and education early in life can improve a child's development and help to establish SSNRs to create a positive pathway throughout the lifespan. Policies and practices must address the need for quality childcare options, preschool enrichment and family engagement, and improved licensing and accreditation of childcare and preschool programs. These opportunities can enhance a child's ability to succeed academically and socially. A key approach to preventing child abuse and neglect is equipping parents with the necessary skills and tools to promote healthy child development.

Several evidence-based early childhood home visitation programs (e.g., Healthy Families, Nurse-Family Partnership) have been shown to be effective in reducing child abuse and neglect by providing information and resources, support, training about child development, health, and discipline in the caregiver's home. Parents/ caregivers and families at greater risk of child maltreatment should have access to parenting skill development and positive relationship development programs in the community. Not only do these home visiting programs address issues related to child abuse and neglect but also can also protect children from other forms of violence (Knox et al., 2011; Portwood et al., 2011).

Child Maltreatment Prevention Models

Home Visiting Programs

Various models of child maltreatment prevention have been developed over the years, with the most common and most studied being home visitation. Home visiting programs have existed for decades, and in 2010 the Congress established the Maternal, Infant, and Early Childhood Home Visiting Program (MIECHV) to provide federal funds to states and tribal entities to support voluntary, evidence-based home visiting services to at-risk families. These programs, although varied, typically involve a professional (nurse or social worker) who meets regularly with an expectant parent or a parent of an infant in their home to provide information and support with parenting skill development, child development, and accessing resources and supports in the community. Home visitation programs differ in terms of the populations they serve (e.g., expectant mothers, parents, new mothers), who conducts the home visit (e.g., nurse, volunteer, peer, other professional), when the program is offered (prenatally, postnatally), and for how long (e.g., 3 months, 18 months); however, evidence has shown that this type of intervention improves child and maternal well-being and can prevent child maltreatment.

There are multiple evidence-based programs delivered across the United States, including the Nurse-Family Partnership and Healthy Families. These programs individually share similar core components and offer flexible and specific programming based on the population they serve. Studies have examined specific program areas (e.g., timing, topics of visits, use of assessments and screening tools, training for visitors) to determine what key quality components show positive outcomes. The Administration for Children and Families (ACF) along with its partners conducted a systematic review of early childhood home visiting research most recently in December of 2019 (HomVEE), which outlines the effectiveness of the most common home visiting programs available (Sama-Miller et al., 2019). They examined program outcomes in eight domains: (1) maternal health, (2) child health, (3) positive parenting practices, (4) child development and school readiness, (5) reductions in child maltreatment, (6) family economic self-sufficiency, (7) linkages and referrals to community resources, and (8) reduction in juvenile delinquency, family violence, and crime. Of the 50 models reviewed, 21 met the criteria set forth by the United States Department of Health and Human Services for an evidence-based home visiting program, including Healthy Families America, Nurse-Family Partnerships, SafeCare, and Parents as Teachers. Within these models, research continues to improve services and increase engagement (e.g., Beasley et al., 2018). There are promising practices being developed that address specific groups, such as engaging fathers (e.g., Guterman et al., 2018).

Practice Highlight

Examples of Child Maltreatment Prevention Programs

Triple P – Positive Parenting Program: a primary prevention strategy that provides parenting support for those with children ages 0–16 to prevent and manage behavioral and emotional issues through parenting skill development and empowerment.

Period of Purple Crying: aims to assist new parents and caregivers in understanding infant crying while offering support and tips for managing prolonged infant crying.

Parents as Teachers: is a home visiting program for parents beginning during pregnancy up until the age of 5. It helps parents to understand child development and positive parenting practices, while preventing child maltreatment and promoting school readiness.

Incredible Years: targets parents, teachers, and children (ages 4 to 8) through curricula that promote social and emotional competence and address behavioral or emotional concerns.

Safe Care: is an in-home program that supports parents how to positively interact with their children, deal with difficult behaviors, and respond when a child is in need.

Parent Education Programs

Parent education provides caregivers the resources, knowledge, and support to be the best parent they can while enhancing the parent-child relationship and promoting well-being. Parenting practices can promote child well-being and child development (e.g., Longo et al., 2017). Parent education programs focus on enhancing parenting practices and behaviors, including increasing knowledge about child development and positive discipline, promoting positive play and interaction between parents and children, and assisting with identifying and accessing community resources and supports.

Several elements of parent education programs have been shown to promote positive parenting and child well-being. These programs highlight mutual support among parents, promote father engagement, and recognize that parents have individual needs that need to be addressed in a culturally relevant way. Parent education programs may be just one component of a larger child maltreatment prevention approach (e.g., home visiting, Triple P); however many adopt strategies that promote protective factors, are tailored to the parents' cultural and community needs (e.g., Effective Black Parenting Program, Positive Indian Parenting), and utilize qualified and trained professionals as teachers and facilitators. Further, Wilder Research (2016) describes several program elements to reinforce protective factors, such as early and active parent engagement, availability of frequent and ongoing classes, and the promotion of family routines and activities.

When examining the evidence for parent education programs, several stand out as preventing maltreatment and promoting healthy children and families, for example, the Incredible Years, Nurturing Fathers Program, Parent-Child Interaction Therapy, SafeCare, Triple P (Positive Parenting Program), and the Nurturing Parenting Program (Child Welfare Information Gateway, 2019). Ongoing evaluations of parenting programs specifically for parents who are involved with the child welfare system are necessary, especially to determine if changing parents' behaviors persists and if child maltreatment is reduced (Akin et al., 2017) and if the parents find the interventions acceptable and appropriate (Lewis et al., 2016).

Community-Level Interventions

There are benefits of using a community-level approach to preventing child maltreatment to reach families who may not be connected to services and resources already and extend beyond the individual level. Many community-level programming focuses on under-resourced neighborhoods and communities that experience multiple challenges such as violence, lack of healthy food options and transportation, and environmental barriers. Community-level prevention strategies target those risk factors associated with child maltreatment risk, such as a lack of affordable childcare and health care and economic, housing, and employment stability. Community-based prevention requires collaboration among multiple system levels, including the community members, local service providers, and government agencies.

Research Brief

Community Prevention

What do efforts to promote child well-being in a community look like? One project identified that children from low socioeconomic status often have lower language development than their peers in higher socioeconomic statuses. To address this, an intervention that would occur in supermarkets was developed; signs were placed in supermarkets that encouraged adult-child dialog (Ridge et al., 2015). Evaluation of the project found that when the signs were present quality and amount of talking between adults and children in in the supermarkets serving low socioeconomic communities. This simple, cost-effective strategy may improve children's language development.

Specific strategies using a community-level approach include promoting social norms through public awareness campaigns and education and addressing the unique needs of the community through services, resources, and support. Community-level approaches to prevention are typically primary prevention strategies; however, they also include some secondary strategies in the form of services and supports for at-risk families. Common community-based efforts include public service announcements related to issues such as shaken baby syndrome/abusive head trauma, guidance for safe sleeping practices for baby, child sexual abuse, and corporal punishment. Such media campaigns involve radio announcements, television ads, bulletin boards, widespread distribution of pamphlets and literature, and newsletters.

Child maltreatment prevention efforts at multiple targets (individual, family, and community) are continuing to improve and expand, benefitting many families who are in need. However, there continues to be challenges to the current approaches

Practice Highlight

Child Abuse Prevention Month

April is **National Child Abuse Prevention Month**. This month and throughout the year, the child welfare agency and other businesses and organizations encourage all individuals and organizations to play a role in making their communities a better place for children and families. Information about child maltreatment is shared along with ways to promote healthy child and family well-being.

Pinwheels for Prevention® In 2008, Prevent Child Abuse America (PCA) introduced the Pinwheels for Prevention® campaign. Pinwheels represent childlike whimsy and lightheartedness. PCA's vision is for a world where all children grow up happy, healthy, and prepared to succeed in supportive families and communities.

in theory and in practice. For example, prevention programs are not a one-size-fits-all, and families differ in their makeup, needs, and culture. Many communities lack the financial means or support to implement prevention programs. Further, there are many programs to choose from, and it may be difficult to find one that fits the family or community, or it is not available to the family or community. Research continues to show that a multipronged approach is needed to benefit the most families. Research should continue to study the impact of current programs and explore new ways to prevent child maltreatment.

Research Brief

Promoting Social Norms in the Community to Prevent Child Maltreatment

In order to increase safe, stable, and nurturing relationships and environments, we must also focus on obtaining broad engagement across multiple groups, including parents, teachers, day care providers, and coaches. There needs to be a change in social norms at the community level as well if child maltreatment is to be prevented (Fleckman et al., 2019). Norms refer to values, beliefs, attitudes, and behaviors that are shared among most people in a group. In order to promote social norms, it is important for these group members to have an investment in the outcome, for example, child well-being. Research shows that perceptions about norms can be strong predictors of behaviors. Therefore, if a parent believes that it is common practice for a child should enroll in school at age 5, they will more than likely comply with this norm. They must see the benefits and have a general consensus to behaving accordingly while seeing others also behaving accordingly. Changing someone's core values and beliefs however can be challenging, and it takes time. For example, in the past several decades, public health specialists have changed the norm around cigarette smoking and wearing seatbelts. With regard to child maltreatment, scholars and practitioners have begun to change the norm around corporal punishment. A recent study found that people in the United States believe that child maltreatment is a serious problem and the prevention of child abuse and neglect is possible (Klika et al., 2019). This same study found that people may not be comfortable in taking action to prevent child abuse and neglect due in part to a lack of knowledge. Thus, while norms may be changing, considerable work remains to be done.

Policies Supporting Child Maltreatment Prevention

In addition to federal policies mentioned earlier in the chapter (e.g., CAPTA, FPSSPA, MIECHV), more recent legislation has also authorized funding and guidance related to child maltreatment prevention, most notably the Family First Prevention Services Act of 2018 (Family First). This legislation changes the way Title IV-E funds can be spent by states. With the Family First Act, states, territories, and tribes with an approved Title IV-E plan have the option to use funds for prevention services to allow children to remain in home or with relatives while funding programs and services to facilitate this (e.g., substance abuse or mental health treatment). Family First also has provisions about reducing the use of congregate care and extends support for youth aging out of care.

Family Preservation

Many child welfare agencies engage in primary prevention strategies as part of their role in the community by initiating public service announcements, providing services and supports to all families in the community, and partnering with local organizations focused on maltreatment prevention (e.g., Healthy Families, Prevent Child Abuse America). However, as child welfare professionals, we use a prevention lens when working with families primarily at the secondary and tertiary levels. Child welfare professionals may be working to provide intact family services or family preservation services for families who present a low or medium risk of maltreatment or maltreatment reoccurrence or with families whose children are in care who receive services from the child welfare agency or another child and family-serving agency in the community. The child welfare professional may also not necessarily be the provider of such services, but may refer for services such as parenting classes, mental health support and services, and substance abuse treatment related to child maltreatment prevention.

After the passage of CAPTA, historically when a child was abused or neglected, they were removed from the home to protect them. The philosophy of family preservation services is that the best place for the child is to remain in the home – unless their safety is compromised or that the risk of harm is so great that it is not possible. Family preser-

Practice Highlight

Promoting Safe Sleep Practices

Every year, approximately 3500 babies die in the United States due to Sudden Infant Death Syndrome (SIDS), accidental suffocation, and undetermined reasons.

The American Academy of Pediatrics (AAP) recommends placing babies on their back at all sleep times (naps and night), using a firm sleep surface for the baby (e.g., mattress and crib), keeping soft objects and loose bedding out of the baby's sleep area, and sharing a room with a baby but not the same bed (Task Force on Sudden Infant Death Syndrome, 2016). A recent study led by AAP using the Pregnancy Risk Assessment Monitoring System (PRAMS) showed that 22% of parents reported placing their baby on their side or stomach, 61% shared a bed with their infant, and 39% used soft bedding. They also found that these practices were more common among young, less educated parents who identified as a racial/ethnic minority.

State public health and child welfare agencies have partnered with family-serving organizations to promote safe sleep practices for new parents. However, some of these topics can often be controversial. There are many reasons cited by parents for choosing to sleep with their children, including facilitating feeding (breastfeeding or formula), comforting a fussy or sick infant, improving sleep for mother and child, bonding, cultural traditions, and improving feelings of safety. Some advocacy groups encourage bed sharing to promote longer duration and exclusivity of breastfeeding and state that bed sharing is safe among infants who are breastfed and infants whose parents do not smoke, drink alcohol, or use illicit substances.

vation services are designed for children to remain in their own home while strengthening the ability of the parents to meet their responsibilities in caring for the child.

Further, children need permanency in their family relationships in order to develop into healthy, productive individuals; families should be the primary caretakers of their own children, and the government and social service programs should make every effort to support families in this function. Typically, the state or child welfare agency does not have legal custody of the child and does not take over any of the role functions of the parent.

Certain federal policies, such as the Adoption Assistance and Child Welfare Act (AACWA) of 1980 and the Adoption and Safe Families Act (ASFA) of 1997, prioritize family preservation in cases where child welfare systems become involved with families. AACWA was the first law passed that shifted towards prevention of removal, in place of a reactive response during investigation. It specified that child welfare agencies must develop and implement services to ensure reasonable efforts are made to prevent or eliminate the need for removal of a child from their home. As will be discussed later, this meant assessing a family's needs and responding by providing resources and support. Similarly, ASFA required that states must continue to make reasonable efforts to preserve and reunify families.

The goals of family preservation are rooted in a family-centered and strengths-perspective approach to serving families. The goals are to help parents build on existing strengths in order to reduce the risk of abuse and neglect, prevent the out-of-home placement of children, and enable the family to function without the need for further child welfare system involvement. Statistics show that almost half (49%) of children in care will be reunified with their parent; therefore there is a strong argument for reducing the trauma of removal when possible through the provision of services and supports.

The process and services offered as part of family preservation may look different based on the jurisdiction. Typically, it involves a family assessment, service plan, service provision, a safety plan, ongoing monitoring of progress, and conclusion/case closure within a certain time frame. Levels of intervention can range from no services, where one visit is required to complete an investigation indicating no risk to the child, to regular contact with the child and family, and wraparound services are provided for 90–120 days or more. Community service referrals can be made to reduce the risk of child maltreatment (e.g., food, financial support, assistance with community supports, etc.), as well as short-term services where services and supports can be put in place that will mitigate the risk factors of child maltreatment and that still require a level of supervision and monitoring by the child welfare agency. Some examples that may fit these criteria are environmental neglect, short-term hospitalization, or inadequate supervision. Child welfare professionals meet regularly with their supervisors (weekly) to review the case with regard to safety, assessments, and service provision, make regular in-person visits (weekly at first) with all family members, complete necessary forms and assessments, assess home safety, complete a service plan, and often schedule and hold a child and family team meeting.

In summary, family preservation services are typically short-term, family-focused services designed to assist families in crisis by improving parenting and family functioning while keeping children safe. These in-home services grew out of the recognition that remaining with family is a priority and that separating children from their families is traumatic for them, often leaving lasting negative effects. Family preservation services operate under the premise that many children can be

Note from the Field

Keeping Children in the Home

Jamie, a veteran child welfare professional, was called out to conduct an investigation into a "dirty home," where allegations were made that two children were living with their mother who "drank too much" and the kids sometimes didn't go to school. It was late in the day, but Jamie knew this couldn't wait. She went to the home to talk to the parent and children and planned to talk to other family members, school officials, and neighbors if possible and as appropriate. When she arrived at the door, she noticed two dogs in a fenced in area outside the house. One young child with a diaper hanging on was out front and another preteen was sitting on the door step. The preteen, Muriel, said her mom wasn't home, but would be soon as she had just called to tell her. Muriel had dirty clothes on and looked slim, but not emaciated. Jamie showed her identification and told her who she was and why she was there. Muriel was apathetic and showed her inside the house after retrieving the toddler. She asked when the child's diaper was last changed. Muriel said they had just run out of diapers last night and her mom didn't have enough money to buy more until she got paid. They sat in the kitchen and Jamie noticed they didn't have food in the fridge and there were empty boxes of cereal on the counter. Jamie pulled out an apple, banana, and an orange from her purse and some crackers and asked the kids if they'd like some. Both nodded. Brenda, the kids' mom, arrived home and seemed frazzled and worried. She apologized for the state of the house and started crying. She said her mom died last year in an accident and she was usually the one to help out with the kids and help with rent and other expenses when she didn't have enough from her check. She said she worked full-time at the check-cashing store about 3 miles away. She said she often feels depressed and so tired that she can't clean or tidy the house, finds it hard to make ends meet, and there's nobody to help her. Jamie talked to the kids separately in another room and asked a few more questions. She was convinced that it was not an ideal setting the way it was when she arrived, but thought that with some help, Brenda could provide a safe home for the kids. She asked about family strengths, supports in the neighborhood or her family, and about benefits she might be receiving for food, housing, or cash assistance. Jamie called an agency they worked with and said she would arrange to get some diapers and an emergency food box for the family. She also said she would bring some clothes by the house later along with some applications for financial and housing assistance. She asked that Brenda call her trusted neighbor, Ms. Perkins, to take the kids tonight so she could have some time alone and would refer a cleaning service to help get things started and back on track. Jamie also made referrals for counseling to help her with grief, loss, and depression she has been experiencing. Jamie knows that in some cases, it is the best option to remove kids from their homes to keep them safe. She also knows that the best place for kids is with their family and it's much harder to get them back home once they have been removed. In this case, there were several things she could do to support this family to ensure the children's safety and keep them at home.

safely protected and treated within their own homes when parents are provided with services and support that they need to make the necessary changes.

Conclusion

Child abuse and neglect continue to be a major public health concern; however, communities have made great strides and have shown that preventing child abuse and neglect is possible. Various models and programs have been shown to be effective in addressing child maltreatment at different time points – before it has happened, when it might happen, and after it has happened. Strategies include reducing or removing the risk factors for child maltreatment and promoting protective factors and positive parenting techniques, providing resources and supports, and including community members and systems in supporting child and family well-being. Further family preservation services underscore the importance of keeping families together safely while providing the necessary tools and services to strengthen families.

Discussion Questions

1. How can child welfare professionals engage in child maltreatment prevention?
2. What are three programs that focus on strengthening families to prevent child maltreatment?
3. How can the child welfare system prevent child maltreatment and support families?
4. What are the five strategies the CDC recommends that lead to safe, stable, and nurturing relationships?
5. What services can a child welfare worker recommend when referring for family preservation programs?

Suggested Activities

1. Review materials released as part of child abuse prevention month (April), and practice writing an editorial about raising awareness about child maltreatment.
2. Read essays on why prevention matters: https://preventchildabuse.org/resource/why-prevention-matters/. Write a reflection paper on why you think prevention is important in child welfare work.
3. Preventing child maltreatment includes supporting families and communities to create positive experiences. Watch the video "Building Partnerships in Child Welfare," and write down a list of ideas for activities and resources for families: https://www.youtube.com/watch?v=ES8Vij2CNBA
4. Learn more about the activities that promote child abuse prevention month (April) in the state you live in. Obtain promotional materials, find ways to increase awareness about child abuse prevention, and share information and risk and protective factors.
5. Read the story, "The Fence or the Ambulance" by John N. Hurty, MD, and consider the parallels to child abuse and neglect prevention: https://www.ncbi.nlm.nih.gov/pmc/articles/PMC1558450/pdf/amjphnation00932-0024.pdf

6. Read Lewis et al. (2016). As you read the mothers' insights about their perceptions of acceptability and appropriateness about the Triple P program fit as well
as the barriers to participation, consider how this information can be useful to
child welfare professionals. Discuss with others the importance of engagement
with child welfare-involved families.

> Lewis, E. M., Feely, M., Seay, K. D., Fedoravicis, N., & Kohl, P. L. (2016).
> Child welfare involved parents and Pathways Triple P: perceptions of pro-
> gram acceptability and appropriateness. *Journal of child and family stud-
> ies, 25*(12), 3760-3770. (Available: https://rdcu.be/cbVtZ).

Additional Resources

Child Maltreatment Prevention: A Planning Framework for Action: https://cantasd.
info/wp-content/uploads/Framework_for_Prevention_Planning-
FINAL-10-5-17.pdf

California Evidence-based Clearinghouse for Child Welfare: https://www.cebc4cw.org/

Centers for Disease Control and Prevention, Child Abuse and Neglect Prevention:
https://www.cdc.gov/violenceprevention/childabuseandneglect/index.html

Centers for Disease Control and Prevention, Preventing Child Abuse and Neglect:

https://www.cdc.gov/violenceprevention/pdf/CAN-Prevention-Technical-Package.pdf

Centers for Disease Control and Prevention, Essentials for Childhood: https://www.
cdc.gov/violenceprevention/childabuseandneglect/essentials.html

Child Welfare Information Gateway, National Child Abuse Prevention Month:
https://www.childwelfare.gov/topics/preventing/preventionmonth/

Prevent Child Abuse America: https://preventchildabuse.org/

CO4Kids, Primary Prevention Measurement Guide: https://www.co4kids.org/tools-
and-education/toolkit/prevention-measurement-guide

References

Akin, B. A., Yan, Y., McDonald, T., & Moon, J. (2017). Changes in parenting practices during
Parent Management Training Oregon model with parents of children in foster care. *Children
and Youth Services Review, 76*, 181–191. https://doi.org/10.1016/j.childyouth.2017.03.010

Beasley, L. O., Ridings, L. E., Smith, T. J., Shields, J. D., Silovsky, J. F., Beasley, W., & Bard,
D. (2018). A qualitative evaluation of engagement and attrition in a nurse home visiting program: From the participant and provider perspective. *Prevention Science, 19*(4), 528–537.
https://doi.org/10.1007/s11121-017-0846-5

Caplan, G. (1964). *Principles of preventive psychiatry*. Basic Books.

Centers for Disease Control and Prevention. (2014). *Essentials for childhood: Creating safe, stable, nurturing relationships and environments for all children*. Retrieved from: https://www.
cdc.gov/violenceprevention/childabuseandneglect/essentials.html

Center for the Study of Social Policy. (n.d.) *Strengthening Families*. Retrieved from: https://cssp.org/our-work/project/strengthening-families/#:~:text=The%20Strengthening%20Families%20framework%20is,building%20the%20five%20protective%20factors

Child Welfare Information Gateway. (n.d.). *Framework for prevention of child maltreatment*. Retrieved from https://www.childwelfare.gov/topics/preventing/overview/framework/

Child Welfare Information Gateway. (2014). *Protective factors approaches in child welfare*. Washington, DC: U.S. Department of Health and Human Services.

Child Welfare Information Gateway. (2019). *Parent education to strengthen families and reduce the risk of maltreatment*. U.S. Department of Health and Human Services, Children's Bureau.

Child Welfare Information Gateway. (2018). *Preventing child abuse and neglect*. U.S. Department of Health and Human Services, Children's Bureau.

Daro, D. (2016). A public health approach to prevention: What will it take? *Trauma, Violence, & Abuse, 17*(4), 420–421. https://doi.org/10.1177/1524838016658880

Daro, D., Jarpe-Ratner, E., Karter, C., Crane, K., Bellamy, J. & Seay, K. (n.d.). *Child maltreatment prevention: A planning framework for action*. Chapin Hall. Available: https://cantasd.info/wp-content/uploads/Framework_for_Prevention_Planning-FINAL-10-5-17.pdf

Drazen, Y., Guenther, L., & Hansen, J. (2009). Public awareness campaigns. In K. S. Slack, K. M. Jack, & L. M. Gjertson (Eds.), *Child maltreatment prevention: Toward an evidence-based approach* (pp. 17–18).

Fleckman, J. M., Taylor, C. A., Theall, K. P., & Andrinopoulos, K. (2019). Perceived social norms in the neighborhood context: The role of perceived collective efficacy in moderating the relation between perceived injunctive norms and use of corporal punishment. *Child and Adolescent Social Work Journal, 36*(1), 29–41. https://doi.org/10.1007/s10560-018-0581-1

Fortson, B. L., Klevens, J., Merrick, M. T., Gilbert, L. K., & Alexander, S. P. (2016). *Preventing child abuse and neglect: A technical package for policy, norm, and programmatic activities*. https://doi.org/10.15620/cdc.38864

Frieden, T. R. (2010). A framework for public health action: the health impact pyramid. *American Journal of Public Health, 100*(4), 590–595. https://doi.org/10.2105/AJPH.2009.185652

Guterman, N. B., Bellamy, J. L., & Banman, A. (2018). Promoting father involvement in early home visiting services for vulnerable families: Findings from a pilot study of "Dads matter". *Child Abuse & Neglect, 76*, 261–272. https://doi.org/10.1016/j.chiabu.2017.10.017

Kempe, C. H., Silverman, F. N., Steele, B. F., Droegemueller, W., & Silver, H. K. (1962). The battered-child syndrome. *JAMA, 181*(1), 17–24. https://doi.org/10.1001/jama.1962.03050270019004

Klika, J. B., Haboush-Deloye, A., & Linkenbach, J. (2019). Hidden protections: Identifying social norms associated with child abuse, sexual abuse, and neglect. *Child and Adolescent Social Work Journal, 36*(1), 5–14. https://doi.org/10.1007/s10560-018-0595-8

Knox, M. S., Burkhart, K., & Hunter, K. E. (2011). ACT against violence parents raising safe kids program: Effects on maltreatment-related parenting behaviors and beliefs. *Journal of Family Issues, 32*(1), 55–74. https://doi.org/10.1177/0192513X10370112

Lewis, E. M., Feely, M., Seay, K. D., Fedoravicis, N., & Kohl, P. L. (2016). Child welfare involved parents and Pathways Triple P: perceptions of program acceptability and appropriateness. *Journal of Child and Family Studies, 25*(12), 3760–3770. https://doi.org/10.1007/s10826-016-0526-2

Longo, F., McPherran Lombardi, C., & Dearing, E. (2017). Family investments in low-income children's achievement and socioemotional functioning. *Developmental Psychology, 53*(12), 2273. https://doi.org/10.1037/dev0000366

Phillips, D. A., & Shonkoff, J. P. (Eds.). (2000). *From neurons to neighborhoods: The science of early childhood development*. National Academies Press.

Portwood, S. G., Lambert, R. G., Abrams, L. P., & Nelson, E. B. (2011). An evaluation of the adults and children together (ACT) against violence parents raising safe kids program. *The Journal of Primary Prevention, 32*(3-4), 147. https://doi.org/10.1007/s10935-011-0249-5

Ridge, K. E., Weisberg, D. S., Ilgaz, H., Hirsh-Pasek, K. A., & Golinkoff, R. M. (2015). Supermarket speak: Increasing talk among low-socioeconomic status families. *Mind, Brain, and Education, 9*(3), 127–135. https://doi.org/10.1111/mbe.12081

Sama-Miller, E., Akers, L., Mraz-Esposito, A., Coughlin, R., & Zukiewicz, M. (2019). *Home visiting evidence of effectiveness review: Executive summary*. Mathematica Policy Research.

Stith, S. M., Liu, T., Davies, L. C., Boykin, E. L., Alder, M. C., Harris, J. M., et al. (2009). Risk factors in child maltreatment: A meta-analytic review of the literature. *Aggression and Violent Behavior, 14*(1), 13–29. https://doi.org/10.1016/j.avb.2006.03.006

Strompolis, M., Cain, J. M., Wilson, A., Aldridge, W. A., Armstrong, J. M., & Srivastav, A. (2020). Community capacity coach: Embedded support to implement evidenced-based prevention. *Journal of Community Psychology*. https://doi.org/10.1002/jcop.22375

Task Force on Sudden Infant Death Syndrome. (2016). SIDS and other sleep-related infant deaths: updated 2016 recommendations for a safe infant sleeping environment. *Pediatrics, 138*(5). https://doi.org/10.1542/peds.2016-2938

Walsh, T. B., McCourt, S. N., Rostad, W. L., Byers, K., & Ocasio, K. (2015). Promoting protective factors and strengthening resilience. In D. Daro, A. Cohn Donnelly, L. Huang, & B. Powell (Eds.), *Advances in child abuse prevention knowledge. Child maltreatment (Contemporary issues in research and policy)* (Vol. 5). Springer. https://doi.org/10.1007/978-3-319-16327-7_9

Wilder Research. (2016). *The benefits of parenting education: A review of the literature for the Wilder Parent Education Center*. Retrieved from https://www.wilder.org/wilder-research/research-library/benefits-parenting-education-review-literature-wilder-parent

Chapter 8
Assessment in Child Welfare Practice

Introduction

Throughout child welfare practice, assessment is important. Assessment broadly can be thought of as a professional collecting information for the purposes of making decisions. There are multiple assessments that occur within child welfare. The assessment of parenting ability, the home environment, risk factors, safety, and protective factors are all assessments that child welfare professionals conduct. Likewise, there are assessments for children for trauma, education, and behavioral issues. Associated professionals also assess for health, mental health, substance misuse, and developmental issues.

Assessing Safety and Risk

To ensure children are safe in the future, child welfare professionals need to assess safety and risk. Safety is when the child is in a home and family where there is no threat of danger that could harm a child, or if there is a threat of danger, the family has the ability to protect the child and manage the threat. Risk is the likelihood of child maltreatment occurring in the future. Sometimes the term "imminent risk" used to indicate that the risk of maltreatment is likely. It indicates that the child is not safe. Risk factors are things that increase the changes of maltreatment occurring and include things like intimate partner violence, parental substance misuse, and parental mental health. Child risk factors include those who are young or who have disabilities.

Through the identification of protective factors and risks, child welfare professionals determine to what extent a child is safe in an environment. However, assessments extend beyond looking at risk because protective factors and the context are considered. For example, a risk factor could be a parent drinks heavily, frequently passing out and not supervising or providing basic needs for the child. If the child is

© Springer Nature Switzerland AG 2021
J. M. Geiger, L. Schelbe, *The Handbook on Child Welfare Practice*,
https://doi.org/10.1007/978-3-030-73912-6_8

Table 8.1 Comparing safety and risk

Comparing safety and risk		
	Safety	Risk
Time	Now or very near future	Long-term
Degree of harm	Moderate to severe	Low to severe
Purpose of intervention	To control or stop harm	To reduce or resolve

Fig. 8.1 Risk and safety circles. Safety is a subset of risk where all factors of safety apply to risk. Not all risk factors apply to safety

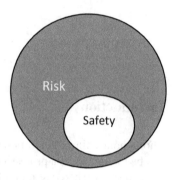

a teenager and grandparents live in the home and provide care for the child, the risk is lessened. However, if the parent lives alone with a young child, there is a greater risk for maltreatment.

A child is considered to be safe when an assessment of available information supports the belief that a child is not in immediate (near future) danger of moderate-to-severe harm. The focus in safety determination is to establish the potential for moderate-to-severe harm that could happen immediately or in the near future (see Table 8.1). If it is determined that a child is not safe, it is necessary to intervene to control and stop any potential harm.

Risk, however, involves the likelihood of any degree of longer-term future harm or maltreatment. To assess risk, child welfare professionals must consider factors in the family including their strengths and limitations as well as the resources available to them. Child welfare professionals make decisions about the potential that children may be abused or neglected in the future. It is important to note that risk does not predict when the future harm might occur, but rather the likelihood that it will happen at all. Further, concerns of risk do not specify a degree of harm or when harm might occur. Safety is a subset of risk. All factors related to safety also apply to risk, but not all risk factors may apply to safety (see Fig. 8.1).

There are differences and similarities between safety and risk. Both are concerned with potential of future harm, both related to conditions of home environment and caregiver or family member behavior, both can change quickly, and both can be controlled. The differences between the two are time (safety is now and near future; risk is longer term), degree of harm, and the purpose of intervention (safety needs to be controlled or managed now; risk can be resolved or reduced to protect a child from potential longer-term harm).

As a child welfare professional, this means that safety must be assessed quickly, often in one visit. Risk is assessed over a longer period of time, allowing time to gather, assess, and evaluate information. Like safety, risk is reassessed whenever there is a recurrence of maltreatment or a change in circumstances (e.g., child returning home). Safety and risks can often be controlled by drawing on family strengths or mitigating circumstances.

There are a number of potential safety threats, defined as specific family conditions that are present and uncontrolled that may likely to result in moderate-to-severe harm to the child. They may be related to child vulnerability (e.g., age, disability, psychological or emotional problems, lack of verbal skills), severity of the abuse or neglect, and history of abuse and/or neglect and/or child welfare system involvement. The child welfare professional must consider the effect any adult or other member of the household could have on a child's safety (e.g., parent's significant other, extended family member). As part of a safety threat assessment, all children residing in the home are to be seen and, if possible, interviewed out of the presence of the caregiver and alleged perpetrator. Interviews should be conducted in a developmentally appropriate manner.

> **Practice Highlight**
>
> **Minimum Parenting Standards**
>
> Often a controversial and difficult concept to grasp for many individuals is the idea of a minimum parenting standard. When we think about parenting, we think about ideal standards and practices that go beyond the basics of ensuring the child's safety. Many states and jurisdictions have a law about what consists of "minimum parenting standards." Although the definition may vary, common elements of this standard are that a parent (or other person responsible for the child's welfare) ensures that the child is:
>
> - Adequately fed
> - Clothed appropriately for the weather conditions
> - Provided with adequate shelter
> - Protected from physical, mental, and emotional harm
> - Provided with necessary medical care and education required by law

If it is determined that the home is unsafe and the parents cannot provide a safe environment for the child, a safety plan needs to be developed. This plan needs to include a time frame for implementation, plan for continued monitoring, a contingency plan if the plan is no longer effective, and requirements for terminating the plan. A safety plan requires signatures of all involved in the plan. Child welfare professionals must then follow up to ensure that the plan is being followed.

Safety Assessment Goals

The goal of safety assessment in child welfare practice is to determine if there is (or not) a threat to the child's safety, to determine if the child is safe or unsafe, and to use our critical thinking skills to analyze and apply the information we collect from our assessment process to planning and intervening to ensure child safety. This means that we go beyond simply identifying whether abuse or neglect occurred or may occur and consider the potential for future abuse and neglect and think about child safety throughout the life of the case. Many child welfare agencies will outline specific and required timeframes to document safety assessments (e.g., every 90 days, within 24 hours prior to the child returning home, etc.). It is also important to note that safety concerns are not always related to parental or caregiver behavior and often include environmental conditions that impact child safety.

Reflection: Safety or Risk Concern or No Concern?

Consider the following case studies, and ask yourself if you think there is a safety concern, risk concern, or no concern by consulting Table 8.1:

1. Emerson,[1] age 10, and her siblings, Elijah (7) and Ezra (6), are children to Mark and Rochelle. Rochelle is in dental assistant school, and Mark is at home with the kids after being laid off. A hotline call was received from a neighbor who overheard yelling and crying from next door. Rochelle was yelling for Mark to stop hitting Emerson. When the police arrived, the younger children ran from the apartment towards them. Mark sat down and started crying, apologizing for hitting Emerson. Rochelle was tending to Emerson and consoling her. She had several cuts on her face and was bleeding. Rochelle also had a bruise on her face. She said it was from Mark when she was trying to stop him from hitting Emerson. Police have responded to numerous calls at their home in the past. When Emerson was younger, they received services from the child welfare agency due to physical abuse.
2. Allison, age 4, was reported by domestic violence shelter staff. She had bruises on both of her arms which she said her mother's boyfriend caused when he grabbed her the previous day when she wouldn't pick up her toys. When Allison told her mother, they had an argument, and the boyfriend was violent with her. Allison's mother left and brought the kids to the shelter where she plans to stay until she can find housing for her and the kids.
3. An investigator finds the Adams' family home in complete disarray. There is animal feces on the floor in several rooms and rotting food in the kitchen and kids' bedroom. There are roaches in the kitchen. April (age 2) and Addison (age 3) are sitting on the living room floor eating yogurt while their mother watches television in the kitchen. Ms. Adams was reported to the child welfare agency twice in the past for leaving her children alone in the home.

- Is there a concern for safety now or the near future (time)?
- Is the degree of harm moderate to severe (degree of harm)?
- Is the purpose of intervention to control or stop harm or to reduce or resolve (purpose of intervention)?

If yes is the answer for any of these questions, there is likely a concern for the child's safety.

---

[1] All names and other personal identifiers in cases and examples throughout this book have been changed to protect privacy and confidentiality.

Assessment Tools

There are multiple assessment tools used within child welfare. States have adopted different models. Child welfare professionals must become experts on the tools used in their jurisdiction. It is central that whatever tools are used is relevant for the population on which they are used. It must be emphasized that assessment tools all have limitations. Something to take into consideration is that risk and safety assessment tools typically identify discrete factors, yet there are always interactions among factors that likely contribute to outcomes child welfare professionals seek to prevent (i.e., child fatalities, reoccurring violence; Pecora et al., 2013). Remember, there is not a full understanding of the etiology of child maltreatment, and there is no perfect predictor of maltreatment or other outcomes.

Practice Highlight

Examples of Screening and Assessment Tools

The US Department of Health & Human Services Administration for Children and Families (2012a, b) created a list of screening and assessment instruments to measure well-being and trauma. Within the chart, they provide details about the domains the tool assesses (i.e., behavioral/emotional, social, other/cognitive/physical), targeted ages, the type of assessment (e.g., parent/caregiver report, direct child assessment, child/youth report), and any training, administration, and costs required to use the instrument. Additionally, information is provided about which measurements are used in various national data collection and which are recommended by experts who were consulted in the development of the list of screening and assessment instruments. Below are some of the instruments that are described in the report:

Early childhood

- Ages and Stages: Social-Emotional (ASQ:SE; Squires et al., 2002)
- Bayley Infant Neurodevelopmental Screener (BINS; Aylward, 1995)
- Child and Adolescent Needs and Strengths (CANS & CANS-0–3; Lyons et al., 2004)
- Devereux Early Childhood Assessment for Infants and Toddlers (DECA--I/T; Powell et al., 2007)
- Family Map of the Parenting Environment of Infants and Toddlers and Family Map of the Parenting Environment in Early Childhood 4 (IT-Family Map; EC-Family Map; Whiteside-Mansell et al., 2013)
- Infant Toddler Social Emotional and Brief Infant Toddler Social Emotional Assessment (ITSEA; BITSEA; Carter & Briggs-Gowan, 2006)
- MacArthur-Bates Communicative Development Inventories – Second Edition (CDIs; Fenson et al., 2007)
- Peabody Picture Vocabulary Test. Fourth Edition (PPVT-4, Dunn & Dunn, 2007)
- Trauma Symptom Checklist for Young Children (TSCYC; Briere, 2005)

Middle childhood and adolescent

- Child and Adolescent Needs and Strengths; Child and Adolescent Needs and Strengths – Mental Health (Lyons et al., 1999; CANS-MH).
- Child Behavior Checklist, Teacher Report Form, and Youth Self Report Form (CBCL, TRF, YSR; Achenbach, 1999).
- Child PTSD Symptom Scale (CPSS; Foa et al., 2001).
- Children's Depression Inventory (CDI 2; Kovacs, 2003).
- Loneliness and Social Dissatisfaction Scale (Cassidy & Asher, 1992).
- Mood and Feelings Questionnaire (Angold & Costello, 1987).
- Pediatric Symptom Checklist-17 (PSC-17; Jellinek et al., 1999; Jellinek et al., 1988).
- Strengths and Difficulties Questionnaire (SDQ; Goodman, 1997).
- Trauma Symptom Checklist (TSCC; Briere, 1996).

All age groups

- Behavioral and Emotional Rating Scale (2nd Edition) (BERS-2; Epstein, 2004).
- Eyberg Child Behavior Inventory (ECBI; Eyberg & Pincus, 1999).
- Vineland Screener (VSC; Sparrow et al., 1993).
- Social Skills Rating System (SSRS; Gresham & Elliott, 1990).

Actuarial and Clinical-Based Approaches

Two broad categories of approaches within assessment tools are actuarial and clinical approaches. Clinical approaches are likely what first comes to mind with assessment. In these approaches, child welfare professionals through their use of training and assessment tools arrive at decisions based on their professional training and expertise. After weighing all of the evidence they have available, the professional and in many cases their supervisor and team make a decision. While tools are used, the basis of the decision is on clinical knowledge.

With actuarial approaches, clinical knowledge is still relevant; however, the decisions are made using algorithms built to identify likelihood of specific outcomes. Child welfare workers collect all the relevant information and enter into a computer system which generates a recommendation for action. These systems rely on models that are built using extensive knowledge about child maltreatment and a review of what outcomes have previously happened with cases.

One of the strengths of the actuarial approaches of assessment is that through using them bias can be reduced. Bias exists in clinical decision-making because people hold views that are based on stereotypes and prejudices. It is concerning that decisions made by child welfare professionals are based on information other than facts and could be discriminatory. However, one concern is that the modeling may not take everything into consideration and there may be relevant information that cannot be captured in the model. There are limits with all models.

Most child welfare agencies will use a structured approach to decision-making designed to guide, support, and document professional judgment in situations in which children are potentially in danger immediately or in the very near future. In protecting children, the major concern is the potential for harm that is immediate and moderate to severe. There are four stages of

> **Practice Highlight**
>
> **Factors That May Influence Safety and Risk**
>
> - Domestic violence (DV) and intimate partner violence (IPV)
> - History of reports to the child welfare agency, child welfare system involvement, and documented abuse or neglect
> - Substance use and abuse
> - Child's age and vulnerability
> - Excessive violence or out of control behavior
> - Child's fearfulness
> - Caregiver's attitude towards the child is predominantly negative
> - Dangerous expectations of the child
> - Caregiver hides or refuses access to the child

assessment: gathering information (identify factors that pose concerns about immediate safety), analyzing information (assess whether the current circumstances mitigate the identified safety factors), drawing conclusions (determine whether the child is safe or unsafe), and making decisions (developing and implementing interventions to control for safety, if deemed unsafe).

> **Practice Tip**
>
> **Items to Assess for Home Safety**
>
> **Fire and Burn Prevention**
>
> - Working smoke detectors near family's sleeping areas
> - A fire escape plan in case of fire or emergency
> - Access to lighters or matches restricted
> - Stove burners are not used to heat the home
> - Hot water from faucets is not at scalding temperature
> - Electrical appliances are kept out of the reach of young children (e.g., curling irons, hair dryers)
> - Electrical outlets are not overloaded
> - Extension cords are not under rugs or furniture

Sleeping

- Infant sleeps in crib or bassinette
- Infant sleeps with no toys, stuffed animals, or pillows
- Infant is placed on back to sleep

Choking, drowning, and falls

- Small items are kept out of reach of small children (e.g., plastic bags, pins, buttons, coins)
- Younger children only play with toys that are too large to swallow, unbreakable, and without points or sharp edges
- Infants and toddlers are never left alone near bath, pool, bucket, or toilet
- Children are always supervised near water
- Infants and toddlers are never left alone on changing tables, counter-tops, etc.
- Baby walkers are not used

Poison

- Cleaning products, medicine, pesticides, and alcohol are kept out of reach of children
- Paint is not chipping or peeling off the walls
- Rodent traps and poison are kept out of reach of younger children
- Toddlers and younger children do not have access to rotten food or trash

Violence

- Parent knows how to calm a crying infant and knows never to shake a baby
- Firearms and ammunition are stored separately in locked locations

Supervision

- Parent provides appropriate level of supervision considering child's development
- Children are left with an appropriate caregiver when the parent is not home

Illness, medical care, and immunizations

- Parent can recognize signs of illness
- Children have regular physical exams
- Children are up to date on their immunizations

New Ways to Identify Families in Need of Services

Increasingly child welfare systems seek opportunities to address children and families' needs prior to reports to child protective services. Primary prevention and universal services that promote well-being for all families attempt to eliminate the need for child welfare services and to intervene prior to maltreatment occurring. (See Chap. 7 for more information about child maltreatment prevention.)

Predictive analytics is the use of statistical procedures that analyze current and historic data to determine the likelihood of future events. This approach has been used to identify cases that are at risk for child fatalities or reentry into the child welfare system. While not without criticism (Eubanks, 2018), there is momentum that predictive analytics can help identify patterns that are not readily observable and assist with decision-making (Russell, 2015). The use of this strategy to identify families in need of services and at risk for negative outcomes is still developing. There are many practical and ethical considerations that need to be considered (Lanier et al., 2020). Some child welfare systems have embraced the use of predictive analytics.

By Abuse Type

During assessments, specific elements are considered for different abuse types. When a child appears to have experienced physical abuse, the child should be evaluated for injury by a professional healthcare provider. During the evaluation, the healthcare provider will assess the injury and take into consideration multiple factors including consistency of explanation with the injury, feasibility of the injury happening due to an accident, location of the injury, developmental ability of child, and history of injuries.

With child sexual abuse, child welfare professionals with special training are

> **Practice Highlight**
>
> **Family Strengths that Mitigate Safety and Risk Concerns**
>
> - Extended family networks
> - Shared parenting practices
> - Range of individuals as potential resources and supports
> - Tangible resources (e.g., transportation, income, utilities, housing)
> - Willingness to accept help
> - Religion, values, and spirituality
> - Demonstrates love and care for family members

responsible for interviewing and evaluating the child. With child sexual abuse, it is best practice to minimize the number of times a child is interviewed (e.g., Duron & Cheung, 2016), and the number of people conducting interviews should be as small as possible. The interviews are conducted in a way to minimize the traumatization and ensure that information is collected that would be relevant for any court proceedings. In some cases, it may be necessary to have a healthcare provider conduct a physical exam of a child where there are allegations of child sexual abuse.

Emotional abuse is evaluated by trained mental health professionals. Within emotional abuse, as discussed in descriptions of maltreatment types in Chap. 3, it is important that it is documented that the caregivers' emotional abuse directly impacted the child. When assessing emotional abuse, it is important to observe the child and parent interactions to understand the child-parent relationship. The relationship should also be assessed through the interview with both the parent and the child. Other people who interact with the parent and child (e.g., teachers, neighbors, friends) may also provide information helpful in determining the presence of emotional abuse.

Neglect is assessed through examining the extent to which a child's basic needs are met. This includes physical needs such as food, clothing, and shelter. Evidence that the children's needs are not being met would be if the parents are not providing adequate nutrition to the child, if the child does not have appropriate clothing for the weather, or if the child does not have stable housing (i.e., moves frequently). Assessment should determine if the house has hazardous conditions (e.g., exposed wires, holes in floor, missing balcony railing, broken windows, no fence around a pool, medication or cleaning supplies accessible to young children) or unsanitary conditions (e.g., animal feces in home, trash throughout home). Assessing neglect also extends to children's emotional, health, and educational needs. Evidence of neglect could include a parent not getting the child required medical care or not having the child attend school. Within the assessment of neglect, child welfare professionals must also determine if there is appropriate level of supervision based on the child's developmental stage and abilities.

Practice Highlight

The Safety Plan

In cases where the child is considered unsafe, the safety plan may be for the child to enter care with protective custody. However, there are other options to ensure safety even when safety threats have been identified. Identifying family strengths or circumstances that can mitigate the concerns and remove the threat(s) to the child through a safety plan that outlines an agreement with the caregiver and to monitor the situation. Safety is paramount; however, we also want to develop a plan that is least intrusive and disruptive to the child.

The safety plan is typically a written description of what will be done or what actions will be taken to ensure the child's safety, who will be responsible for implementing the plan and its components, and how it will be monitored. Safety plans must be developed alongside the family and explained in detail. The safety plan should also include a time frame for implementation, a contingency plan, and requirements for terminating the plan. A copy of the safety plan should be reviewed and signed by the caregiver and any other party involved, and a copy should be provided to them.

Assessment in Different Contexts

Assessments take place throughout the course of a child and family being involved with the child welfare system. The assessment process conceptually begins when a call is reported to child protective services. If screened in, the initial investigation is the first assessment. However, assessments occur throughout the course of the involvement with child welfare. Once a child enters care, the case manager conducts ongoing assessments. Some are about the child's placement and well-being. Others are about progress that is being made by the parents in the case plan. Some of these assessments are formal and documented with specific assessment tools. Other times, the assessments are somewhat informal as is the case when a case manager conducts routine monthly visits with children in out-of-home care. Assessments are not only performed by child welfare professionals; other professionals involved in the assessment process include healthcare providers, mental health providers, and substance abuse providers.

Skills for Assessment in Child Welfare

Child welfare professionals must have multiple skills to conduct assessments and intakes successfully. The skills for assessment include interviewing, observation, documentation, and critical thinking. Although it must be stressed that the skills alone are insufficient, content knowledge is central to assessment. Child welfare professionals must understand the different types of maltreatment and the various indicators. To conduct assessments, child welfare professionals must also understand a child's capacities, which is based on a deep understanding of development. They should also have knowledge about family systems, trauma, and working with people from various racial and ethnic backgrounds.

In addition to the content-relevant knowledge, the foundation of any assessment is the child welfare professionals' ability to interview and observe. In the interviewing process, child welfare professionals must ensure they are asking appropriate questions and listening. It is important to suspend judgment during an interview so that there can be an understanding of the circumstances. It is dangerous to assume that answers to questions are known. Seeking clarification is important. Within the interviews and observation, child welfare professionals must pay attention to detail.

Protocol directs much of assessment, and each child welfare system has specific tools that are used. Some tools are interview guides or checklists used during observations for the child welfare professional to use to document information. Others are short questionnaires for parents, teachers, or others to complete. Many of the tools that are used in assessments are for specific developmental periods. For example, there are specific assessments for young children as well as specific assessments for adolescents. To administer some tools, sometimes there is an extensive training process for the child welfare professional. With all assessment tools and protocols, documentation, which is discussed later in the chapter, is paramount.

Regardless of how structured an assessment may be, child welfare professionals must always engage in critical thinking. Critical thinking allows the child welfare professionals to interpret what they are seeing and to not accept what they see without applying reason and knowledge. With various assessment tools having actuarial components and the rise of predictive analytics within child protection, it is important that professionals can interpret what the models and assessments produce. As no models are perfect and mistakes can be made, professionals must be able to identify when something may be wrong. When an assessment that determines there is no immediate threat while the child welfare professional is confident that the child's immediate safety is at risk, a professional must be able to think critically and determine if a mistake was made rather than blindly following the assessment.

Family Engagement in Interviewing

Interviewing occurs every time a child welfare professional meets with a client, and their family and purposeful conversations should occur at each interaction. There should always be a plan and a reason for contact with the family. It is also important to note that interviewing is not interrogating – it is an interactional exchange for sharing information and developing solutions collaboratively. The context by which child welfare professionals keep the client engaged is through the relationship or the rapport that has been cultivated over time. It is important to establish trust through honesty and full disclosure. Dishonesty and failure to disclose information can lead to a breakdown in trust and disillusionment on the client's part.

There are several stages in an interview: social, needs identification, focus, and closure. The social stages mainly involve establishing rapport, promoting engagement, and making the individual(s) being interviewed feel comfortable, safe, and open to talking. Individuals who feel safe and able to talk about issues that they have in common or something nonthreatening (e.g., weather, news, etc.) are more likely to be open to other topics in discussion. Examples include small talk about current events and something in the home (e.g., artwork, furniture, etc.) while also engaging family members in conversation about everyday matters (e.g., school, routine). This stage is often brief, but all members should be invited to participate, if possible. It allows the interviewer to appear more approachable, relatable, and genuine. The second stage, needs identification, involves questions about the purpose for the interview or visit and obtaining information about strengths and needs from the perspective of individuals in the family. Once this information is obtained, action-oriented questions related to how these needs will be met should follow, for example, "what needs to happen in order for your family to get there?" when referring to needs and desires. The purpose of this stage is to allow families to express their perspective and to get their input about the issue(s) and possible solutions. A strengths perspective and family-centered approach should always be used to merge individual and family strengths that will address the family's needs. The purpose of the focus stage is to encourage family members to talk to each other about the changes they want for their family. It is important to use language around safety and well-being that is action-oriented. For example, a worker could ask the family members, "what do each of you think needs to happen in order for the children to be safe?" During this phase, the child welfare professional serves as the facilitator of the conversation and should be prepared to ensure all topics are covered and addressed and that all members of the family have had an opportunity to contribute to the conversation. The closure stage is intended for reviewing the information gathered and summarizing the plan developed. It is important to also identify any agreements, commitments, and next steps.

Conducting Family and Home Assessments

Child welfare professionals conduct family and home assessments. At their foundation, these assessments are to identify risk and to determine if the caregivers can
ensure a child's safety in the home environment. Family assessments examine the
child's family and determine their ability to care for the child and meet the child's
needs. Comprehensive family assessments are considered best practices in child
welfare as they provide both a broad and in-depth examination of the child's and
family's situation (Smithgall et al., 2015). These assessments are multifaceted and
look at all family member's strengths, functioning, and needs as well as the context
of the problems.

When assessing the household functioning, it is important to critically examine
a broad range of aspects starting with who is in the home. Beyond the people present, child welfare professionals need to understand the roles of the people including
who cares for the children; who provides income; and who is responsible for the
upkeep and cleaning of the house. When examining who cares for the child, it is
important to identify those who have significant caregiver responsibilities. Who is
providing the daily care for the child and responsible for the safety and well-being
of the child? This may not be only those who are legally responsible (i.e., birth parent, adoptive parent, legal guardian); it also may include paramours or other adults
living in the home. Understanding the household dynamics and family culture is
important as is having a complete picture of the support system outside of the home.
The assessment should generate an understanding of household operates.

Practice Tip

Observations of the Home Environment and Parent-Child Interactions

Your observations as a child welfare professional are extremely important
while assessing the family and the current circumstances. Some questions to
consider when making observations include the following verbal and nonverbal behaviors:

- Are they calm, relaxed, gentle, and confident about their parenting role?
- Do they seem to be anxious, easily frustrated, inattentive, indifferent, or
  detached?
- How do they look at, touch, and attend to the child?
- What is their tone of voice and responsiveness to the child's needs?
- Do they provide the child with appropriate stimuli?
- Do they enhance the child's sense of security and meet their basic needs?
- Do they rely on the child to meet their needs? (Role reversal)
- Are their expectations developmentally appropriate for the child?
- Is the home safe and equipped to meet the child's basic needs?
- What are the safety and risk factors present in the caregiver and home?
- How does the child respond to the parent or caregiver?

Understanding Families

To properly conduct assessments, child welfare professionals should understand families. There is a wide range of family structures, and none are inherently bad. Families can be nuclear or extended. Within nuclear, it is the parents and children. Extended families include additional generations and go outside the nuclear parents and children structure. Grandparents, aunts, uncles, and cousins are part of a child's extended family. While nuclear and extended families are two structures, there are additional patterns to take into consideration. Some families are interdependent and prioritize the good of the family over individual family member's needs and desires. Other families are more independent, meaning family members' individual identities are seen and people are not expected to only prioritize the needs of the family. Different cultures often prioritize and value different family structures. It is the job of the child welfare professional to understand the family's structure and functioning.

Families are all unique with different dynamics and patterns. Some of these are overt and easily observed by outsiders, while others are covert and not readily apparent to someone outside the family. Family patterns are based on the values and norms in the family. They are the ways that family members engage with one another and behave. Within families, people have roles. (See Chap. 3 on information about family roles.) Understanding the roles of the family can provide valuable insights about a family's strengths as well as risks for maltreatment.

All families have strengths. (See Chap. 6 on information on strengths-based practice.) Assessments are needed to identify the strengths and needs of families. The assessments take into consideration the uniqueness of each family. There are various instruments that are used to assess families, some of which are used by child welfare professionals. Some assessments require advanced training, and child welfare professionals must collaborate with professionals with the specialized expertise in assessing children and adults for health, mental health, substance misuse, and developmental issues. For these assessments, child welfare professionals often partner with community agencies. This is typically done with referrals to agencies. In some communities there are limited resources, and it may be challenging to have assessments done in a timeline manner. This can create challenges for child welfare professionals who need the information as well as the caregivers who are trying to meet their case plan goals. It is important to recognize these stressors for families and to collaborate with other professionals to ensure the assessments are conducted.

Child Assessments

In assessing children, child welfare professionals have a range of tools to use. Different agencies have different assessments that are used, but what most have in common is that they are multidimensional and take a child's development into consideration. One such tool that widely is used is the Child and Adolescent Needs and Strengths (CANS) which not only assists with assessment but also can assist with monitoring outcomes. CANS, as the name indicates, examines both the needs and strengths of the children. It does so on scales that indicate the strength or need is not identified or evident, the strength is a centerpiece strength, and the need requires immediate/intensive action. Through using CANS or other assessments, child welfare workers can determine how to best serve children.

Practice Tip

Interviewing Children and Youth

The child welfare professional's approach to interviewing is key in obtaining important information and assessing for safety. When interviewing a child, be gentle, reassuring, and supporting when asking questions. Avoid blaming or judging the parents in the child's presence. Child welfare professionals need to emphasize that they are there to help the family and information they provide will help to accomplish this. It's also important to know when it is time to cease questioning, take a break from questioning, and resuming if appropriate. When the interview is completed, it is good practice to thank them for taking the time to talk and provide reassurance without making any promises that cannot be kept.

There are often questions where the child may be hesitant to share information with the child welfare professional. Consider the following when conducting interviews:

Culture: It's possible that parents may have to give their permission for the child to speak with you.

Dependency: Children may have an allegiance to their parents and may be distrustful of the child welfare professional, the child welfare professional's role, or the child welfare system.

Coaching: Parents or caregivers may have coached the child regarding what they should or shouldn't say to the child welfare professional.

Consequences: Children may fear punishment if they reveal problems in their home or family.

Personality and temperament: The child may be naturally quiet, timid, or unable to communicate effectively, and these elements should be taken into consideration.

Forensic Interviewing

Child welfare professionals are often the first to interview a child and their family when a report of child maltreatment is investigated. Guidance regarding this first interview to assess safety, risk, and needs for the family is further discussed in Chap. 6. This section provides an overview of forensic interviewing with children and research-based strategies used during a forensic interview, usually conducted by a professional when further investigation is required when a criminal legal matter is being pursued. These interviewing considerations and tools are helpful for child welfare professionals when interviewing a child as well, when child maltreatment is suspected. It is important to be aware of and make plans regarding the setting, interview structure, language, introducing the topic of abuse, rapport development, and strategies for discussing details. Research shows that a child's memory of an event is quite accurate, with some omissions (e.g., Paz-Alonso et al., 2009). The accuracy of these verbal accounts in interviews is dependent on the child's age, the event, and the setting of the interview/retrieval of information (Bottoms et al., 2009). Further, children are more accurate in their recall of events that involve familiar individuals than unfamiliar individuals (e.g., Cordón et al., 2016).

Several evidence-based protocols have been developed to standardize the forensic interviewing process and to ensure its accuracy of reports (e.g., cognitive interview, narrative elaboration interview, NICHD protocol, and Lyon's 10-step interview). As with other interviews, forensic interviews involve multiple steps, which include an initial preparatory phase (introductions, instructions, rapport development), information gathering, and closure. Guidelines typically recommend a private space, age-appropriate, and quiet setting for an interview. The setting should minimize distractions and additional unnecessary individuals and be child-friendly. Research shows that interviewers that approach questioning in a more supportive way can elicit an improved flow to the conversation and improve accuracy of responses (Bottoms et al., 2007). Interviewers who provide positive feedback, smile, and are friendly can reduce a child's resistance during an interview. Questions should be phrased in a way and with language that the child can understand. Interviewers should gauge understanding by asking for clarification on certain words or phrases and avoid introducing difficult concepts, especially legal terms or ones that are too abstract. Questions should be open-ended and not leading, and children should be permitted to say they don't know the answer to the question.

There are a number of organizations that provide in-depth training to conduct forensic interviewing, and with experience, interviewers improve their practice. These types of interviews are extremely important when dealing with cases where the criminal justice system becomes involved. It is also important to consider avoiding re-traumatizing a child who has experienced maltreatment and has had to answer questions with multiple individuals regarding the incident. Some interviewers prefer or are required to follow an interview protocol, while some can be somewhat flexible depending on the case and circumstances.

Documentation

A good rule for child welfare professionals to live by is "if it is not documented, then it did not happen." Child welfare professionals must keep documentation current. Completing documentation in a timely manner increases the likelihood that information is not lost. Child welfare workers may believe that they will remember important salient details, yet relying on memory of what someone said is not ideal.

Human memory is notoriously unreliable. As the details of a case may be needed long after a child welfare professional learned of them, it is always best to have the information clearly documented to ensure the information is preserved. No child welfare professional wants to have to testify in court on their memory alone.

Every agency has specific guidelines for documentation and forms that are required. There are timelines about when documentation must be completed in a case. Increasingly, states have transitioned to electronic case notes which has the potential to increase efficiency, decrease redundancy, increase communication across workers, increase standardization, and improve opportunities for communication across agencies. Some agencies provide laptops or tablets for workers to use during home visits or when meetings outside the office. This may facilitate timely documentation, although in order to build rapport and engage families, it is often not possible for workers to complete documentation when they are with a child or a family. Additionally, in some geographic areas, there may not be cell phone service or Wi-Fi needed to access cloud-based forms and databases where case notes are completed. Workers must dedicate time to paperwork.

Writing Effective Case Notes

While there is variation in the format and process of writing effective case notes, there are best practices. Child welfare professionals must use facts including details of who was involved, what happened, where did something happen, and how did it happen. Within documentation, child welfare professionals should describe behavior rather than label behavior. For example, labeling behavior is "SJ was upset by the update." To write this in describing the behavior, "When at SJ's home, I told her the shelter hearing was scheduled for Tuesday; she covered her face with her hands, stood up, and left the room crying." Effective documentation quantifies information as much as possible, meaning giving concrete numbers within descriptions. For example, "There was a hole in the kitchen wall that was approximately two feet in diameter that exposed electrical wiring" is stronger than writing "There was a big hole in the kitchen wall." It is the responsibility of the child welfare professionals to capture details through documentation as ultimately this is the information used to determine how cases proceed.

Case notes are the chronological record of interactions, observations, and actions involving a specific person and/or family. They provide a record of all the things that have happened during a family's involvement with the child welfare agency, including phone calls, face-to-face contacts, contacts with service providers, team meetings, court hearings, and visits. Case notes are also important for case continuity, for legal discovery purposes, and for historical record. Information

Practice Tip Writing Good Case Notes
• Be concise
• Be accurate (facts vs. opinions)
• Nonjudgmental/without your appraisal
• Avoid slang/inappropriate language
• Check spelling, grammar, sentence structure, etc.
• Avoid jargon

recorded in case notes about a person or family should be impartial, accurate, and complete. Documentation should be objective, descriptive, clear, concise, accurate, and relevant. The language used in documentation should be nonjudgmental. The information included in the documentation should be relevant and detail the context in which the information was collected. Information that is not directly relevant to the case should not be included in the documentation.

Good case notes include several important elements, including the reason for involvement, reason for contact, the gathering of information and conversation, who was present and seen, observations, interactions and underlying factors, and services, intervention, and safety plan. Table 8.2 describes each of these elements and provides concrete examples.

Table 8.2 Case note examples

Part of case note	Description	Example
Reason for involvement	• Related to referral/report/ allegation of abuse or neglect • Provides context	Caseworker is currently involved with the Brown family because of a recent mandated report to DCFS that Johnny has been absent from school for more than 2 months. Caseworker is required to follow up in assessing Johnny's reason for failing to attend school and monitor his attendance
Reason for contact	• Related to the reason for involvement, but more specific to the interaction • Stating the reason keeps you focused on the service goals to be accomplished	Caseworker made a home visit with Ms. Brown today to address Johnny's failure to attend school for the past 2 months.

Gathering of information/ conversations	• Information from the child, family, and collateral sources is a key task as a caseworker
	• Assessment of the family must be family-focused and highlight the strengths, specific needs, and functioning of each family member
	• At the first meeting, it is helpful to get a full family history
	• Other notes related to gathering of info:
	  School records, interview with principal (or staff that handles attendance)
	  Medical report
	  Reports of other kids' attendance records
	  Schedule a meeting with homeroom teacher to investigate story of child in class
		Caseworker met with Ms. Brown and all the children (Mary, age 16; Johnny, age 15; and Jonathan, age 2) at Ms. Brown's home on 10/2/19. Caseworker asked Ms. Brown and Johnny about the reason he has missed 2 months of school. Ms. Brown said she was not aware of the absences until DCFS called because he leaves the house every day and comes home at the same time every day. Johnny claims he has been attending school, but he has not been going to his homeroom class because a boy in that class has been picking on him. According to Ms. Brown, Johnny does not have a history of truancy; this is the first occurrence. Johnny also said that he has not been truant before

(continued)

Table 8.2 (continued)

Who was seen?	• Since you are assessing for safety and risk factors related to child abuse or neglect, it's important to document *who* you saw and the *location* of the visit	Present at the home today was Ms. Brown, her three children (Mary, Johnny, and Johnathan), and her live-in partner, Mr. turner. We all met in the living room of the home, and I toured the home to see the children's bedrooms, bathrooms, and kitchen
Observations	• It's important to use your knowledge about what you know about child development, family dynamics, social behavior, mental health, and culture to record your observations • Record physical, social-emotional, and cognitive development and health, financial well-being, and environmental issues. • Pay attention to affect, appearance, dress, behavior, interactions, mannerisms, and home conditions	Ms. Brown looked tired and yawned frequently. She stated that she was tired because she worked late the night before. The children's hair looked dirty and unkempt. They were dressed in cotton shorts and t-shirts that were stained and soiled, but appropriate for the weather. The children looked healthy and well-fed. No bruises or scars were observed. According to Ms. Brown, they were seen by a medical provider for well check appointments the summer prior
Interactions	• Note how the family members interact with each other and with you • Qualify with examples	Ms. Brown met caseworker at the door and did not invite the CW in the house. She smiled and responded briefly to questions. She seemed distracted and not very engaged in the conversation. The older children only spoke when they were asked a question. The children appeared tense and anxious in the presence of Mr. Turner
Underlying factors	• Assess for mental health concerns, domestic violence/intimate partner violence, developmental disorders, substance abuse, and trauma histories • Assess for strengths, values, and beliefs	Ms. Brown stated that she rarely leaves the house. She experiences anxiety and is fearful about going out. She said the problem started a year ago and recently got worse
Services/ intervention/ safety plan	• Identify goals and service needs related to the presenting or emerging issues. • The services and interventions should address underlying conditions and contributing factors that may place children at risk of abuse/neglect. • Include short- and long-term goals to help stabilize and support the family	Caseworker explained to Ms. Brown that her teenage children are old enough to help with household chores and showed her how to set up a chore schedule

Conclusion

Assessment is a central skill in child welfare practice. Child welfare professionals are responsible for continuously assessing safety and risk through assessment. Additionally, they must determine the strengths and needs of children and families. While there are a range of tools that child welfare professionals use and the protocols vary among agencies, assessments are consistently used in child welfare. The assessments and interactions that child welfare professionals have with children and families must be documented. Child welfare professionals must master writing effective case notes that are concise, accurate, and judgment-free.

Discussion Questions

1. What are three things to assess while conducting a home safety assessment?
2. How are risk of child maltreatment and safety concerns different and similar?
3. What is an example of a tool to assess for strengths and needs? What are some advantages to using this tool?
4. What are two tips to keep in mind when writing effective case notes?
5. What information should be included in case notes?

Suggested Activities

1. Explore what assessment tools used at the child welfare agency where you live. Are they actuarial tools and assessments? How much do the assessments rely on professional knowledge and expertise? Who is the process for assessment?
2. Use one of the case studies offered in this chapter and practice writing case notes for different points in time (e.g., investigation, monthly home visit, case closures).
3. Download and review the Child and Adolescent Needs and Strengths (CANS) manual   (https://www.nctsn.org/measures/child-adolescents-needs-strengths). Write down some of the strengths and limitations of using this type of assessment with children and families.
4. Read Lanier et al. (2020) and discuss with others your thoughts about using predictive analytics in child welfare. What are the strengths? What concerns do you have about child welfare agencies using predictive analytics to make decisions?
Lanier, P., Rodriguez, M., Verbiest, S., Bryant, K., Guan, T., & Zolotor, A. (2020). Preventing infant maltreatment with predictive analytics: applying ethical principles to evidence-based child welfare policy. *Journal of family violence, 35*(1), 1–13. (Available: https://rdcu.be/cbVsb).

Additional Resources

American Professional Society on the Abuse of Children: Forensic Interviewing training clinics and institutes: https://www.apsac.org/forensicinterviewing

CDC Home Safety Checklist: https://www.cdc.gov/steadi/pdf/check_for_safety_brochure-a.pdf

Child Welfare Information Gateway, Assessing Risk and Safety: https://www. childwelfare.gov/topics/responding/iia/investigation/safety-risk/

Child Welfare Information Gateway, Child Neglect: A Guide for Prevention, Assessment, and Intervention: https://www.childwelfare.gov/pubPDFs/neglect.pdf

NC Division of Social Services, Documentation in Child Welfare: Effective Practices for County DSS Agencies: https://fcrp.unc.edu/files/2017/09/documentation_webinar.pdf

Florida's Center for Child Welfare, Developing Safety Plans: http://centerforchildwelfare.org/Preservice/ActionBoosterTrainings/SafetyPlanning/Developing%20Safety%20Plans%20Training%20Fall%202014%20PG%2010-21.pdf

Kids Health, Household Safety Checklist: https://kidshealth.org/en/parents/household-checklist.html

References

Achenbach, T. M. (1999). The child behavior checklist and related instruments. In M. E. Maruish (Ed.), *The use of psychological testing for treatment planning and outcomes assessment* (pp. 429–466). Lawrence Erlbaum Associates Publishers.

Angold, A., & Costello, E. J. (1987). *Mood and feelings questionnaire (MFQ)*. Developmental Epidemiology Program, Duke University. https://doi.org/10.1037/t15197-000

Aylward, G. P. (1995). Bayley infant neurodevelopmental screener. *San Antonio*. https://doi.org/10.1037/t14989-000

Bottoms, B. L., Najdowski, C. J., & Goodman, G. S. (Eds.). (2009). *Children as victims, witnesses, and offenders: Psychological science and the law*. Guilford Press.

Bottoms, B. L., Quas, J. A., & Davis, S. L. (2007). The influence of interviewer-provided social support on children's suggestibility, memory, and disclosures. In *Child sexual abuse* (pp. 145–168). Psychology Press.

Briere, J. (1996). *Trauma symptom checklist for children* (pp. 00253–00258). Psychological Assessment Resources. https://doi.org/10.1037/t06631-000

Briere, J. (2005). *Trauma symptom checklist for young children (TSCYC)*. Psychological Assessment Resources.

Carter, A. S., & Briggs-Gowan, M. J. (2006). *Manual for the Infant-Toddler Social & Emotional Assessment (ITSEA)-Version 2*. Psychological Corporation. https://doi.org/10.1037/t14990-000

Cassidy, J., & Asher, S. R. (1992). Loneliness and peer relations in young children. *Child Development, 63*(2), 350–365. https://doi.org/10.2307/1131484

Cordón, I. M., Silberkleit, G., & Goodman, G. S. (2016). Getting to know you: Familiarity, stereotypes, and children's eyewitness memory. *Behavioral Sciences & the Law, 34*(1), 74–94. https://doi.org/10.1002/bsl.2233

Dunn, L. M., & Dunn, L. M. (2007). Peabody picture vocabulary test-revised. *Pearson*. https://doi.org/10.1037/t15144-000

Duron, J. F., & Cheung, M. (2016). Impact of repeated questioning on interviewers: Learning from a forensic interview training project. *Journal of Child Sexual Abuse, 25*(4), 347–362. https://doi.org/10.1080/10538712.2016.1161687

Epstein, M. H. (2004). *BERS-2 Behavioral and emotional rating scale* (2nd ed.). PAR, Inc., London.

Eubanks, B. (2018). *Artificial intelligence for HR: Use AI to support and develop a successful workforce*. Kogan Page Publishers, New York, NY.

Eyberg, S., & Pincus, D. (1999). *Eyberg child behavior inventory & Sutter-Eyberg student behavior inventory-revised: Professional manual.* Psychological Assessment Resources.

Fenson, L., Marchman, V. A., Thal, D. J., Dale, P. S., Reznick, J. S., & Bates, E. (2007). *MacArthur-Bates communicative development inventories.* Paul H. Brookes Publishing Company. https://doi.org/10.1037/t11538-000

Foa, E. B., Johnson, K. M., Feeny, N. C., & Treadwell, K. R. (2001). The child PTSD symptom scale: A preliminary examination of its psychometric properties. *Journal of Clinical Child Psychology, 30*(3), 376–384. https://doi.org/10.1207/S15374424JCCP3003_9

Goodman, R. (1997). The strengths and difficulties questionnaire: A research note. *Journal of Child Psychology and Psychiatry, 38*(5), 581–586. https://doi.org/10.1111/j.1469-7610.1997.tb01545.x

Gresham, F. M., & Elliott, S. N. (1990). *The Social Skills Rating System.* Circle Pines, MN: American Guidance Service.

Jellinek, M. S., Murphy, J. M., Little, M., Pagano, M. E., Comer, D. M., & Kelleher, K. J. (1999). Use of the pediatric symptom checklist to screen for psychosocial problems in pediatric primary care: A national feasibility study. *Archives of Pediatrics & Adolescent Medicine, 153*(3), 254–260. https://doi.org/10.1001/archpedi.153.3.254

Jellinek, M. S., Murphy, J. M., Robinson, J., Feins, A., Lamb, S., & Fenton, T. (1988). Pediatric symptom checklist: Screening school-age children for psychosocial dysfunction. *The Journal of Pediatrics, 112*(2), 201–209. https://doi.org/10.1016/S0022-3476(88)80056-8

Kovacs, M. (2003). *Children's depression inventory (CDI).* Multi-Health System.

Lanier, P., Rodriguez, M., Verbiest, S., Bryant, K., Guan, T., & Zolotor, A. (2020). Preventing infant maltreatment with predictive analytics: Applying ethical principles to evidence-based child welfare policy. *Journal of Family Violence, 35*(1), 1–13. https://doi.org/10.1007/s10896-019-00074-y

Lyons, J., Griffin, E., Fazio, M., & Lyons, M. B. (1999). *The child and adolescent needs and strengths: An information integration tool for children with mental health challenges and their families.* Northwestern University Institute for Health Services Research and Policy Studies. https://doi.org/10.1037/t02500-000

Lyons, J. S., Weiner, D. A., & Lyons, M. B. (2004). Measurement as communication in outcomes management: The child and adolescent needs and strengths (CANS). (p. 461–476) in (Ed. Mark E. Maruish). The use of psychological testing for treatment planning and outcomes assessment. Volume 2: Instruments for children and adolescents. Third Edition. Laurence Erlbaum Associates, Publishers. doi:https://doi.org/10.4324/9781410610621-17.

Paz-Alonso, K., Ogle, C. M., & Goodman, G. S. (2009). Children's memory and testimony in "scientific case studies" of sexual abuse. Issues in investigative interviewing, eyewitness memory, and credibility assessment, 143–172. doi:https://doi.org/10.1007/978-1-4614-5547-9_6.

Pecora, P. J., Chahine, Z., & Graham, J. C. (2013). Safety and risk assessment frameworks: Overview and implications for child maltreatment fatalities. *Child Welfare, 92*(2), 143–160.

Powell, G., Mackrain, M., LeBuffe, P., & Lewisville, N. C. (2007). *Devereux early childhood assessment for infants and toddlers technical manual.* Kaplan Early Learning Corporation.

Russell, J. (2015). Predictive analytics and child protection: Constraints and opportunities. *Child Abuse & Neglect, 46,* 182–189. https://doi.org/10.1016/j.chiabu.2015.05.022

Smithgall, C., Jarpe-Ratner, E., Gnedko-Berry, N., & Mason, S. (2015). Developing and testing a framework for evaluating the quality of comprehensive family assessment in child welfare. *Child Abuse & Neglect, 44,* 194–206. https://doi.org/10.1016/j.chiabu.2014.12.001

Sparrow, S. S., Carter, A. S., & Cicchetti, D. V. (1993). *Vineland screener: Overview, reliability, validity, administration, and scoring.* Yale University Child Study Center.

Squires, J., Bricker, D., & Twombly, E. (2002). *Ages and stages questionnaires: Social-emotional.* Brookes. https://doi.org/10.1037/t11524-000

U.S. Department of Health & Human Services, Administration for Children and Families, Administration on Children, Youth and Families, Children's Bureau. (2012a). Well-being instruments for early childhood. https://www.acf.hhs.gov/cb/grant-funding/well-being-instruments-early-childhood

U.S. Department of Health & Human Services, Administration for Children and Families, Administration on Children, Youth and Families, Children's Bureau. (2012b). Well-being instruments for middle childhood and adolescence. https://www.acf.hhs.gov/cb/grant-funding/well-being-instruments-middle-childhood-and-adolescence

Whiteside-Mansell, L., Johnson, D., Bokony, P., McKelvey, L., Conners-Burrow, N., & Swindle, T. (2013). Supporting family engagement with parents of infants and toddlers. *NHSA Dialog, 16*(1).

Chapter 9
Foster Care Placement

Introduction

In 2018, approximately 250,000 children were removed from their homes and placed into out-of-home placements (US DHHS, 2020a). Over 400,000 children were in foster care on September 30, 2019, and over 670,000 children are in foster care annually (US DHHS, 2020b). There are various types of placement to meet children's unique needs and circumstances. What all out-of-home placements have in common is that there are people who are caring for a child to meet the child's daily needs during a time when it has been determined that the child cannot safely remain in the home. Not all children who are involved in the child welfare system are in out-of-home placements, but foster care play a central role in child welfare.

Child Removal and Placement Process

The decision to remove a child from their caregivers is made only after it is determined that a child cannot safely remain within the home. Removing a child from the home is not the preferred option, but will be done when it is necessary to keep the child safe. Child welfare professionals do not make the decision to remove a child from their home in isolation; they must get a court order to remove children from their caregivers. Each jurisdiction has slightly different procedures; however, the overarching process is the same.

When child welfare professionals determine a child is not safe and is at imminent risk during an investigation, they may petition the court to temporarily remove a child from the home. The child will be placed in an appropriate out-of-home setting. There will be a shelter hearing where the child welfare professionals, who are joined by the agency attorneys, present information about the maltreatment and safety. The caregivers, who have the right to have their own attorney, can challenge the petition

© Springer Nature Switzerland AG 2021
J. M. Geiger, L. Schelbe, *The Handbook on Child Welfare Practice*,
https://doi.org/10.1007/978-3-030-73912-6_9

for the child's removal. A judge determines if the child is to remain in out-of-home care or returned to the caregiver. (See Chap. 2 for more details about the process.)

The courts oversee the out-of-home placement, and the judges approve the case plan and oversee the case including placements and visitation. Review hearings are regularly scheduled to monitor the process on the case plan. Children are not reunified with their caregivers unless the case plan has been completed successfully. After a year in out-of-home placement, a permanency hearing determines the permanency for the child. At this point, the courts may seek to terminate parental rights as per the Adoption and Safe Families Act of 1997 (ASFA).

Trauma of Removal

Being removed from their home and placed in out-of-home care can be traumatic for children. The disruption of relationships and daily routine can negatively impact a child. The process is foreign to children who may not understand why they must leave their family and may desperately wish to remain with their caregivers despite the maltreatment. Children may be given little information about the process, being removed with little warning and without the opportunity to say goodbye or pack personal belongings to take with them (Mitchell, 2018). Being removed from their home may be alarming, and the presence of law enforcement could make them feel that they have done something wrong. Children often experience loss and grief after being removed from their caregivers and placed in foster care. This may be amplified when the process does not take children's needs into consideration, for example, information is poorly communicated to the child, the process described to the child is not followed, or siblings are separated (Mitchell, 2018). (See Chap. 5 for information about trauma-informed child welfare practice.)

Note from the Field

Always Ready

In foster parent training, they always said to be ready at any time – even in the middle of the night – for a call from the child welfare agency to have a child placed with us. We didn't have any kids of our own and were hoping to have a child placed with us long term. We thought we were ready for anything. One cold December night, we received a call that they needed to place a 3-year-old child. He was left alone in a car while his mother went to work at a nightclub. He had been put to sleep with a bunch of blankets in the backseat. This was in southern California, so it wasn't freezing temperatures, but it got cold at night. A passerby noticed him in the car alone and didn't see anyone come back to the car for 15 minutes, so they called the police. Police tried to locate mom, but the child, being so young, could not verbalize who or where his mother was.

The child was placed in protective custody and they were on their way to our house. I quickly tidied the house up and got the bed ready for the child. His name was Andrew, and he looked so tired and afraid. The investigator tried to hand him to me; he flinched and started wailing. I felt terrible. Once he was able to calm down a bit, I offered him a snack and showed him where he would be sleeping. His clothes were soiled and didn't smell great, so I also offered him a bath. He seemed excited about that, so I let him pick out some bubbles and gave him eat a granola bar, which he gobbled up. He still seemed very apprehensive and would have short crying spells asking for his mom. I did my best to stay calm and reassure him. I wrapped him up in a towel and got some warm pajamas. We read a book together, and I held him in the rocker. He was not yet verbal, but he would keep looking up at me and then back down. I went to put him in the bed and he cried again and said "home" over and over. It broke my heart. It must have been so confusing for him. I told him he would stay here tonight to stay warm and safe. We rocked in the chair for 2½ hours until he fell asleep well enough to be put down in the bed. He awoke several times crying. I rubbed his back and he fell back asleep. In these situations, we try to understand how the child must feel. He missed his mom and didn't know where he was or why. He didn't know me, but I hope that he could feel that I cared and that I was gentle and kind.

Placement Ideals

Removing children from their caregivers should be considered a last resort. Careful considerations must be made to ensure that children are in the best placement available to meet their needs. Children should be in the least restrictive environment. In most cases, it is ideal for children to be placed with family or kin, and sibling groups should be kept together. Placements should be culturally appropriate and have close proximity to the child's family to facilitate visitation and maintain relationships with peers and continuity of education. There should be frequent assessments of the suitability of the placement for children who remain in care.

Least Restrictive Environments

The principle of least restrictive environments states that children should be put in a placement that is most family-like and able to meet the child's needs. The least restrictive environment continuum can be envisioned as remaining with birth family to kinship placement to foster care to congregate care. Within some of these broad categories, subcategories exist. Foster care includes therapeutic foster homes, which is considered more restrictive than another foster home setting due to the additional structure and requirements. Within congregate care, the least restrictiveness in descending order are group homes, institutional settings, and lockdown facilities. While some children may need more restrictive settings to meet their needs and ensure their safety, the goal is to ensure that the environment is only as restrictive as it must be and that ultimately children will "step down" to a less restrictive environment. Although it happens, children should not be placed in a restrictive environment because there are no other placement options.

Normalcy

Within the foster care placements, especially those which are more restrictive, children and youth are often prohibited from engaging in activities that their "typical" peers who are not involved in care participate in. In placements, youth may feel the rules are restrictive and not developmentally appropriate (e.g., Rauktis et al., 2011). "Normalcy" refers to allowing children and youth who are in care to be involved in developmentally appropriate activities that are considered "routine." This could be playing sports, taking music lessons, attending dances or school functions, volunteering, going to friends' homes, attending camp, or attending community events. With teenagers, normalcy can include getting a job and learning how to drive.

The idea behind normalcy is that children and youth in foster care need to have the experiences that promote growth and connection. While typical activities may carry some risks (i.e., a child could get hurt playing sports; a friend's home is not a controlled environment), children and youth need to have the experiences that help them gain responsibilities, develop skills, and build relationships. Traditionally, the child welfare system has not always supported normalcy because of the risks and liability inherent in some of the activities. Some jurisdictions required extensive background checks including fingerprinting for a child in care to be involved in routine activities; and although normalcy is considered an ideal for children and youth in care, some agencies still require cumbersome documentation and background checks. Increasingly there is a shift towards promoting normalcy, especially for adolescents in care.

Family/Kin

Increasingly there is a push to place children who need to be removed from the home with relatives. The logic behind this practice is that there have be continuity in relationships with family members with whom have long-term relationships with children. Relative care can preserve family relationships and may be less traumatic as a child is not removed from their caregiver and placed with strangers. There is typically more permanency with the use of relative placements as children do not move among placements as much. One of the concerns about the use of relative care is that payments to caregivers providing relative care may be inadequate; some agencies pay smaller stipends to caregivers of relative placements as compared to nonrelative placements. Thus, the child may not be adequately provided for. Critics of relative care have also raised concerns that relatives of the children may not be screened and trained as rigorously as nonrelative foster parents because of the assumption that the familial relationships have prepared them to care for the children placed in their care. However, this may not be the case. In some cases, family members' relationships with the caregivers could lead to issues such as the child may not be adequately protected from the caregiver if the relative does not adequately supervise visitation.

Note from the Field

Kinship Placements

Ashley Wilfong, MSW

As a child protective investigator, I felt like my biggest successes and failures were around kinship placements. In one case, I removed a 6-month-old baby from a home where her mother and father were manufacturing methamphetamines. The child was placed with her maternal grandparents. The grandparents had seen a huge shift with their daughter's behavior and parenting over the year before the child was placed with them. They knew there were drugs involved and tried to intervene on their own. They cared so much for the child and the mother. They encouraged the mother to come to their home as much as possible for supervised visits. They picked her up and took her to the child's doctor's appointments. The mother even helped them pick out a daycare when they placed their grandchild in daycare. The mother remained involved in her child's life while having the space to work on herself and create a safe home for the child to come back to. Addiction to methamphetamines is not an easy thing to overcome, but she did it with time and support from her family.

It took the mother a little over two years to reunify with her child. If her child was placed in foster care, I do not think that would have happened. Because of the kinship placement, lasting and meaningful change was able to happen for the mother which, in the end, meant that the child got to go home safely and long term.

In another case I worked, I removed two children from their mother for physical abuse and domestic violence. The mother had a huge family who were all willing to take the children in. In the beginning of the case, I was excited about this because I know kinship placements are more successful. That changed as I started interviewing family members. Everyone in the family seemed to know exactly what was happening to the two children. Most of them not only were present when abuse took place but also did not seem to see a problem with what was happening. It was normal for them. Many of the adults in the family either had violent criminal histories or records for child abuse. It became clear that they did not understand why the children were in danger and would not monitor the children's contact with the mother appropriately.

I made the decision to deny multiple home studies for various family members. I put the two children in foster care. They were placed in a great foster home and thrived there. The oldest child bloomed in that house. The children became incredibly social and tried new things; their favorite being going to the gym with the foster parent. They liked to go so they could hype people up to do their best at the gym. The children made friends and did well academically. Finally, they were in a house where there was no volatility. They had structure and support. The foster parent was very communicative with the mother and family, so visitations were frequent. The mother was informed about school and doctors' appointments. While she was encouraged to be a part of those things by the foster parent, she was resistant.

I got a lot of pushback from case management and the mother's attorney. As an investigator, my time with any case was limited to 60 days. Once I was off the case, the case manager approved one of the home studies I had denied. The children were moved out of the county. They had to switch schools and lost the friends they had made. Visitations were difficult because the mother and family member lacked transportation. The children had a hard time making appointments because of this as well. The foster parent attempted to stay in contact and help as much as possible, but the family would not allow it.

Kinship placements are more likely to be the right call for children when they are removed for their parents but not always. Sometimes there is just no one available, and sometimes those that are available are just as entrenched as the children's parents in the maltreatment. My advice is to try as hard as possible to find a kinship placement, but not to put the children in another dangerous situation.

Siblings

It is considered a best practice to keep siblings together in placement. In doing so, siblings are able to maintain some of their central relationships. Research has also found that siblings not only can provide support and stability but also contribute to development. Siblings who are placed together have higher levels of placement stability. Placing siblings together is often a challenge, especially with larger sibling groups or when siblings have complex or a diverse range of needs. When different siblings have specific needs, it can be challenging to find a single placement that can adequately address diverse needs. This may often be the case when there is a large range of age. Another barrier to placing siblings together is the siblings may not enter out-of-home care at the same time.

Sometimes workers have concerns that in a sibling group an older sibling has assumed the role of the parent, and this could be difficult to handle in a foster home. Another concern is when there are tension-filled relationships among siblings. Despite these concerns – which some experts say are myths and unfounded – sibling placement remains best practice. Foster homes that can accommodate sibling sets are in high demand. When siblings cannot be kept together in placements, it is important for siblings to visit and communicate regularly with one another. Some states have established sibling visitation as a right for children in out-of-home care.

Note From the Field

Sibling Bonds

Early in my career, I would volunteer for a nonprofit organization that provided grants to families who cared for children in foster care. Every year, they would put on a sibling reunion day event for brothers and sisters to get together and play games, talk, and spend quality time together. As a new social worker, it seemed so strange to me that there were siblings who were not able to be placed together. I reflected on my own relationships with my siblings and how important they were in my story and my childhood. To think that some siblings don't grow up together and see each other every day seemed unfathomable. Volunteers worked to reach caseworkers across the city to find out who would benefit from this event and then coordinated the activities and logistics. One year we had over 500 kids. Many of whom hadn't seen their brother or sister in months. Most of the kids just wanted to sit under a tree, share a meal, and talk with each other. Others played games and ran around. Others didn't know what to say or do. At the end of the day, there were a lot of tears. It was hard to say goodbye.

Siblings are an important part of the fabric of "us." They know us and our history better than anyone. They share our DNA and our memories – good and bad. I know that sometimes kids cannot be placed together; however we must do everything we can do to make sure they are placed together and/or see each other regularly. They deserve that. They need that.

Culturally Appropriate Settings

With the sordid history of child protection for children who are racial and ethnic minorities, there must be an acknowledgement of the need for culturally appropriate settings for children in out-of-home care. (See Chap. 1 for details about the history.) Federal policies have several mandates for serving children who are racial and ethnic minorities. In addition to following these policies, it is important to make sure the placement addresses the cultural needs of a child in foster care. For example, children should be able to attend the religious ceremonies and celebrate the holidays of their choice. They should never be forced to convert to another religion. Foster parents and congregate care staff should receive training and support to be culturally competent. While they may not be of the same background as the child, they can assist children in the development of positive self-regard and respect for their culture while allowing the child to maintain a connection to their culture while in out-of-home placement. Child welfare professionals need to prioritize placements that are culturally appropriate for children and select the best placement for the child with regard to language, religion, national origin, and race/ethnicity. Some states have very specific policies regarding the process of selecting and placing a child in out-of-home care regarding their culturally needs. Some of the ways child welfare professionals can understand and support children in maintaining cultural ties are to ask questions about cultural and religious traditions and practices they engage in and/or are interested in participating in and seek out events, individuals, and information to better meet these needs.

Proximity

A placement in or near the neighborhood where the child previously lived can reduce the disturbances in a child's life. Such placements can avoid the disruption of relationships with friends, classmates, and neighbors. Staying in the same community means that there may be a familiar environment, even if the home and the people providing for the children are different. An out-of-home placement that is geographically close to the caregivers may facilitate more frequent visitation. Likewise, it may make it possible for a child to remain in the same school, ultimately providing more stability and permanence. This can reduce the stress and trauma of being in an out-of-home placement for a child.

Types of Placement

When parents and caregivers cannot ensure the safety of their children, children may be removed from their homes and placed in a foster care placement. The U.S. federal government defines foster care as "24-hour substitute care for children placed away from their parents or guardians and for whom the Title IV-E agency has placement and care responsibility" (45 C.F.R. § 1355.20, 2012). The Title IV-E agency is the child welfare authority within a given jurisdiction. The goal of foster care is to keep children safe by providing temporary out-of-home care when necessary until the child can be safely returned home, permanently placed with a relative or adoptive family, placed in a legal guardianship, or another permanency arrangement is determined. While a child is in a placement, the person (e.g., foster parent, relative) or congregate care facility who is responsible for the daily care of the child typically receives a stipend from a child welfare agency. The options for placement largely fall into the categories of relative/kinship, nonrelative family/family foster care, and congregate care. Within these categories there are other distinctions. Additionally, some children are in pre-adoptive homes or in supervised living settings. In an effort to not remove a child from their home, some receive family preservation services in their homes and are not removed from their caregivers.

Relative/Kinship

Kinship care is "A licensed or unlicensed home of the child's relatives regarded by the Title IV-E agency as a foster care living arrangement for the child" (45 C.F.R. § 1355, Appendix A, 2012). Adults who are related to the child through blood, marriage, or adoption and tribal or clan members or others who are determined to have a kinship bond with the child may provide kinship care. Prior to placing a child in out-of-home placement, efforts are to be made to determine if a child's kin are an appropriate placement. Kinship care increasingly is the preferred substitute placement option as it is considered the least restrictive and facilitates children maintaining their cultural and familial connections. Additionally, kinship care is understood as a more normative living arrangement and carries less stigma than other forms of placement.

In the past decade, the percentage of children in kinship care increased from 25% in 2007 to 32% in 2019 (U.S. DHHS, 2020a). Grandparents of low socioeconomic status with lower levels of educational attainment provide the majority of kinship care (e.g., Ehrle & Geen, 2002). There are concerns about kinship providers having the resources needed to care for children who often have substantial needs. Historically, child welfare agencies have offered kinship providers fewer supports and less training than caregivers in nonrelative placements (e.g., Sakai, Lin, & Flores, 2011). To address the challenges kinship caregivers face, agencies increasingly have offered support programs and services targeting kinship caregivers. There is a need to better understand the nuances and complexity of kinship placements, and child welfare agencies must consider the variability among the kinship arrangements (Berrick & Hernandez, 2016). Despite some disadvantages, a review of 62 studies found that compared to children in other types of placement, children in kinship placements experienced greater placement stability and fewer behavioral and mental health problems (Winokur, Holton, & Valentine, 2014).

There are a number of advantages of having children and youth placed with relatives or kin, as well as some disadvantages, all depending on the circumstances of the case. Children and youth often feel more comfortable living with family members they are familiar with and can continue to practice family traditions and share common values and interests. They may also be able to continue to reside in the same neighborhood and continue to see other extended family members. However, placement with family can also be challenging for some children and their relative caregivers. For example, biological parents may often resent their family members for becoming involved with the case and having to enforce limits on contact and visitation, which is difficult for many. Many kinship caregivers may lack the financial ability to take the children into the home or struggle with how to access services and navigate the child welfare and/or behavioral health systems. Some caregivers may not be physically able to care for the children and feel extreme guilt about not being able to care full-time for their relative in need. Kinship care and placement is often complex, despite the services and supports available. In most circumstances, youth do well when living with kin providers who are ready and able to temporarily or permanently care for them in their home.

Nonrelative Family Placement

The federal government defines nonrelative family foster care as "A licensed family foster home regarded by the Title IV-E agency as a foster care living arrangement" (45 C.F.R. § 1355, Appendix A, 2012). With nonrelative family placements, or family foster care, children are placed in a home of nonrelative adults to care for them. Next to kinship care, family foster care is the preferred placement option as it allows children to live in a family-like environment. In 2019, 46% of children in out-of-home lived in a nonrelative family foster home; it was the most common type of placement (U.S. DHHS, 2020b).

Family foster care may be a preferred placement for younger children when kinship care is not an option and for foster youth with less severe behavioral and mental health problems. Studies have found that children in family foster care are adopted and reunified with their families at higher rates than children in kinship care (e.g., Bell & Romano, 2015). The Family First Prevention Services Act clearly prioritizes the family setting, as it has placed limitations on the reimbursement to states for children placed in group homes.

Therapeutic Foster Placements Therapeutic foster care, sometimes called treatment foster care, is a family foster care setting where the foster parents have received specialized training to meet the needs of children who have significant medical needs or emotional or behavioral issues. These complex needs may be due to past trauma, ongoing health concerns, or a combination of reasons. In many regards therapeutic foster homes are like other nonrelative placements. The reimbursement rate for the foster parents may be higher, and additional support to the foster family may be provided. There are also additional restrictions such as limitations such as a lower number of children allowed in the home to ensure there is adequate time to provide the needed care for the children with special needs.

Congregate Care

Group homes and institutions are nonfamily settings out-of-home placements that are referred to as congregate care. A group home is "a licensed or approved home providing 24-hour care for children in a small group setting that generally has from seven to twelve children." An institution is defined as "a child care facility operated by a public or private agency and providing 24-hour care and/or treatment for children who require separation from their own homes and group living experiences" (45 C.F.R. § 1355, Appendix A, 2012). In 2019, 10% of children in out-of-home care were placed in some form of group care or institution (U.S. DHHS, 2020b). In the last decade, group care and institutional placements have declined by over a third (37%; Children's Bureau, 2015).

Due to the high costs, restrictiveness, possible iatrogenic effects, and weak evidence supporting their benefits for children, congregate care has been criticized. Yet group care is the appropriate placement option for the children in care who need more intensive or structured care than less restrictive settings can offer (Barth, 2005;

Children's Bureau 2015). There is interest in strengthening the evidence base of congregate care and improving outcomes of children who are in congregate care (Boel-Studt & Tobia, 2016). Compared to children in other out-of-home settings, children in congregate care are older on average, more likely to be male, and exhibit more severe behavioral and mental health problems (Children's Bureau, 2015). Studies on effectiveness of residential group care have mixed findings (Bettman & Jasperson, 2009); however, there is evidence group homes contribute to positive behavioral and emotional outcomes for some youth (e.g., Hooper et al., 2000; Lyons et al., 2001), as well as prosocial skills and family functioning (e.g., Hooper et al., 2000).

Pre-adoptive Homes

A pre-adoptive placement is defined as "a home in which the family intends to adopt the child. The family may or may not be receiving a foster care payment or adoption subsidy on behalf of the child" (45 C.F.R. § 1355, Appendix A, 2012). Pre-adoptive homes may overlap with foster home placements, as foster families may adopt a child in foster care after reunification is no longer a goal and parental rights have been terminated. In 2019, on a single day, fewer than one in 20 (4%) of children in foster care were in pre-adoptive placements (U.S. DHHS, 2020b). Almost a quarter (26%) of children in foster care are adopted; however, rates vary greatly by age. Of children who are adopted from foster care, almost a quarter (22%) are by relatives; the majority of children adopted are by nonrelative families (Malm, Vandivere, & McKindon, 2011).

Supervised Independent Living

Supervised independent living (SIL) is "an alternative living arrangement where the child is under the supervision of the agency but without 24-hour adult supervision, is receiving financial support from the child welfare agency, and is in a setting which provides the opportunity for increased responsibility for self-care" (45 C.F.R. § 1355, Appendix A, 2012). SIL is designed to serve youth preparing to age out with APPLA as a goal of their permanency plan. SIL supports youth who are transitioning into adulthood by providing holistic psychosocial, educational, employment, and vocational supports and supervision. The Fostering Connections to Success and Increasing Adoptions Act allowed states to increase the age limit for youth to remain in care from 18 to 21, allowing them continued access to support services including SIL. In 2019 an estimated 2% of youth in foster care lived in SIL (U.S. DHHS, 2020b).

SIL is considered a promising practice, but there is great variation in the provision of services, and limited studies have examined its effectiveness. SIL has been found to improve youths' daily living skills and self-sufficiency, which are necessary as youth transition to adulthood and leave care. (See Chapter 11 working with special populations for more information about working with transition-aged youth.)

Emergency Foster Care

Occasionally child welfare professionals determine a child is an imminent risk and must be removed from their home immediately. This may be due to an unexpected arrest or death of a caregiver or other situation where a caregiver cannot care for the child. A child's removal from their family can happen at any day or time in these emergencies. In emergency foster care cases, a child may be placed in a foster home for a short period of time, typically between 72 hours and 30 days. Efforts are made during this time to find a more permanent placement for the child, which may be a different type of placement.

Reflection

Determining the Least Restrictive Placement

Read the following brief scenarios, and consider the advantages and disadvantages of the placement types.

Example 1: The case involves a 5-year-old child with health issues who has experienced physical abuse from his mother, who is a single parent and struggles with opioid use.

Placement options: Child placed in a nonrelative foster home; kin placement with elderly grandmother

Example 2: Thirteen-year-old who has been sexually abused by stepfather

Placement options: Child placed with father and stepmother who live out of state and have not seen the child for eight years; in a group home; with her boyfriend's parents

Example 3: Five siblings ranging from ages 2 to 14 who experienced neglect

Placement options: Children placed with an aunt and uncle who both work full-time at entry-level positions to support their four school-age children; divide the siblings with the older two going to one foster home, the youngest going to another, and the other two children going to a third

---

Placement Trends

Within the last decade, the number of children in foster care has been fairly stable and consistently has been around 400,000 children in care, with numbers rising slightly over the last 5 years (US DHHS, 2020a). Over 690,000 children were served by the foster care system in FY 2019, which also is an increase over the last 5 years (US DHHS, 2020a). On June 23, 2020, the average age of children in foster care was 8.4 years, and just over half (52%) were male (US DHHS, 2020b). Over 30,000 children under the age of 1 entered foster care, comprising 7% of the children who entered foster care in FY 2019 (US DHHS, 2020b). Of the children in the foster care system, 44% were White/Caucasian, 23% were Black or African American, 21% were Hispanic, and 2% were American Indian/Alaskan Native (US DHHS, 2020b). It should be noted that this highlights the racial disparities in the child welfare system, especially with Black or African American children and American Indian/Alaskan Native children. The average length of time in foster care was 19.6 months in FY 2019, which has decreased since 2010 (US DHHS, 2020b).

Children with certain characteristics are less likely to receive timely permanency. Children who are younger, Caucasian, and without a mental health diagnosis are more likely to exit care within ASFA's guidelines (Becker et al., 2007). Older children, children in a sibling group, and children with a disability or physical or mental issues are more likely to remain in care (Akin, 2011; Glisson et al., 2000). African American children are less likely to achieve reunification or adoption and have longer stays in foster care (Cheng, 2010). Children who remain in foster care without achieving permanency may have poorer behavioral outcomes than those who achieve timely permanency (Lawrence et al., 2006; Lloyd & Barth, 2011). Long stays in out-of-home care places children at risk for poorer developmental outcomes.

Note from the Field

Child Welfare and Juvenile Justice Dual System Involvement

Carly B. Dierkhising, PhD

Naomi[1] was first referred to child protective services at age 3 for severe neglect and caretaker absence. Only the allegation of caretaker absence was substantiated, and the family engaged in voluntary family maintenance services. The case closed shortly after. What the social worker did not know was that Naomi's stepfather was abusive towards her mother and her mother was physically abusive towards her brothers. Around age 6, Naomi's school records indicated that she began getting into fights at school, and when she was nine years old, there were additional child protection referrals for general neglect, emotional abuse, and an at-risk sibling which were all found to be inconclusive.

When Naomi was in middle school, she experienced bullying which eventually led to a fight on school grounds and a referral to the probation department, per school policy. She was assigned a court date and released to go home. Before her court date came up, things became more abusive in the household, and another referral to child protection was made for physical abuse, an at-risk sibling, and general neglect: only the neglect allegation was substantiated, and a case was opened. During this time, Naomi began running away to get away from the chaos in the home. She would stay at her friend's house, began skipping school, and accidently missed her court date. Missing her court date triggered an automatic warrant being issued for her arrest. When she and her mother came to court, her mother told the judge that Naomi was "out of control," and when the judge recommended community probation with an ankle monitor, Naomi's mother told the judge she didn't want her in the house because she believed she couldn't take care of her. The judge, then, sent Naomi to a group home and placed her on probation for 9 months.

At 13 years old, Naomi began living at a group home with ten other girls. In the group home, she was somewhat receptive to the therapeutic services and seemed to get along with one particular staff member at the group home. Three months later, Naomi left the group home without permission with another one of the girls who lived there. The group home staff reported this to her probation officer who charged her with a violation of her probation which extended her probation term 3 more months. Two months after this, Naomi was supposed to get a family visit with her brothers and mother, but her mother canceled telling Naomi she didn't want her sons to be around Naomi since she was a bad influence. Naomi became distraught, began yelling at the group home staff, and threw her phone across the room which struck one of the group home staff. The staff member insisted on calling her probation officer and urged the probation officer to charge Naomi with assault. Naomi was detained until her court date because the group home, per policy, couldn't let her stay in the home due to the pending assault charge. It was at this court hearing that the judge discovered that Naomi also had a case open in the child welfare system, and she referred Naomi to the dual system unit for a multidisciplinary assessment.

Naomi is a more typical case for dual system youth. Group homes tend to push these youth "deeper into the system," and almost always the court doesn't know that the youth are dually involved. Youth like Naomi pay the costs when systems to not work together and there is little understanding that youth in the juvenile justice system may have experienced child maltreatment which contributed to their juvenile justice system involvement.

---

[1] All names and other personal identifiers in cases and examples throughout this book have been changed to protect privacy and confidentiality.

Relevant Policies

There are multiple policies informing foster care placement options and decision-making. After CAPTA was passed in 1974, the number of children in foster care drastically increased as record numbers of children were removed from their homes. To address concerns about the number of children placed in foster care, legislation was passed. The Indian Child Welfare Act of 1978 (ICWA) was passed with aims of reducing the high numbers and inappropriate removals of American Indian and Alaska Native children through awarding tribal courts' jurisdiction over child maltreatment cases regarding American Indian and Alaska Native children.

The federal government passed the 1980 Adoption Assistance and Child Welfare Act (AACWA) to address the issue of the children remaining in foster care for extended periods of time. The legislation required states to make reasonable efforts to keep children in their homes, to reunite families, and required each child in foster care to have a permanency plan.

In 1994, the Multi-Ethnic Placement Act (MEPA) was passed to decrease the time that children remained in out-of-home care. The key elements of the MEPA prohibit child welfare agencies from considering race, color, or national origin when approving a foster or adoptive parent and likewise cannot refuse to delay foster care placements or adoption due to a child's or parent's race, color, or national origin. Also, the MEPA requires agencies to recruit foster and adoptive parents from diverse racial and ethnic backgrounds that reflect the diversity of children in care. The

> **Practice Highlight**
>
> **Foster Care Awareness Month**
>
> May is National Foster Care Month, a time to consider how we can each play a part in enhancing the lives of children and youth in foster care. Since 1988, leaders across the United States issue proclamations in recognition of National Foster Care Month to show appreciation and gratitude to foster parents across the nation.
>
> Throughout the years, the purpose and focus of Foster Care Awareness Month has changed. Recently, activities have focused on increasing the visibility of the needs of children and youth in foster care and ways to recruit and retain foster caregivers.

Interethnic Placement Act (IEPA) amended the MEPA to clarify language about cultural considerations and specified that race, color, or national origin could not be used in any placement decisions. Additionally, the IEPA added an exception in individual cases where it could be demonstrated that considering race, color, or national origin was in a certain child's best interest.

Despite the AACWA's mandates, the number of children in out-of-home care continued to increase. To address this, the Adoption and Safe Families Act (ASFA) was passed in 1997. The primary goals of the ASFA are child safety and timely permanency. The legislation prioritizes reunification and identifies adoption as the preferred alternative permanent plan. The ASFA shortens the timeframes for case plans and defines reasonable efforts required to preserve and reunify families, including placing children within a timely manner. Reunification is to occur within 12 months of removal, and adoption within 24 months. ASFA endorses the use of concurrent planning where there is a primary and an alternative plan simultaneously being addressed. The provisions remain minimally changed since the legislation was passed. Funding has been reauthorized, and in 2001, amendments were made to address the increase in minority children awaiting adoption.

In 2008, the Fostering Connections to Success and Increasing Adoptions Act (Fostering Connections Act) was passed with the goal of increasing the number of adoptions and guardianships through improved incentives. The Fostering Connections Act also sought to improve services to youth aging out through provisions extending foster care to age 21. The legislation also increased support for American Indian and Alaska Native children in the child welfare system.

Landmark legislation Family First Prevention Services Act (Family First) was passed in 2018 that changed how states could use Title IV-E funds and included prevention services. Relevant to foster care, Family First emphasizes family foster homes and seeks to reduce the use of congregate care facilities for out-of-home placements. States may not be reimbursed by the federal government for children placed in group care for more than 2 weeks, and the settings must be approved using a trauma-informed care model and employ nursing and licensed clinical staff.

While it is technically a public education policy, the Every Student Succeeds Act (ESSA) has mandates for states regarding children in foster care. Passed by the U.S. Congress in 2015, the legislation requires that children can stay at their school of origin unless it is not in the best interest of the child. The school districts and child welfare agencies must have agreements about how to provide and fund transportation for foster children to remain in their school of origin. If a child changes schools, the enrolling school must contact the previous school to get the current records. State education agencies are required to have a point of contact for child welfare agencies, and at the local level, schools must have a point of contact for child welfare if the child welfare agency has designated a point of contact for the schools.

Services for Children in Foster Care

Many children who enter foster care require services due to the maltreatment and trauma they experienced. Child welfare professionals collaborate with professionals in other systems to make sure that the children's needs are met. A wide range of services are provided to children in foster care to meet their needs including their health and mental health concerns. There could be early interventions to address developmental delays, such as speech, occupational, and/or physical therapy (see Chap. 3 for other examples). There may also be services to address behavioral concerns. Visitation with family is also provided to children in foster care. All of these services are child-specific, and appropriate assessments should be made to determine their needs and corresponding services.

It is estimated that a third of the children in foster care have a chronic medical condition such as asthma, severe allergies, repeated ear infections, and eczema (Ringeisen et al., 2008). While not all of the medical conditions may be life-threatening, some are. The mortality of children in foster care is higher than children in the general population (Chaiyachati et al., 2020). Children in foster care also frequently have dental problems, with an estimated one in five children entering care having significant dental issues (Szilagyi et al., 2015). Children in foster care are more likely than their peers to have developmental delays, many of which can be traced back to the maltreatment. The state is required to meet the medical and dental needs of children. Initial assessments as well as ongoing treatments are needed. Case managers work with the foster parents or congregate care facility to facilitate the appropriate services.

An estimated 40–80% of children in foster care have a major behavioral or mental health condition requiring treatment (Clausen et al., 1998; Garland et al., 2000; Halfon et al., 1995; Stahmer et al., 2005). Common diagnoses are attachment disorders, depression, and anxiety. Like with physical health, services are provided to children in foster care to address their behavioral and mental health needs. There are various interventions that have been found to have positive outcomes for addressing the needs of children in foster care. Unfortunately, in some communities there may be limited availability and difficulty accessing services. Interventions should be developmentally and culturally appropriate.

Visitation with biological parents, siblings, and other family members is also offered and is a critical component to a case. In almost all cases, with the exception of some extenuating circumstances, all children are provided with visitation at a minimum of once a week, sometimes more. Visitation is not only an opportunity

Practice Highlight

Psychotropic Medication and Youth in Foster Care

Doctors prescribe children in foster care psychotropic medications at rates 3.5 to 11 times higher than their peers not in care (Dos Reis et al., 2005), and they often prescribe children in foster care multiple types of psychotropic medications and higher doses than the maximum recommended (Zito et al., 2008). The rates of antipsychotic medication for children in foster care remains high, although in the last decade there has been a decrease in the antipsychotic polypharmacy (Matone et al., 2012). Interventions can reduce the prescribing of psychotropic medication for children in foster care (Cohen et al., 2013).

for children to see their siblings and parents, but for parents to demonstrate changes in their parenting behavior and receive guidance and advice from a parent aide or case manager who is present at the visit. Visits can take place in a number of different locations, including the agency office (least desirable), in-home, or in public spaces such as visitation centers, libraries, restaurants, and local parks. The latter locations are preferred so that children and their parents can be observed in more natural settings. Visitation can change over time and depending on circumstances, with increases in time together as a case moves towards reunification. Visitation time can also be decreased if a parent is inappropriate during the visits or it has been deemed detrimental to the child's well-being.

Services for Foster and Kinship Care Providers

Foster and kinship care providers provide for the daily needs of children who have been placed into their care. Due to the maltreatment and other traumas, many children in foster care have significant behavioral and physical needs that can be emotionally, physically, and financially demanding for the families who care for them (Hayes et al., 2015). Recognizing this, foster parents are required to complete extensive training before they are licensed to provide foster care. There are different standards for kinship care providers, and in many cases, there is not the same extensive training and support of family members who are providing care for a child in an out-of-home placement. Foster and kinship care providers express the need for appropriate, ongoing training support from formal and informal sources, child welfare agencies, and other foster and kinship care providers (Geiger et al., 2013), as well as advocacy and having their voice heard (Geiger et al., 2014). There are various national and local organizations that promote education, advocacy, and support for families caring for children in the foster care system. Foster and kinship care providers may need assistance in dealing with the child's trauma and health, mental health, and behavioral needs. There are interventions such as KEEP (Keeping Foster Parents Trained and Supported) that are promising practices (Price et al., 2015). In addition to training and guidance, the providers also may need concrete supports (e.g., crib, booster seat, medical apparatus) as well as reimbursements for the costs of taking care of the child (e.g., clothing, school supplies, transportation costs, recreation activities). Most foster care providers receive some financial support from a child welfare agency. This varies depending on the state, the child's needs,

---

Practice Highlight

Assessing and Supporting Older Kinship Caregivers

The number of both older caregivers and the children placed in their care has risen in recent years. The number of children who have achieved permanency with older caregivers has risen significantly since 1997 as a result of the Adoption and Safe Families Act. However, adoptions and subsidized guardianships with older caregivers have disrupted because caregivers die, become ill, or for other reasons are unable to provide for the children long term.

There are a number of challenges for older caregivers for children including the following:

- Caregiver's ability to meet the child's need for safety, well-being, and permanency
- Caregiver's mobility, transportation, and health
- Increased need for attention and resource delivery involving older caregivers
- Developing viable long-term care plans for the child(ren) in care
- Ability to access services for caregivers and/or other adults for whom they provide care (spouses, parents, siblings) through the statewide aging network

When working with older caregivers as placement for a child, we consider several things, including the caregiver's current status and the changing developmental needs of the child. If the assessment suggests there may be factors which could impact the safety and stability of the placement over the life of the placement, caseworkers may request further assessment through trained geriatric caseworkers licensed by the departments on aging. It is important to consider a long-term plan as well as a backup plan.

The long-term care plan identifies a permanency goal for the child, includes services and supports needed for the child's safety now and in future, and identifies a viable and reliable backup caregiver and contingency care plans. Backup plans should be developed for all cases. Closing to adoption or guardianship, a backup caregiver must be identified – regardless of the age of the caregivers. The backup plan is developed for ongoing care for the child if the time comes when the older caregiver can no longer care for the child. It should be detailed enough to cover any predictable contingencies, and the identified backup caregiver should be informed about limiting factors in the older caregiver's situation so he/she can make a fully informed decision about their agreement to be the backup caregiver and their ongoing role in the life of the child.

licensure, and cost of living. The foster and kinship care providers' ability to provide the necessary care for the child is connected to availability and access to services for the child.

Respite care is one service that may be available to foster and kinship care providers. With respite care, a child is sent to another placement short term for a set period of time before returning to the original foster or kinship placement. Respite care, sometimes called "short-term foster care," may be used for various reasons including giving the foster and kinship care providers a break from a child's demanding health needs or behavioral problems or when the providers may have to attend to specific obligations (e.g., death in the family, out-of-town business trip). It often

Note from the Field

Advocating for Therapy and Academic Supports

Libby Fakier, MBA

Most of the children who have been placed in our care struggle academically, either because of the circumstances in their birth home or due to changes in school placement as a result of moves from placement to placement. Exacerbating the issue is that many children in care have learning disabilities, psychosocial challenges, and generalized anxiety that inhibit their ability to learn.

When a child comes into our home, we meet with the case management team to assess grades, individualized educational programs (IEPs), learning disabilities, psychological evaluations, and supports that are currently in place. Often, we find that the child has not been evaluated for services or that evaluations were not followed up with approvals and implementation of therapeutic services. We see that children go years without services and suffer academically, psychologically, and physically because by the time they are evaluated at one placement, they are moved again before services are implemented. At the outset of receiving a new placement in our home, I advocate for my children to immediately receive psychological counseling with a professional that I have worked with for years. This creates the foundation of care for my kids on which we can build supports for all the other areas where the child needs help.

Wading through the bureaucracy is not for the faint of heart and requires a determined and unrelenting mindset to ensure that children in care get the services and support they need and deserve. Foster parents must be vigilant about advocating for their children's needs and not give up when the case management team or public school system either denies services or drags their feet about getting evaluations completed and services implemented. Daily calls, weekly emails, and constant follow-up with everyone on the case management team is essential to securing services in a timely manner.

There's a very small window to address children's psychological or therapeutic (physical therapy, occupational therapy, and speech therapy) needs to get them back on track. Medication evaluation and management must be streamlined so children have continuity of care and mental health issues are addressed before the child decompensates. Time is of the essence. Foster parents have the moral obligation and responsibility to ensure that their children's needs are met as quickly as possible. They must remain unconquered in their fight to advocate for the support services their children need to grow, heal, and succeed.

takes place over a weekend and rarely lasts more than a couple of weeks. Some families who are not able to make a commitment to being foster care parents provide respite care for children in foster care.

Services for Parents with Children in Foster Care

In most instances when child protective services remove a child from their parents, there is a case plan developed that details what must be done before a child can be reunified with their parents. These case plans are individualized for each family and take into consideration the family's needs and circumstances related to the maltreatment. Federal legislation requires child welfare agencies to make "reasonable efforts" to remedy the circumstances that led to a child being removed from their family.

Depending on the reasons that a child entered foster care, services should be offered to the parent that are consistent with the parents' needs and the reasons the child entered care and the parents' needs. In many cases, the services are mandatory, and it is only after there is documented successful completion may the child return home. Services which are commonly offered include visitation, case management, substance abuse treatment, transportation assistance, housing assistance, counseling, psychological evaluation, parenting education, anger management, and vocational training. There is variation in the availability and offering of services by state and agency. Some services the parents must pay for, while others are provided for them at no cost, although there may be costs to them such as transportation, child care (for children who are not in foster care), and missed work.

While parents are required to participate and complete services outlined by the case plan and court decision, services may be unavailable or inaccessible. A lack of funding is largely the reason this occurs. In some communities there may not be services, or the services available are inadequate to meet the demands, and there may be lengthy waitlists. As case plans require a parent to complete a service (e.g., parenting education, anger management, job training) in a certain timeframe to ensure that the agency is in compliance with the ASFA guidelines, troubles arise when services are not readily available. This can cause frustration and confusion for the parents and may delay reunification. In some cases, the difficulty in accessing services can lead to children not being reunified with their parents who were unable to complete the requirements for reunification outlined in a case plan. Additionally, the AFSA mandates a specific timeframe, which may be shorter than a timeline to complete treatment (e.g., substance abuse treatment) and specific tasks (e.g., obtaining housing and employment) which the case plan specifies.

In order to have successful reunifications, it is paramount that services provided to parents with children in foster care are delivered in a timely and appropriate manner. Parents must be able to access the services and to feel comfortable receiving them. Concerns exist that services provided to child welfare-involved families are not always appropriate and do not match the specific needs of the family (e.g., Bolen, McWey, & Schlee, 2008). There are concerns about parents being referred to unnecessary services. Care should be taken in developing case plans to make sure the servicesrequired will meet the specific needs of the parents and children. Ultimately, the services offered to parents with children in foster care should be designed to help the parents be able to provide for their children and family and address the reasons that the child was placed in foster care.

In-Home Services and Family Preservation Services

Not all children involved in the child welfare system are removed from their care-givers and enter foster care. Some children living in families reported to child pro-tective services for allegations of abuse and neglect receive in-home services. In these cases, child welfare professionals determine there is a low risk for future mal-treatment and determine a child can safely remain in the home while addressing the conditions that led to the allegations of maltreatment. Services are provided in-home when children can remain safe to avoid potential traumas of removal. The fact that most children are reunified with families further supports the arguments to make efforts to keep children in their own homes.

When children remain in the home, services still may be provided to ensure child safety and well-being. Sometimes the services are voluntary, while other times the cases are supervised by the courts. These community-based services assist parents in their caregiver role and can address the maltreatment or risks of maltreatments through an array of services. Services offered may include counseling, financial support, parenting education, case management, housing assistance, and referrals for services. The goal of the services is to prevent child maltreatment and to strengthen and support families. (See Chap. 7 for details about family preservation services.)

Child welfare agencies may provide intensive family preservation services to families in crisis where an imminent risk of out-of-home placement exists. With family preservation services, children remain in the home, but child protection pro-fessionals monitor cases. Often voluntary in nature, the family support and preser-vation services often face challenges in engaging families. Vast differences exist across programs; however, many programs have smaller caseloads, quick start (within 24 hours of referral), more frequent contact and visits, after-hours availabil-ity, short duration (4–6 weeks), concrete supports (e.g., financial, food, transporta-tion), and a strengths-based approach. Family preservation services attempt to address crises, improve family functioning, and encourage the use of families' for-mal and informal social support systems. Family support and preservation programs are often voluntary and may have difficulties engaging families

Findings on program effectiveness in preventing out-of-home placement are mixed. In a meta-analysis of 20 intensive family preservation programs, overall, programs were found to have a medium and positive effect on family functioning but were generally not effective in preventing out-of-home placement for families experiencing maltreatment (Al et al., 2012). Several design and methodological rea-sons may contribute to the inconsistency of family preservation services' efficacy; however, the practices continue to be used to prevent out-of-home placement (Tyuse, Hong, & Stretch, 2010), and clients report overall positive family impact and expe-riences with family preservation services (e.g., Lietz, 2009; Mullins, Cheung, & Lietz, 2012).

Recruiting, Training, and Licensing Foster Parents

With more than half of all children residing in nonrelative foster homes, it is important for child welfare professionals to understand best practices in collaborating with foster caregivers while also understanding the process for becoming a foster parent and their experiences as foster parents. Further, many foster parents go on to adopt the children in their home and serve as a critical member of the child welfare team, as they provide care every day, all day to children in need. Foster parents become the point person for many of the child's needs, including their healthcare, education, and social-emotional development. They ensure that their basic needs are being met and that they are on task developmentally.

Despite their critical role, there is often a shortage of foster parents available to meet the needs of the child welfare agency, partly due to failure to recruit adequate numbers of foster caregivers for various reasons, a lack of training and support, and issues related to retention. In fact, it was estimated that the median length of service of foster parents in three states was 8–14 months (Gibbs & Wildfire, 2007). The shortage of foster parents is of great concern to child welfare agencies as foster parents provide the daily care for children in the system. There are many efforts to increase the number of foster homes.

Foster parents become licensed foster caregivers for a number of reasons. Most foster parents say they became licensed to become foster parents to help kids and provide a loving home, while many say they had a calling to care for kids in need. Some choose to foster with the hopes of later adoption, sometimes due to their inability to have children or more children, or because their children were grown and no longer in the home (Geiger, Hayes, & Lietz, 2013). Many have a desire to give back to the community or know a child or family in need and went on to become licensed.

Foster parent training and licensure requirements vary by state and jurisdiction. One of the most commonly adopted training models is PRIDE (Parents' Resources for Information, Development, and Education). This training model is designed to strengthen the quality of family foster care and adoption services by providing a standardized, structured framework for recruiting, preparing, and selecting foster and adoptive parents. The majority of states and jurisdictions will have a standardized recruitment and training program for all foster caregivers. As part of the PRIDE program, all foster caregivers must successfully complete nine sessions (27 hours) of pre-service training before they can be licensed. To maintain the license, they must participate in ongoing training, and most licenses are valid for 3–5 years unless there is a reason to revoke the license or the foster caregiver chooses to end the license. Relatives are also encouraged to pursue licensure as additional financial and social support is often provided along with licensure. Goals of PRIDE are to ensure that children are protected and nurtured and have their developmental needs met; relationships between children and their families are supported; children are connected to long-term, safe, nurturing relationships; and foster caregivers are members of the child welfare team.

Training emphasizes several areas regarding roles and responsibilities of the foster caregivers and the child welfare agency; helps new foster caregivers to understand the importance of parents and families involved with child welfare, managing loss, and teamwork; and assists with understanding the value of diversity and cultural competence and the various protocols and policies that occur with cases (e.g., mutual family assessment and informed decision-making).

In addition to pre-service training, foster caregivers pursuing licensure will also have a home and family assessment which occurs in the home and through the gathering of documents, reports, and forms. This process ensures that a family is prepared, appropriate, and safe when trusted to care for a child. A home study is conducted to help the child welfare professional and the agency decide if adoption or foster care is right and identify the type

Practice Highlight

PRIDE Training Session Topics

- Session 1: Connecting with PRIDE
- Session 2: Teamwork towards permanency
- Session 3: Meeting developmental needs: attachment
- Session 4: Meeting developmental needs: loss
- Session 5: Strengthening family relationships
- Session 6: Meeting developmental needs: discipline
- Session 7: Continuing family relationships
- Session 8: Planning for change
- Session 9: Taking PRIDE – making an informed decision

of child or children who will be the best match for the family. The process includes interviews, home visits, documentation of key information, and reference checks with people who know the family members well, criminal record check, and a home inspection. One this assessment is complete, a recommendation is made regarding fitness and the number and ages of children a foster caregiver's license includes.

Unfortunately, foster caregiver retention continues to be challenging for many child welfare agencies. In fact, it is estimated that up to 40% of foster families discontinue fostering during the first year and 20% plan to do so (Rhodes, Orme, & Buehler, 2001). Some of the reasons provided when a family chooses to discontinue fostering are encountering issues with the child welfare agency/navigating the system, concerns about a child's behavior, stressful interactions with birth parents, problems between foster children and birth children, and being named in allegations of abuse. Foster parents were more likely to discontinue fostering if they were dissatisfied with agency relationships or had poor communication with workers (Rhodes et al., 2001). In studies comparing foster parents who chose to stop fostering and those who plan to continue, many point to adequate training, mentorship from seasoned foster parents, and support from the agency and other parents (Geiger et al., 2013). Foster parents have identified the need for strong relationships with child welfare professionals (Geiger, Piel & Julien-Chinn, 2017).

Note from the Field

Saying Goodbye

Kris Jacober

It's the first thing we heard as a foster family. "I could never do that. It would be too hard to have to say goodbye." And yet, over 15 years we did it over and over and over again. Saying goodbye, and then sometimes saying hello again, to 18 children who shared our home.

We'd cared for our first placement, two little girls, for more than 2 years. They were moving 100 miles away with an aunt they, or we, had barely met. She seemed nice enough and, over time, has proven to be a wonderful woman, but on the day those two girls rode away, new pet goldfishes in their laps, van piled high with toys and clothes, it was the end of our world. Next up, a brother and sister who stayed for 3 months and then moved in with their aunt, 100 miles in a different direction. Three months is not 2 years, but these two likewise left their mark on our family. By now we had a little ritual. Dinner at Chuck E. Cheese. Letters from every member of our family. Photo book of our adventures. "Oh, the Places You'll Go" book with all of our autographs and, most important, our home phone number. Over the next years, more children, more painful goodbyes. We dropped off one little boy who we'd cared for 2 years at his home, all of us wearing sunglasses so he couldn't see us cry. We cared for the next little boy for 2 years, as well, and he was adopted by our friends. One day he was with us. The next day he was with them.

In the days before a child leaves, you sit in their room packing up all of their clothing and toys. You hug them extra hard when you put them down to bed for the last time. Your biological kids lay on the floor and cry, and you wonder over and over if you're doing the right thing. Three little girls were with us for more than a year. Two were adopted by a new "forever family." One, with a different father, was adopted by her aunt. The scene when we dropped off two of the sisters, but not the third, still haunts me. The two sisters in their "new bedroom" at their new home, us walking away with their sister who would be with us for a few more weeks until she moved in with her aunt. Two sisters, laying on their beds, crying about where their sister is going. Those are the days when you feel complicit in a crime. You've done the best you can, but the system is not designed for children. It's designed so that adults who interact with children can check the boxes and break difficult decisions into manageable bites.

Over the years we've said "goodbye" in many different ways. Meeting new families in fast-food restaurants halfway between their homes and ours. Dropping children off at their new adoptive homes. After many years of experience, here's what I say to people who say they could never do this because it's too hard. It is hard. And sad. And the losses pile up, one on top of another, each time a child leaves.

It's tough but we're the adults here. Kids need us to be strong and to not be afraid of the loss. We do the best we can while the children are with us. And when they leave, inside the front cover of "Oh, the Places You'll Go," they'll find our home phone number. We've never changed it because, who knows someday they may call and need us again.

Conclusion

When a child is removed from their parents and placed in out-of-home care, there are various types of placement options: relative/kinship, nonrelative family placement, in-home, and congregate care. Children in foster care should be placements that are in least restrictive environments, with siblings, with family/kin, culturally appropriate settings, and in homes closest to a child's neighborhood and school. When it is possible to keep a child in their home, in-home perseveration services should be offered. Placement stability is important for the well-being of children in care. As such child welfare professionals should prioritize recruiting and training foster parents so that they will be prepared to care for children. Various services should be provided to children in care, parents providing foster care, and the parents who have children in care.

Acknowledgments The authors thank Ashley Wilfong, MSW; Carly B. Dierkhising, PhD; Libby Fakier, MBA; and Kris Jacober for their contributions to Chapter 9.

Discussion Questions

1. What types of placements are considered "least restrictive" and why?
2. What are two benefits to placing children with kin/relatives when they are removed from their family of origin?
3. How can child welfare professionals promote cultural ties for children and youth in care?
4. How can child welfare professionals ensure the medical, educational, and mental health needs of children are being met?
5. What types of training do prospective foster parents engage in order to become licensed?

Suggested Activities

1. Review this document from the American Bar Association regarding culture among children in foster care: https://www.americanbar.org/groups/public_interest/child_law/resources/child_law_practiceonline/january%2D%2D-december-2019/supporting-cultural-identity-for-children-in-foster-care/
   On your own or with a classmate, think about ways you can promote culture with children in care. Are current state and federal policies enough? Why or why not?
2. Review the case of "Baby Veronica" (Adoptive Couple v. Baby Girl, 570 U.S. 637 (2013)) http://nulawreview.org/extralegalrecent/2020/9/16/challenging-the-narrative-challenges-to-icwa-and-the-implications-for-tribal-sovereignty. Consider the ways in which this case is different than others.
3. Watch the video "Big Mama", which won an Academy Award for Best Short Documentary in 2001. Consider the implications for placing Walter with his grandmother. What services could have been put in place to support her and the family?

4. Read Geiger, Piel & Julien-Chinn (2017). Discuss with others how child welfare agencies and child welfare professionals can incorporate the ideas of foster care provides shared in the article.
   Geiger, J. M., Piel, M. H., & Julien-Chinn, F. J. (2017). Improving relationships in child welfare practice: Perspectives of foster care providers. *Child and Adolescent Social Work Journal, 34*(1), 23–33. (Available: https://rdcu. be/ccaPL).

Additional Resources

Child Welfare Information Gateway, National Foster Care Awareness Month: https://www.childwelfare.gov/fostercaremonth/

Child Welfare Information Gateway Podcast: Supporting Kinship Caregivers Part 1: https://www.acf.hhs.gov/cb/resource/child-welfare-podcast-supporting-kinship-caregivers-part1.

Child Welfare Information Gateway Podcast: Supporting Kinship Caregivers Part 2: https://www.acf.hhs.gov/cb/resource/child-welfare-podcast-supporting-kinship-caregivers-part2

Annie E. Casey Foundation. Engaging Kinship Caregivers with Joseph Crumbley: https://www.aecf.org/blog/engaging-kinship-caregivers-with-joseph-crumbley/

Child Welfare Information Gateway, Sibling Issues in Foster Care and Adoption: https://www.childwelfare.gov/pubs/siblingissues/

References

Akin, B. A. (2011). Predictors of foster care exits to permanency: A competing risks analysis of reunification, guardianship, and adoption. *Children and Youth Services Review, 33*(6), 999–1011. https://doi.org/10.1016/j.childyouth.2011.01.008

Al, C. M., Stams, G. J. J., Bek, M. S., Damen, E. M., Asscher, J. J., & van der Laan, P. H. (2012). A meta-analysis of intensive family preservation programs: Placement prevention and improvement of family functioning. *Children and Youth Services Review, 34*, 1472–1479. https://doi.org/10.1016/j.childyouth.2012.04.002

Barth, R. P. (2005). Residential care: From here to eternity. *International Journal of Social Welfare, 14*(3), 158–162. https://doi.org/10.1111/j.1468-2397.2005.00355.x

Becker, M. A., Jordan, N., & Larsen, R. (2007). Predictors of successful permanency planning and length of stay in foster care: The role of race, diagnosis and place of residence. *Children and Youth Services Review, 29*(8), 1102–1113. https://doi.org/10.1016/j.childyouth.2007.04.009

Bell, T., & Romano, E. (2015). Permanency and safety among children in foster family and kinship care: A scoping review. *Trauma, Violence & Abuse, 18*(3), 268–286. https://doi.org/10.1177/1524838015611673

Berrick, J. D., & Hernandez, J. (2016). Developing consistent and transparent kinship care policy and practice: State mandated, mediated, and independent care. *Children and Youth Services Review, 68*, 24–33. https://doi.org/10.1016/j.childyouth.2016.06.025

Bettman, J. E., & Jasperson, R. A. (2009). Adolescents in residential and inpatient treatment: A review of the outcomes literature. *Child & Youth Care Forum, 38*, 161–183. https://doi.org/10.1007/s10566-009-9073-y

Boel-Studt, S. M., & Tobia, L. (2016). A review of trends, research, and recommendations for strengthening the evidence-base and quality of residential group care. *Residential Treatment for Children & Youth, 33*(1), 13–35. https://doi.org/10.1080/0886571X.2016.1175995

Bolen, M. G., McWey, L. M., & Schlee, B. M. (2008). Are at-risk parents getting what they need? Perspectives of parents involved with child protective services. *Clinical Social Work Journal, 36*, 341–354. https://doi.org/10.1007/s10615-008-0173-1

Chaiyachati, B. H., Wood, J. N., Mitra, N., & Chaiyachati, K. H. (2020). All-Cause Mortality Among Children in the US Foster Care System, 2003–2016. *JAMA Pediatrics.* https://doi.org/10.1001/jamapediatrics.2020.0715

Cheng, T. C. (2010). Factors associated with reunification: A longitudinal analysis of long-term foster care. *Children and Youth Services Review, 32*(10), 1311–1316. https://doi.org/10.1016/j.childyouth.2010.04.023

Children's Bureau. (2015). *A national look at the use of congregate care in child welfare.* U.S. Department of Health and Human Services.

Clausen, J. M., Landsverk, J., Ganger, W., Chadwick, D., & Litrownik, A. (1998). Mental health problems of children in foster care. *Journal of Child and Family Studies, 7*, 283–296. https://doi.org/10.1023/A:1022989411119

Cohen, D., Lacasse, J. R., Dan, R., & Senglemann, I. (2013). CriticalThinkRX may reduce prescribing to foster youth: Results from an intervention trial. *Research on Social Work Practice, 23*, 284–293. https://doi.org/10.1177/1049731513477691

Dos Reis, S., Zito, J. M., Safer, D. J., Gardner, J. F., Puccia, K. B., & Owens, P. L. (2005). Multiple psychotropic medication use for youths: a two-state comparison. *Journal of Child and Adolescent Psychopharmacology, 15*, 68–77. https://doi.org/10.1089/cap.2005.15.68

Ehrle, J., & Geen, R. (2002). Kin and non-kin foster care-findings form a national survey. *Children and Youth Services Review, 24*, 15–35. https://doi.org/10.1016/S0190-7409(01)00166-9

Garland, A. F., Aarons, G. A., Saltzman, M. D., & Kruse, M. I. (2000). Correlates of adolescents' satisfaction with mental health services. *Mental Health Services Research, 2*, 127–139. https://doi.org/10.1023/A:1010137725958

Geiger, J. M., Hayes, M. J., & Lietz, C. A. (2013). Should I stay or should I go? A mixed methods study examining factors influencing foster parents' decision to continue or discontinue fostering. *Children and Youth Services Review, 35*, 1356–1365. https://doi.org/10.1016/j.childyouth.2013.05.003

Geiger, J. M., Julien-Chinn, F. J., & Lietz, C. A. (2014). *Foster Parent Satisfaction Survey.* Center for Applied Behavioral Health Policy, School of Social Work, Arizona State University.

Geiger, J. M., Piel, M. H., & Julien-Chinn, F. J. (2017). Improving relationships in child welfare practice: Perspectives of foster care providers. *Child and Adolescent Social Work Journal, 34*(1), 23–33. https://doi.org/10.1007/s10560-016-0471-3

Gibbs, D., & Wildfire, J. (2007). Length of service for foster parents: Using administrative data to understand retention. *Children and Youth Services Review, 29*(5), 588–599. https://doi.org/10.1016/j.childyouth.2006.11.002

Glisson, C., Bailey, J. W., & Post, J. A. (2000). Predicting the time children spend in state custody. *Social Service Review, 74*(2), 253–280. https://doi.org/10.1086/514479

Halfon, N., Mendonca, A., & Berkowitz, G. (1995). Health status of children in foster care: The experience of the Center for the Vulnerable Child. *Archives of Pediatrics & Adolescent Medicine, 149*, 386–392. https://doi.org/10.1001/archpedi.1995.02170160040006

Hayes, M. J., Geiger, J. M., & Lietz, C. A. (2015). Navigating a complicated system of care: Foster parent satisfaction with behavioral and medical health services. *Child and Adolescent Social Work Journal, 32*, 493–505. https://doi.org/10.1007/s10560-015-0388-2

Hooper, S. R., Murphy, J., Devaney, A., & Hultman, T. (2000). Ecological outcomes of adolescents in a psychoeducational residential treatment facility. *American Journal of Orthopsychiatry, 70,* 491–500. https://doi.org/10.1037/h0087807

Lawrence, C. R., Carlson, E. A., & Egeland, B. (2006). The impact of foster care on development. *Development and Psychopathology, 18*(1), 57–76. https://doi.org/10.1017/S0954579406060044

Lietz, C. A. (2009). Examining families' perceptions of intensive in-home services: A mixed methods study. *Children and Youth Services Review, 31,* 1337–1345. https://doi.org/10.1016/j.childyouth.2009.06.007

Lloyd, E. C., & Barth, R. P. (2011). Developmental outcomes after five years for foster children returned home, remaining in care, or adopted. *Children and Youth Services Review, 33*(8), 1383–1391. https://doi.org/10.1016/j.childyouth.2011.04.008

Lyons, J. S., Terry, P., Martinovich, Z., Peterson, J., & Bouska, B. (2001). Outcome trajectories for adolescents in residential treatment: A statewide evaluation. *Journal of Child and Family Studies, 10,* 333–345. https://doi.org/10.1023/A:1012576826136

Malm, K., Vandivere, S., & McKlindon, A. (2011). *Children adopted from foster care: Child and family characteristics, adoption motivation, and well-being.* Office of the Assistant Secretary for Planning and Evaluation, U.S. Department of Health and Human Services.

Matone, M., Localio, R., Huang, Y. S., Dosreis, S., Feudtner, C., & Rubin, D. (2012). The relationship between mental health diagnosis and treatment with second-generation antipsychotics over time: a national study of US Medicaid-enrolled children. *Health Services Research, 47*(5), 1836–1860. https://doi.org/10.1111/j.1475-6773.2012.01461.x

Mitchell, M. B. (2018). "No one acknowledged my loss and hurt": Non-death loss, grief, and trauma in foster care. *Child and Adolescent Social Work Journal, 35*(1), 1–9. https://doi.org/10.1007/s10560-017-0502-8

Mullins, J. L., Cheung, J. R., & Lietz, C. A. (2012). Family preservation services: incorporating the voice of families into service implementation. *Child & Family Social Work, 17,* 265–274. https://doi.org/10.1111/j.1365-2206.2011.00777.x

Price, J. M., Roesch, S., Walsh, N. E., & Landsverk, J. (2015). Effects of the KEEP foster parent intervention on child and sibling behavior problems and parental stress during a randomized implementation trial. *Prevention Science, 16*(5), 685–695. https://doi.org/10.1007/s11121-014-0532-9

Rauktis, M. E., Fusco, R. A., Cahalane, H., Bennett, I. K., & Reinhart, S. M. (2011). "Try to make it seem like we're regular kids": Youth perceptions of restrictiveness in out-of-home care. *Children and Youth Services Review, 33*(7), 1224–1233. https://doi.org/10.1016/j.childyouth.2011.02.012

Rhodes, K. W., Orme, J. G., & Buehler, C. (2001). A comparison of family foster parents who quit, consider quitting, and plan to continue fostering. *Social Service Review, 75*(1), 84–114. https://doi.org/10.1086/591883

Ringeisen, H., Casanueva, C., Urato, M., & Cross, T. (2008). Special health care needs among children in the child welfare system. *Pediatrics, 122*(1), e232–e241. https://doi.org/10.1542/peds.2007-3778

Sakai, C., Lin, H., & Flores, G. (2011). Health outcomes and family services in kinship care: Analysis of a national sample of children in the child welfare system. *Archives of Pediatrics & Adolescent Medicine, 165*(2), 159–165. https://doi.org/10.1001/archpediatrics.2010.277

Stahmer, A. C., Leslie, L. K., Hurlburt, M., Barth, R. P., Webb, M. B., Landsverk, J., & Zhang, J. (2005). Developmental and behavioral needs and service use for young children in child welfare. *Pediatrics, 116,* 891–900. https://doi.org/10.1542/peds.2004-2135

Szilagyi, M. A., Rosen, D. S., Rubin, D., & Zlotnik, S. (2015). Health care issues for children and adolescents in foster care and kinship care. *Pediatrics, 136*(4), e1142–e1166. https://doi.org/10.1542/peds.2015-2656

Tyuse, S. W., Hong, P. P., & Stretch, J. J. (2010). Evaluation of an intensive in-home family treatment program to prevent out-of-home placement. *Journal of Evidence-Based Social Work, 7,* 200–218. https://doi.org/10.1080/15433710902911063

U.S. Department of Health & Human Services, Administration for Children and Families, Administration on Children, Youth and Families, Children's Bureau. (2020a). Child Maltreatment 2018. Available from https://www.acf.hhs.gov/cb/research-data-technology/statistics-research/child-maltreatment

U.S. Department of Health & Human Services (2020b). The AFSCARS Report. https://www.acf.hhs.gov/sites/default/files/documents/cb/afcarsreport27.pdf

Winokur, M., Holtan, A., & Batchelder, K. E. (2014). Kinship care for the safety, permanency, and well-being of children removed from the home for maltreatment. *Cochrane Database of Systematic Reviews, 2014*, 1–239. https://doi.org/10.1002/14651858.CD006546.pub3

Zito, J. M., Safer, D. J., Sai, D., Gardner, J. F., Thomas, D., Coombes, P., Dubowski, M., & Mendez-Lewis, M. (2008). Psychotropic medication patterns among youth in foster care. *Pediatrics, 121*, e157–e163. https://doi.org/10.1542/peds.2007-0212

Chapter 10
Permanency in Child Welfare Practice

Introduction

Permanency, or a permanent plan for a child's legal placement and relationships, is a priority of the child welfare system. It is considered at every stage of the case. Federal legislation has been enacted to increase permanency of children involved in the child welfare system. Permanency refers to having nurturing relationships with adults who provide support to children and youth in their care. Ideally, permanency takes the form of a long-term relationship that includes a legal component. The child welfare system is charged with finding a permanent placement for each child who enters the foster care system, one that is stable and healthy. In most cases, children will be reunited with their biological parents/caregivers. However, many children may not be able to return home, and a plan for guardianship or adoption must be made and carried out.

In the most recent Adoption and Foster Care Analysis and Reporting System (AFCARS) report for children in care, 55% of children had a case plan goal of family reunification, and 28% had a goal of adoption (US DHHS, 2020). Of the children who had exited during the same time period, 47% had been reunited with their parents, 26% had been adopted, 11% had entered in a permanent guardianship, 8% had emancipated, and 6% were living with other relatives (US DHHS, 2020).

Permanency Planning

There are several factors that child welfare professionals must balance when making decisions and plans for permanency. For example, the reason for the child entering care – is this an issue that can be resolved within a timely manner so that a child can safely return home? There are a number of legal timelines and guidelines that child welfare professionals must consider with permanency, such as laws and

© Springer Nature Switzerland AG 2021
J. M. Geiger, L. Schelbe, *The Handbook on Child Welfare Practice*,
https://doi.org/10.1007/978-3-030-73912-6_10

policies regarding time, caregivers, and expectations, which will be discussed below. All efforts in preventing a family from becoming involved with the child welfare system are made through family preservation services/intact family services to alleviate issues among families who are considered low-risk. These families may be in need of resources (educational, medical, financial, housing, food, etc.) and psychoeducation about discipline or parenting skills or require supports such as childcare or health insurance.

Permanency planning begins at the first contact with a family and extends through the life of a case (intake, investigation, case management, closure). Effective permanency planning requires uniform implementation of basic social work practice fundamentals and permanency principles. Family reunification (discussed in Chap. 7) is the preferred outcome and is always the case plan goal for families becoming involved with the child welfare system, with exceptions for cases involving aggravated circumstances that require expedited termination of parental rights (e.g., "when the maltreatment of children is so egregious that efforts should not be made to preserve the family"). Focus is always placed on having children return home as soon and safely as possible. When this is not possible, child welfare professionals identify other families, particularly relative or kinship caregivers, as well as nonrelative licensed caregivers (foster parents) who will care for the child or children while family reunification is pursued. Permanency is not only an outcome but a process. It involves making decisions about placement, services, time frames, goals, and the responsibilities of all parties involved. Parents are often asked to complete a series of services, tasks, and/or work towards building skills related to caring for the child or children involved in order for family reunification to occur.

Practice Highlight

Guiding Principles in Permanency Planning

1. Base decision-making on the child's sense of time and urgency

2. Focus service on achieving health, well-being, and safety for children

3. Respect child's family and value the importance of family connectedness

4. Prioritize ongoing, thorough, and complete assessments of children and families.

5. Embrace shared decision making

6. Ensure full disclosure

7. Conduct frequent reviews

8. Ensure thorough assessment and services that match

9. Involve child welfare professionals as change agents working with families, children, and service providers

Principles Guiding Permanency Planning

Child welfare professionals lead perma- nency planning efforts, in collaboration with parents, family, children and youth, and service providers. There are several principles guiding permanency planning to consider in child welfare practice. First, child welfare professionals must be sure to base their decision-making on the needs of the child in terms of time and urgency. For example, the law designates specific time frames for service completion. As soon as it appears that reunification may not occur, and that it is no longer an appropriate or achievable goal, it is the child welfare pro- fessional's responsibility to consider chang- ing the permanency goal to meet the needs of the child or children. Second, the child welfare professional should prioritize ser- vices that specifically address the needs of the parent(s) and child that caused the child to be placed in out-of-home care. Services provided to the parent and/or the child should focus on the child's health, safety, and well-being. Family is extremely impor- tant in permanency planning. Immediate and extended family should be involved in the case and planning and considered as placement when children cannot be placed with their parents. Family members should always be treated with respect and con- sulted when important decisions are made. Child welfare professionals must determine the conditions that children can safely return home. Ongoing, thorough, and complete family and child assessments are critical in making these decisions. This also allows one to ensure safety and minimize risk to the well-being of the child. Shared decision- making is key when determining the options

Policy Highlight

Examples of Aggravated Circumstances that May Require Expedited Termination of Parental Rights

The parent committed murder of another child of the parent.

The parent committed voluntary manslaughter of another child of the parent.

The parent aided or abetted, attempted, conspired, or solicited to commit such a murder or volun- tary manslaughter.

The parent committed a felony assault that resulted in serious bodily injury to the child or another child of the parent.

The parental rights of the parent to a sibling of the child were termi- nated involuntarily.

The parent abandoned the child.

The parent was convicted of the crime of trafficking in persons.

The parent has sexually exploited or allowed the sexual exploitation of the child.

The child was removed from the home previously due to abuse or neglect and was removed again due to a subsequent incident of abuse or neglect.

The parent was convicted of a sex- ual offense that resulted in the child's conception.

for placement and permanency for children. When interdisciplinary teams work together to support children and families, children and their parents are more likely to access more services and are more motivated to work towards their goals while feeling sup- ported in the process. Child welfare professionals should be honest about how the case is progressing and provide clear, concise information about the case to all parties in the case (parents, children [as appropriate], caregivers, and service providers). This is not always easy as decisions made can often not be what everyone would like to see happen (e.g., termination of parental rights); however, when approached honestly, with empathy and sensitivity, parents and other parties can better understand how decisions are made, especially when they are kept apprised of changes and communicated with regularly. Child welfare professionals should conduct frequent reviews to evaluate progress, make any necessary changes, and determine the continued appropriateness of the plan, relevance of the services, and frequency and duration of child-parent visitation. Throughout the case, assessment and subsequent recommendations should always inform and match services provided as well as the child's placement.

Practice Highlight

Actions Speak Louder than Words!

Parents' behavior is the ultimate determinant of permanency outcomes. However, a child welfare professional can also positively impact the case outcomes and child and family well-being, especially when providing appropriate, timely, and culturally sensitive services within the mandated time limits.

Permanency: Policies and Laws

A number of federal and state level policies have been enacted to improve permanency outcomes for children and youth involved in the child welfare system. Over the last century, child welfare in the United States has shifted between a focus on safety to one of family preservation. In the 1970s, there was an increased focus on reducing the time a child spent in foster care and less time towards permanency. In 1997, the Adoption and Safe Families Act (ASFA, P.L. 105-89) was the first legislation that addressed permanency by highlighting the need for both safety and permanency for children and families to achieve child well-being. The AFSA provided a clear definition and guidelines for permanency for children in care. This groundbreaking legislation required states to improve the safety of children, promote adoption and permanent placements for children, and support families. It also required child protection agencies to offer timely assessments and services (e.g., substance abuse, psychological assessment and treatment, parenting, etc.) to children and families involved in the child welfare system. Following the AFSA, states were required to report "reasonable efforts" to provide services, find permanent homes and families for children, and conduct concurrent planning for permanency (secondary goal for permanency if reunification was not possible). If child protection agencies/states did not demonstrate reasonable efforts, they were subject to fines and/or other legal sanctions. This is particularly relevant for child welfare professionals, who are responsible for identifying the needs of the family to meet permanency goals and offering services to parents and children in a timely and consistent manner. Court proceedings will involve the reporting of findings for reasonable efforts for each case.

In 2008, the Fostering Connections to Success and Increasing Adoptions Act (P.L. 110–351) amended the Social Security Act to improve outcomes for children in foster care, connect and support relative caregivers, and offer incentives for adoption. Fostering Connections enhanced services for youth aging out of care and created new programs to help children and youth in or at risk of entering foster care to reconnect with family members. Through this legislation, permanency was prioritized.

More recently, the Family First Prevention Services Act (Family First Act) was signed into law as part of Division E in the Bipartisan Budget Act of 2018 (HR 1892). It provides additional guidance and funding to reduce the number of children entering foster care through prevention services, supporting families, and promoting family-based care for children in care. With regard to permanency, the law promotes permanent families for children by establishing an electronic interstate case-processing system to help states expedite interstate placement of children (ICPC) in care, adoption, or guardianship. It also extends the Adoption and Legal Guardianship Incentive Payment program for 5 years so that states can receive incentives for increasing the number of children leaving care through adoption or guardianship. Family First also outlines steps to ensure that states are investing in post-adoption services to decrease the number of children re-entering foster care.

Permanency Goals

Reunification with the biological parents/caregivers is the preferred initial permanency goal when children enter care, except in cases where aggravated circumstances exist. When this is not possible, other permanency goals must be considered concurrently or after a reasonable amount of time has elapsed, as a new goal. As a case moves forward and parents have been unable to remedy the circumstances for which a child entered care within a reasonable time frame, the child welfare professional and legal counsel may make a recommendation for the termination of parental rights (TPR) and adoption. In these circumstances, it is preferred that a child is already placed in a permanent placement with a family who wishes to adopt them. However, it is not always the case that a family has been identified and the child welfare professional, often one who specializes in adoption, will work towards identifying a family that meets the needs of the child or children and begin working towards a transitioning to a permanency placement with this family.

> **Practice Highlight**
>
> **Types of Permanency Goals**
>
> **Reunification** with the parent
>
> **Termination of parental rights (TPR)** and **adoption**
>
> **Guardianship** with a permanent guardian
>
> **Guardianship** with a "fit and willing relative" while remaining in the state's legal custody
>
> **Another planned permanent living arrangement (APPLA)** while remaining in the state's legal custody

Other permanency goals include guardianship with a permanent guardian and guardianship with a "fit and willing" relative while remaining in the state's custody. Guardianship is a permanent arrangement that involves a court order appointing a specific caretaker for the child without having to terminate parental rights. Guardianship accounts for approximately 11% of case outcomes in the United States (US DHHS 2020). Appointed guardians have similar rights and duties of a biological or adoptive parent (e.g., health care, educational, etc.). Plans of guardianship are often used when children are placed with kinship caregivers and in situations where permanency options of adoption and family reunification have been ruled out. Finally, revocation of guardianships can be requested by a parent at any time, with court involvement and review.

The least desirable permanency goal is "another planned permanent living arrangement" or APPLA. This goal is the least frequently used and mostly used among older youth in care for which an adoptive or legal guardian permanent placement was not identified. It is possible in these circumstances that a parent's rights were not terminated, therefore ruling out adoption. Additionally, it is possible that a youth is choosing not to be adopted or enter into a legal guardianship. The case manager will work with the older child to identify another planned permanent living arrangement when reunification, adoption, and guardianship are not appropriate options. In this scenario, the child welfare professional attempts to build upon and foster permanent supports and connections and to provide independent living services that help prepare the youth for self-sufficiency in adulthood.

Case Study: Adoption with a Kinship Caregiver
Maria,[1] 7, had been in foster care for 1 year. The courts had just changed her case plan from family reunification to adoption. Her mother and father had not been able to successfully complete the case plan tasks to have them reunited with Maria. Maria had been living with her aunt, Susanna, since being removed from her parents' care. Susanna was willing to adopt Maria and provide a permanent placement with her. Once her parents' parental rights were terminated by the courts, Susanna worked with an attorney to file for adoption. Within 3 months, Maria was adopted by Susanna.

[1]All names and other personal identifiers in cases and examples throughout this book have been changed to protect privacy and confidentiality.

Regardless of the older youth's permanency plan, any child 16 years of age or older should receive an independent living assessment and services while they are living in any type of foster care. They may be working towards achieving any of the permanency goals (i.e., reunification, adoption, guardianship, or APPLA). Independent living services generally include assistance with money management skills, educational assistance, household management skills, employment preparation, and other life skills services. A case plan of APPLA typically involves older youth who will most likely age out of care at the age of 18 or 21, depending on their state of residence. The process of aging out and special considerations for working with older youth are discussed further in Chap. 11.

Reunification, adoption, guardianship, and APPLA are general permanency goal options used within federal guidelines; however, states and tribal communities often use more specific options or more expansive permanency goals. For example, in Illinois, permanency goals are expanded within family reunification. Options include reunification after 5 months, 12 months, and pending status hearing, among others.

Case Study: APPLA: Another Planned Permanent Living Arrangement

Jeremiah was 16 when he entered foster care after his mother died. He had not known his father and did not have any family able to care for him. Jeremiah lived in two different group homes before moving to live with a foster family when he was almost 17 years old. The foster family was an older couple living in his neighborhood. It was a perfect living arrangement and fit for Jeremiah. Jeremiah struggled with the death of his mother and was not ready to be adopted by another family. Given his age and his wishes, he chose to continue his case plan as APPLA. His caseworker would have preferred that he have more of a legal permanency plan of adoption or guardianship; however, Jeremiah was not willing to consider those options. He continued to have an excellent relationship with his caregivers, Anna and Joseph, into adulthood.

Adoption

The goal of adoption is selected when the parental rights of both parents are terminated or relinquished through adoptive surrenders or consents, including consents to adoption by specified persons. In 2019, 26% of children exiting foster care were adopted (US DHHS, 2020). The court must first terminate parental rights following a motion to the court from a party to the case, most often the child welfare agency and/or their legal representative. Adoption needs to be determined to be in the best interest of the child or children. Many jurisdictions also consider the consent of older youth in their own adoption.

Practice Highlight

National Adoption Month

November is National Adoption Month, a month set aside to raise awareness about the need for adoptive families for children and youth in foster care and celebrate adoptions across the country. National Adoption Month began in 1976 when Massachusetts Governor Mike Dukakis announced the first Adoption Week. The idea of having time set aside to create awareness around adoption grew in popularity and spread nationwide. In 1984, President Ronald Reagan proclaimed the first National Adoption Week, and in 1995, under President Bill Clinton, the week was expanded to the entire month of November.

Adoption is a common concurrent case plan goal, after family reunification. Adoption is promoted to ensure a child's relational and legal permanency. When placing a child, a child welfare professional should always consider the case and likelihood of reunification and whether the current placement is one that would consider adoption. These circumstances, however, are very difficult to predict, and planning and having options will help guide the case as it moves forward. When parental rights are severed, a child is free for adoption. Ideally, there should already be a family that is identified who will adopt the child when legal proceedings to sever the parents' rights occur.

There are a number of agencies that specialize in promoting and facilitating private adoptions and adoptions from foster care. For example, AdoptUsKids is an initiative to connect children in foster care who are awaiting adoption with families interested in adoption (Adopt Us Kids 2020). Child welfare professionals who specialize in cases at the adoption phase rely on foster and adoptive agencies, kinship care providers, and foster care providers as the case moves along from foster care to adoption. To ensure a successful adoption, child welfare professionals can do several things. In addition to ensuring that all legal steps have been taken to move forward, caseworkers should consider the fit of the current caregivers as long-term adoptive parents. They should consider whether this is a placement with caregivers who are physically, financially, and emotionally able to care for the child. The child welfare professional should think about what the child and family

Practice Tip

How to Facilitate a Healthy Adoption

- Create a "Lifebook" to help the child understand their past and placement history
- Identity and enlist important attachment figure (e.g., family, caregivers, mentors, etc.)
- Acknowledge the child's preferences and give permission to love another caregiver
- Acknowledge the past and its impact on the future
- Honor and support racial and cultural identity

Practice Tip

Talking to Children About Adoption

- Talk about adoption with *all* children – not just those who are adopted.
- Tell the truth.
- Use age-appropriate language.
- Follow the child's lead and let them ask questions.
- Seek professional help if needed.
- Start talking about adoption as early as possible and as much as necessary.
- Express excitement about the possibility of adoption.

may need during the transition and in the long term to ensure a stable and healthy placement for the child and the caregiver. This requires a thorough assessment and talking with the various players involved (biological parents, potential adoptive parents, providers, the child, and family members). There are benefits to considering foster parent adoption where the child is currently placed, such as maintaining the secure relationship already established; promoting a psychological shift in a sense of identity, connection, and belonging by making the placement permanent; remaining in a familiar school, community, and neighborhood; and having a shorter time to permanency (adoption). It is also important to consider the positive and negative changes that may occur when adoption occurs and the child welfare agency is no longer responsible for monitoring the case. For example, decision-making shifts from the child welfare agency (i.e., caseworker) to the adoptive parents, children and families may lose some of the resources and supports, they no longer have contact with the biological family, and the parents become financially responsible for the child. This points to the need to be forthcoming, honest, and prepared throughout this process.

Child welfare professionals considering placement for adoption with a new family should be honest and open and assist with a thoughtful transition from foster care to adoption. Foster and adoptive parents should talk with children about the transition and use resources available to assist with this process. They should provide all of the information about the child's past, current needs, and resources available during the transition and after the adoption. For all adoptive parents, child welfare professionals should provide information about expectations and the potential impact on their current family unit and extended family, the legal steps, access to the adoption assistance subsidy, federal adoption tax credit, family counseling, and making decisions about maintaining contact with the biological family.

Guardianship

Guardianship involves the transfer of guardianship for the children from the state (or tribe) to an individual or couple. This permanency goal may be selected if reunification and adoption have been ruled out as permanent goals, the children reside with relatives or foster home caregivers with whom they have formed emotional attachments, and these caregivers are willing to accept legal responsibility for the child or children and assume commitment to a permanent relationship that meets the child's or children's needs. The court will typically have to approve and/or order guardianship as a goal for permanency.

Case Study: Guardianship
Eloise, age 15, lived with her grandmother since she was 12. She just became a ward of the court when the temporary power of attorney her mother signed to have her grandmother care for her expired and her mother was unable to be located. Cheryl, her grandmother, wanted Eloise to be reunited with her mother, but her mother did not participate in the services offered by the child welfare agency within the time allotted. Eloise wanted to stay with her grandmother but was always hopeful her mother would return to care for her. She still called occasionally, and Eloise deeply cared for her mother. After several child and family team meetings, it was decided that they would pursue guardianship as the case plan so that Eloise could have permanency and maintain the relationship with her mother.

Practice Highlight

Best Interests of the Child

This term refers to the factors that courts consider when deciding what type of services and actions are needed to best serve a child as well as who should do them. "Best interests" determinations are made by taking into account the child's circumstances as well as the parent or caregiver's circumstances and capacity to parent, with the child's safety and well-being the most important concern.

Some factors considered are as follows:

- The emotional ties and relationships between the child and his or her parents, siblings, family and household members, or other caregivers
- The capacity of the parents to provide a safe home and adequate food, clothing, and medical care
- The mental and physical health needs of the child
- The mental and physical health of the parents
- The presence of domestic violence in the home
- Child's wishes
- Maintaining sibling and other close family bonds
- Federal and/or state constitution protections

Concurrent Permanency Planning

Even when the child welfare agency is working with the family on reunification, it may also implement concurrent planning to ensure that permanency is achieved for the child in as timely a manner as possible and within ASFA guidelines. Concurrent planning involves identifying and working towards a child's primary permanency goal, such as reunification, while simultaneously identifying and working on a secondary goal, such as adoption or guardianship. This practice, when implemented correctly, can shorten the time to achieve permanency because progress has already been made towards the concurrent goal if efforts towards the other goal prove unsuccessful. This provides caseworkers with a structured approach to move children quickly from foster care to the stability of a safe and continuous family home.

It is important to remember that although the child welfare professional and agency are responsible for providing and monitoring service participation and the case, there is also a legal side to permanency planning. When it is determined that the case plan goal should change, child welfare professionals should consult with legal counsel about the grounds for doing so based on state laws and policies. The legal department will make the ultimate decision based on evidence, timing, and case progression. Legal screenings or legal staffings occur when a petition or motion needs to be filed (related to case plan goal changes, placement, etc.). The child welfare professional is responsible for documentation regarding services offered and the parent's progression or lack thereof towards case plan goals. Decisions about these legal processes are often made in consultation with all parties to the case (e.g., guardian ad litem, parents' attorneys, court appointed special advocate [CASA]).

Achieving Permanency

Permanency must be a priority due to the many negative consequences (e.g., health, development, behavior disorders, substance abuse, neurological functioning) when it is not achieved (Fisher et al., 2013). Permanency planning will look different depending on the child and their family. For example, permanency planning is different for older youth. Planning can vary depending on the number of children in the family and their ages and the child's needs. There may be different cultural backgrounds (e.g., Austin et al., 2020). Difference in the child's experiences can also shape planning and options for permanency. For example, some variables that are considered when considering long-term placement options are the number of children in the home, pets, proximity to services (medical and behavioral health), proximity to family, educational needs and preferences, age of caregiver (if a child is very young), age of child, contact with biological family, and social-emotional needs of the child. Every child and caregiver is different; however, best practice is to consider all of the factors and talk to all of the parties about all options to ensure that permanency is successful. The administrative approach and process to achieving permanency is similar across age groups; however there are different strategies to promote permanency among children across age groups.

Practice Highlight:

The Importance of Creating Therapeutic Transition Plans

Libby Fakier, MBA

Over the past 3 ½ years, my family has fostered four sibling sets for periods ranging from 9 months to 2 years. At the outset of our placements, we created a therapeutic environment to help children address their trauma resulting from unpredictable parenting responses, sudden or frequent placement changes, and a sense of general isolation, insecurity, and helplessness. We created a stable, structured home with a predictable routine, clear communication, and plenty of time to adjust to any changes we were told the child would encounter. In addition, we have partnered with members of our faith community and paired our children with supporting mentors who invest time in the kids, take them on outings, act as an additional layer of support, and instill in the child the belief that they are loved, special, and worthy.

Our children's response has been nothing short of miraculous. We've watched them transform from dissociative, frightened, frenetic, detached children to happy, carefree, trusting human beings. Because of the documented success we've experienced, I believe it is imperative that the case management team set up structured, predictable transition periods that allow children to slowly let go of the family they've bonded with while creating healthy bonds with their forever family or birth family. This plan recognizes the child's innate need to hold on to the bonds they've created with the families and mentors who have supported them during their time in care. A successful model includes scheduled communication between the children and the prior foster families and mentors and constant reinforcement from the new family that the children are welcome to reach out to their support systems as often as they need to until they adjust to their new placement or permanency option.

Our experience is the kids want to call and FaceTime daily for the first week or two, and then the frequency slowly subsides in weeks two through five. What makes this model so successful is that it reinforces to the child that he or she has a voice and some element of control over his or her situation. This alone sets the child up psychologically and emotionally to view transition and permanency in a positive, healthy way. This approach is essential to repairing a child's ability to trust and create healthy attachments in the future.

For frontline child welfare professionals, it is important to have adequate training about the community-specific needs that are being served, including culture, history, and the community's relationship with the child welfare system. Child welfare professionals must know who the community includes, what their needs are, and what resources are available to them. Collaboration among multiple systems (education, health care, behavioral and mental health care, etc.) is key when improving permanency outcomes for children in care. (See Chap. 6 for detailed information about collaboration.) A focus on prevention through timely and quality services and supports to parents and children before child welfare system involvement must be considered in permanency. (For further discussion, see Chap. 7 on child maltreatment prevention and family preservation.)

Obtaining permanency for every child can be a challenge in general, and certain populations have a more difficult time with achieving permanency. Older youth, children from racial/ethnic minority groups, children with disabilities and significant health needs, and immigrant/refugee children and youth are populations with lower rates of permanency. Parents working towards reunification may need additional resources and services that are specific to their child or children. This should be a priority for child welfare professionals. Further, as child welfare professionals, there are multiple ways to promote permanency among all children, particularly those identified at risk for not achieving timely permanency when reunification is not possible. For example, child welfare professionals can begin early with permanency planning and concurrent permanency planning options. Children should be placed with families that are a good match for the child's needs as early as possible. Communication with caregivers and youth about permanency options early is important when determining options for the child's permanency. Child welfare agencies can work to recruit and retain a diverse group of foster parents and adoptive parents that are representative of the children and youth in care in their state or jurisdiction.

Factors Influencing Permanency

There are several child- and system-level factors that have been shown to influence permanency outcomes. With regard to children, age, race, physical and mental health, and disabilities are strong predictors. For example, older youth are less likely to achieve permanency compared to younger children (Courtney & Wong, 1996; Snowden et al., 2008). African American children are less likely to be reunified with their biological parents than white children (Connell et al., 2006; Romney et al., 2006). Among older youth, factors such as truancy, running away, and gang membership negatively influence permanency outcomes (Orsi et al., 2018). Family structure and experiences, such as single parenthood, poverty, parental mental health, and substance abuse, have also been shown to play a role in permanency outcomes. Families experiencing mental health and intimate partner violence have been shown to have negative permanency outcomes (Risley-Curtiss et al., 2004), and single parents take longer to reunify when compared with married couples (Courtney, 1994). Some studies have examined the influence of system-level factors such as child welfare professional turnover as well as the influence of substitute caregivers on permanency outcomes. For example, higher turnover rates among case managers have been associated with lower rates of reunification and slower permanency (Davis et al., 1996; Ryan et al., 2006). A recent study conducted by Katz et al. (2018) showed that when respite was available for out-of-home caregivers and communication was positive between child welfare professionals and substitute caregivers, permanency was more likely.

Permanency Planning for Older Youth

Youth represent a subgroup of children involved in the child welfare system that may require a different approach when developing and implementing plans for permanency. Adolescents are less likely to be adopted than children under the age of 5. In 2019, 56% of the adoptions were of children under age 5, and only 10% of adoptions involved children over the age of 13 (US DHHS, 2020). Youth are also more likely to spend more time in care, have more placements while in care, and are more likely to live in congregate care settings. This might be due to systemic issues and agency policies that may not fully promote permanency among older youth. This, however, does not minimize the need for permanency among youth. Research has found that permanency is critical to youths' mental well-being (e.g., McGuire et al., 2018). In fact, youth are in great need for relational and legal permanence through adoption, guardianship, and/or kinship care. Youth in care will benefit from strong relationships, including those with peers (Hu et al., 2020).

Older youth are closer to "aging out of care," meaning many will leave care within a relatively short period of time and will need the guidance and support of caring adults to help prepare them for this transition and equip them with skills to care for themselves independently. In addition, all youth require those long-lasting relationships with family members, caring adults, and peers to rely on when in need. Chapter 11 discusses working with special populations, including older youth in care in more depth; however, this section will focus on permanency for older youth in care.

Several policies focus on promoting permanency and stability for older youth in care, including the Preventing Sex Trafficking and Strengthening Families Act (PSTSFA) of 2014, the Family First Prevention Services Act (FFPSA) of 2018, and, most comprehensively, the Fostering Connections to Success and Increasing Adoptions Act of 2008 (Fostering Connections). Further PSTSFA limits the use of another planned permanent living arrangement (APPLA) to youth age 16 and older, and when used, places certain requirements.

There are numerous barriers to achieving permanency among youth in care. For example, there are myths about older youth in care, such as they might be more likely to have behavioral problems or to run away. On a systems level, caseworkers and administrators might have difficulty in identifying and supporting family-like placements, a lack of resources for youth in care and their providers, and/or a need for education and involvement of youth, staff, and providers about permanency and youth in care.

In order to increase permanency among older youth, agencies should do what they can to involve youth in the permanency planning process. The most important component to consider is involving youth

Policy Brief

Fostering Connections Act and Permanency Among Older Youth

- Requires Title IV-E agencies to identify and notify all adult relatives within 30 days of removal of their option to become a placement resource for a child

- Creates a new plan option to provide kinship guardianship assistance payments under Title IV-E on behalf of children who have been in foster care and have a relative who is taking legal guardianship

- Allows youth who leave foster care for kinship guardianship or adoption after age 16 to receive services under the Chafee Program

- Permits states to extend Title IV-E assistance to otherwise eligible youth remaining in foster care after reaching age 18 and to youth who at age 16 or older exited foster care to either a kinship guardianship or adoption and are in school, employed, or incapable for a medical reason

in the permanency planning process. This helps both the caseworker and the youth with youth bringing ideas to the table while enhancing their self-esteem, self-efficacy, and decision-making skills. Child welfare professionals should prioritize these conversations with youth early and frequently, as appropriate. Similarly, child welfare professionals should begin exploring options with concurrent plans in place and expose youth to various options and individuals they already have or can develop strong, long-lasting relationships with. Caseworkers should allow youth to set their own permanency agenda, including deciding who is invited to meetings, establishing long- and short-term goals, and determining how they want to participate in their case and court hearings.

Child welfare professionals can also strengthen reunification services for youth. Return to family is the preferred case plan goal for most children and youth, and more than half of children in care have a case plan goal of family reunification. Therefore, child welfare professionals can work toward this goal through regular parent-child visits, family and individual therapy, and providing critical services to facilitate family reunification. Further, consider that factors leading to family reunification related to safety are often different for older youth than they are for young children. Even if reunification is not possible while youth are in care, it is possible the youth will return to stay with their biological parents after they leave care. Therefore, it is important to provide services while the child welfare agency is involved to prepare youth and biological parents for this.

> **Practice Highlight**
>
> **Reasons to Adopt a Teen**
>
> - No diapers to change.
> - They sleep through the night.
> - They will move out sooner, but can still visit.
> - Parents don't just get a child; they get a friend.
> - They will keep parents up to date on the latest fashion.
> - No more carpools – they can drive others places!
> - No bottles, formula, or burp rags required.
> - They can help around the house.
> - They can learn from parents.
> - They can help to operate the computer and other devices.

Legal permanency is important to ensure there is a plan for permanency and that all of the formal steps are being taken with court proceedings. However, research shows that relational permanency – connections with caring adults – is paramount to youth well-being (e.g., Salazar et al., 2018). These relationships with caregivers, family, peers, and others are often fractured or discontinued when a child enters care. Child welfare workers can help to establish new and maintain existing relationships through mentoring programs, reducing placement instability, providing opportunities to visit family and friends, and communicating with them regularly. This not only helps with improving youth's mental health and well-being but also provides a group of individuals that support the youth and their permanency through placement, guidance, and relationships.

Child welfare professionals can also promote relationships with kin and fictive kin to optimize permanency options and decisions. By promoting communication and contact with kin, relationships develop further and can become options for placement, deeper connections, and permanency for youth. One method to seek out relatives is called Family Finding, where youth work with their caseworker to identify family members and explore relationships with them. Child welfare professionals can also promote guardianship as a permanency option vs. only viewing adoption as the optimal permanency option. Many youth would prefer not to be adopted as a teenager or choose to have less formal arrangements in their placement.

Systemically, the child welfare system can improve how they establish permanency for youth. For example, child welfare agencies can work toward recruiting more nonrelative foster and adoptive families for older youth. Older youth may have different needs and have different skills and qualities to bring to that relationship that should be highlighted. Agencies can specifically recruit a different demographic or group of foster parents who choose to foster older youth. Further, educating the workforce and the public about the needs of older youth in foster care, an opportunity to foster and adopt older youth, and about some of the ways we have discussed how approaching permanency differs for older youth is a step toward improving permanency for this subgroup in care. Child welfare agencies can work toward evaluating policies that impact youth and work closely with personnel in the court system (e.g., judges, attorneys, CASAs, etc.) to determine best practices when working with older youth and prioritizing relational and legal permanency.

Family-Centered Practice

Family-centered practice in child welfare, as discussed in Chap. 6 at length, is a theoretical framework that informs practice with families (Briar-Lawson et al., 2001; Epley et al., 2010) and sets forth a set of principles guiding prevention, assessment, and intervention with families identified at risk for child abuse and/or neglect. Family-centered practice provides guidance during various stages of child welfare practice that involves establishing a relationship and rapport with families, ensuring safety, permanency, and well-being that prioritizes the family in terms of its strengths and needs. Adopting a family-centered approach means focusing on the family unit, engaging and preserving the family when possible, and drawing on the family's strengths and resources to assist with change.

The permanency options and strategies discussed earlier are consistent with a family-centered approach. When the family is prioritized, planning and decision-making involves all family members, and the professional-family relationship is critical in creating healthy change. Implementation of family-centered practice is often cited as the foundation to child welfare agencies' missions; however, family-centered practice is not always infused into child welfare practice due to a variety of conflicting policies and protocols, lack of training, and other organizational factors. In order for child welfare professionals and the agencies they work with to truly adopt a family-centered approach to practice in general and in matters of permanency, a major shift will require federal and state policies, court systems, and approaches to case management, and the provision of services will have to be reinforced on multiple levels.

Practice Tip

Talking to Youth in Care About Permanency

Begin planning early and keep conversation going

Use words youth understand

Explain the meaning of adoption and permanency

Assess and be aware of your own thoughts and attitudes

Keep in mind that the word "adoption" can be perceived as negative

Support youth in understanding and exploring options

Consider engaging family and team members in planning

Involve youth in their own recruitment for caregivers

Consider whether everyone has done everything they can to support permanency

---

Foster Care Re-entry

Foster care re-entry refers to the recurrence of child maltreatment after an earlier episode of out-of-home care that resulted in reunification with biological family. Federal mandates require that states track and report the percentage of children who re-enter foster care within 12 months of reunification with their biological families. Although varying, estimates for foster care re-entry show that 10–30% of children will come back into contact with the child welfare system within 12 months of reunification (U.S. DHHS, 2020; Wulczyn et al., 2000 Wulczyn et al., 2020). Risk for re-entry is greater among infants and older youth (Wulczyn et al., 2020).

There are a number of child, parent, and environmental factors that increase the risk of a child re-entering foster care following reunification with biological parents. For example, child's age (younger children, preteens, and teenagers) and the presence of a disability and educational, mental health, developmental, or behavioral problems increase the risk of foster care re-entry as well as parental substance abuse and mental health conditions (Lee et al., 2012). Further, factors such as receipt of benefits and placement with relatives were associated with lower risk of re-entry (Lee et al., 2012).

Foster care re-entry is unpredictable, and many factors play a role in the likelihood of its occurrence. Foster care re-entry can be extremely traumatic and harmful for a child (Berrick et al., 1998; Rzepnicki, 1987). There are, however, some things that child welfare professionals and child welfare agencies can do to reduce the likelihood of foster care re-entry, such as ensuring proper family assessment, case planning, and follow-up with families. Professionals can assess for parental readiness and ambivalence about reunification while finding ways to increase engagement and stability. Child welfare agencies can provide intensive services during the reunification stage to support the transition home and ensure all of the families' needs are being met.

Practice Highlight

Returning to Foster Care

As a child welfare professional, a big part of the job is helping a child achieve permanency. While they are in care, they experience a lot of changes and often feel confused and uncertain about what will happen next. People often think of permanency as adoption, but permanency is really finding a permanent home or placement. It is legal permanency – the court orders, but also relational permanency – the people and the relationships. This could be adoption with a relative, a foster-adopt family, guardianship with a relative or fictive kin, or reunification with one's family of origin. The goal is not just finding a good permanent placement for the child. It is fostering relationships that will create the right circumstances for the placement to be permanent. That means getting the right services in place before an adoption and making sure the transition home is a healthy one.

One of the hardest things to see when working in child welfare is having a child come back into foster care after going home after being reunited or having an adoption or guardianship not work out. We can't judge the caregiver's decision or choices that caused this to happen, but we see the hurt and disappointment in the child's eyes. These circumstances often leave a child feeling shame, blame, hurt, confused, and at fault. There are many reasons this happens and these feelings often linger. The best we can do is get it right the first time and be as supportive as possible during the transition. There are going to be times when we can't control the circumstances or the hurt. Recognizing the impact of these events on children is critical, and reassuring them we will work to make it better does make a difference.

Conclusion

Ensuring timely permanency for all children and families is critical in child welfare. There are different options for permanency outcomes that vary depending on the case, the child, and the family. The child welfare professional can promote permanency by understanding the child and their needs and making sure the parents have access to services to be able to achieve reunification. In cases where reunification is not possible and when another option is appropriate for permanency, the child welfare professional can use various strategies in helping a child and family prepare for the transition.

Acknowledgments The authors thank Libby Fakier, MBA, for the contribution to Chap. 10.

Discussion Questions

1. What are the two most common permanency outcomes for children in care?
2. What is one federal policy that governs permanency for children in care?
3. What factors are considered in determining the best interests of the child?
4. What are two reasons to adopt a teen from foster care?
5. Under what circumstances should child welfare professionals consider guardianship over adoption?

Suggested Activities

1. Research what your state is doing to promote permanency (reunification and adoption). Think of 2–3 ways that your state and/or child welfare agency could work towards better permanency outcomes in general, for youth, and for children with special needs.
2. Make a list of agencies that recruit and train foster and adoptive parents in your community. What are some services they provide? How could they improve the number of children who need a permanent placement?
3. Read the investigative reporting coverage of "The Child Exchange" https://www.reuters.com/investigates/adoption/#article/part1, and write a reflection paper. Consider exploring how child welfare can learn from the failures of permanency in the international adoptions presented in the report and what we need in society to keep all children safe.
4. Read Austin et al. (2020). Consider the risk and protective factors presented about Alaska Native/American Indian children and non-native children. Write a reflection paper exploring how these factors could be considered in determining permanency for the groups of children.

Austin, A. E., Gottfredson, N. C., Marshall, S. W., Halpern, C. T., Zolotor, A. J., Parrish, J. W., & Shanahan, M. E. (2020). Heterogeneity in risk and protection among Alaska Native/American Indian and non-native children. *Prevention Science, 21*(1), 86–97. https://doi.org/10.1007/s11121-019-01052-y (Available: https://rdcu.be/ccglr).

Additional Resources

Adopt US Kids: https://adoptuskids.org/
Annie E. Casey Foundation: https://www.aecf.org/
Child Welfare Information Gateway, Achieving and Maintaining Permanency: https://www.childwelfare.gov/topics/permanency/

Juvenile Law Center, What is "Permanency" and Why should you Care?: https://jlc.
    org/news/what-permanency-and-why-should-you-care
Child Welfare Information Gateway, National Adoption Month: https://www.
    childwelfare.gov/topics/adoption/nam/
National Center for Youth Law, Promoting Permanency for Teens: A 50 State
    Review of Law and Policy: https://youthlaw.org/wp-content/uploads/2018/02/
    Promoting-Permanency-for-Teens.pdf

References

Adopt Us Kids. (2020). *Information*. Available: https://www.adoptuskids.org/
Austin, A. E., Gottfredson, N. C., Marshall, S. W., Halpern, C. T., Zolotor, A. J., Parrish, J. W., &
    Shanahan, M. E. (2020). Heterogeneity in risk and protection among Alaska Native/American
    Indian and non-native children. *Prevention Science, 21*(1), 86–97. https://doi.org/10.1007/
    s11121-019-01052-y
Berrick, J. D., Needell, B., Barth, R. P., & Jonson-Reid, M. (1998). *The tender years: Toward devel-
    opmentally sensitive child welfare services for very young children*. Oxford University Press.
Briar-Lawson, K., Lawson, H. A., Hennon, C., & Jones, A. (2001). The meaning and signifi-
    cance of families and threats to their well-being. In *Family-centered policies and practices*
    (pp. 21–24). Columbia University. https://doi.org/10.7312/bria12106-003
Connell, C. M., Katz, K. H., Saunders, L., & Tebes, J. K. (2006). Leaving foster care-the influence
    of child and case characteristics on foster care exit rates. *Children and Youth Services Review,
    28*(7), 780–798. https://doi.org/10.1016/j.childyouth.2005.08.007
Courtney, M. E. (1994). Factors associated with the reunification of foster children with their fami-
    lies. *Social Service Review, 68*(1), 81–108. https://doi.org/10.1086/604034
Courtney, M. E., & Wong, Y. L. I. (1996). Comparing the timing of exits from substitute care. *Children
    and Youth Services Review, 18*(4–5), 307–334. https://doi.org/10.1016/0190-7409(96)00008-4
Davis, I. P., Landsverk, J., Newton, R., & Ganger, W. (1996). Parental visiting and foster
    care reunification. *Children and Youth Services Review, 18*(4–5), 363–382. https://doi.
    org/10.1016/0190-7409(96)00010-2
Epley, P., Summers, J. A., & Turnbull, A. (2010). Characteristics and trends in family-
    centered conceptualizations. *Journal of Family Social Work, 13*(3), 269–285. https://doi.
    org/10.1080/10522150903514017
Fisher, P. A., Mannering, A. M., Van Scoyoc, A., & Graham, A. M. (2013). A translational neuro-
    science perspective on the importance of reducing placement instability among foster children.
    Child Welfare, 92(5), 9.
Hu, A., Van Ryzin, M. J., Schweer-Collins, M. L., & Leve, L. D. (2020). Peer relations and delin-
    quency among girls in foster care following a skill-building preventive intervention. *Child
    Maltreatment, 26*(2), 205–215. https://doi.org/10.1177/1077559520923033
Katz, C. C., Lalayants, M., & Phillips, J. D. (2018). The role of out-of-home caregivers in the
    achievement of child welfare permanency. *Children and Youth Services Review, 94*, 65–71.
    https://doi.org/10.1016/j.childyouth.2018.09.016
Lee, S., Jonson-Reid, M., & Drake, B. (2012). Foster care re-entry: Exploring the role of foster
    care characteristics, in-home child welfare services and cross-sector services. *Children and
    Youth Services Review, 34*(9), 1825–1833. https://doi.org/10.1016/j.childyouth.2012.05.007
McGuire, A., Cho, B., Huffhines, L., Gusler, S., Brown, S., & Jackson, Y. (2018). The relation
    between dimensions of maltreatment, placement instability, and mental health among youth
    in foster care. *Child Abuse & Neglect, 86*, 10–21. https://doi.org/10.1016/j.chiabu.2018.08.012

Orsi, R., Lee, C., Winokur, M., & Pearson, A. (2018). Who's been served and how? Permanency outcomes for children and youth involved in child welfare and youth corrections. *Youth Violence and Juvenile Justice, 16*(1), 3–17. https://doi.org/10.1177/1541204017721614

Risley-Curtiss, C., Stromwall, L. K., Hunt, D. T., & Teska, J. (2004). Identifying and reducing barriers to reunification for seriously mentally ill parents involved in child welfare cases. *Families in Society, 85*(1), 107–118. https://doi.org/10.1606/1044-3894.240

Romney, S. C., Litrownik, A. J., Newton, R. R., & Lau, A. (2006). The relationship between child disability and living arrangement in child welfare. *Child Welfare, 85*(6), 965–984.

Ryan, J. P., Garnier, P., Zyphur, M., & Zhai, F. (2006). Investigating the effects of caseworker characteristics in child welfare. *Children and Youth Services Review, 28*(9), 993–1006. https://doi.org/10.1016/j.childyouth.2005.10.013

Rzepnicki, T. L. (1987). Recidivism of foster children returned to their own homes: A review and new directions for research. *Social Service Review, 61*(1), 56–70. https://doi.org/10.1086/644418

Salazar, A. M., Jones, K. R., Amemiya, J., Cherry, A., Brown, E. C., Catalano, R. F., & Monahan, K. C. (2018). Defining and achieving permanency among older youth in foster care. *Children and Youth Services Review, 87*, 9–16. https://doi.org/10.1016/j.childyouth.2018.02.006

Snowden, J., Leon, S., & Sieracki, J. (2008). Predictors of children in foster care being adopted: A classification tree analysis. *Children and Youth Services Review, 30*(11), 1318–1327. https://doi.org/10.1016/j.childyouth.2008.03.014

U.S. Department of Health & Human Services (2020). *The AFSCARS report*. https://www.acf.hhs.gov/sites/default/files/cb/afcarsreport27.pdf

Wulczyn, F., Hislop, K. B., & Goerge, R. M. (2000). *Foster care dynamics 1983–1998*. Chapin Hall Center for Children.

Wulczyn, F., Parolini, A., Schmits, F., Magruder, J., & Webster, D. (2020). Returning to foster care: Age and other risk factors. *Children and Youth Services Review, 116*, 105166. https://doi.org/10.1016/j.childyouth.2020.105166

Chapter 11
Special Populations in Child Welfare Practice

Introduction

There are a number of groups within child welfare that may require a different approach or specialized knowledge, training, or experience to work with effectively. One subgroup is children and youth with disabilities involved with the child welfare system. They may differ greatly when compared to other youth in care. Assessment, services, and permanency may affect children with physical or other disabilities as well as children with complex medical needs differently than other children. Another group that has unique needs are youth aging out or youth who have transitioned from care and have chosen to participate in extended foster programming. They are a subgroup within child welfare that require a special skill set and who also may receive specialized services and supports as youth in care. Immigrant and refugee children and families are another unique group who come in contact with the child welfare system. There are several differences in how child welfare professionals work with children and families who are refugees or immigrants, which can vary based on the state we live it, the culture and nationality of the family child welfare professionals work with, and the needs of the family. Child welfare professionals also may find that working with sibling groups requires a different approach and additional skills. Another group in child welfare that requires special skills and approach is children who have been involved in human and sex trafficking. Within any of these groups, there is going to be great variation, and each child and family should be seen as individuals; yet child welfare professionals understanding commonalities within a subgroup can facilitate a more efficient and appropriate response.

© Springer Nature Switzerland AG 2021
J. M. Geiger, L. Schelbe, *The Handbook on Child Welfare Practice*,
https://doi.org/10.1007/978-3-030-73912-6_11

Children and Youth with Disabilities and Special Needs

Children with disabilities are a subset of vulnerable children involved with the child welfare system. It is estimated that one out of 10 children nationwide and half of the children in the social service system has a physical, mental, emotional, or developmental disability and that half of the children within our country's social service system (Lightfoot et al., 2011). Disabilities are defined as temporary or permanent physical or intellectual disabilities present at birth or acquired later. It is estimated that approximately 50 percent of the 50,000 children available for adoption in the United States have a disability and half of all foster children have developmental delays (Glidden, 2000). Child welfare professionals are in critical positions to recognize the signs of developmental delays, to ensure proper referrals for evaluation, and to help families access related services. It is important for child welfare professionals to have an understanding of the definitions of such disabilities and how specific state and federal statutes treat such a disability or condition with regard to services, case planning, and court proceedings. Child welfare professionals should be prepared to identify and assess for such conditions and refer and monitor services to address those challenges. Interactions, such as interviewing, visiting, meeting, with children with disabilities may also differ, and caseworkers should be adaptable and flexible to such accommodations. They also could benefit from training on how to develop working relationships with agencies that provide early intervention and special education services. Partnering with these agencies and other professionals is important due to their expertise in assessment for children with specific needs. For example, children diagnosed with autism spectrum disorders may have symptoms that are overlapping with trauma symptoms; thus having the ability to differentiate and develop a treatment plan will require professionals with advanced training (Van Scoyoc et al., 2018).

Children with disabilities are more likely to experience maltreatment and have substantiated maltreatment cases than children without a disability. Further, children with emotional and behavioral disorders and children with developmental disabilities are more likely than those with other types of disabilities (Jonson-Reid et al., 2004; Lightfoot et al., 2011). Children with disabilities are more likely to experience neglect than other types of maltreatment, with neglect being related to their disability (e.g., withholding medication or necessary device or equipment).

Especially in the cases where there is a child experiencing developmental delays or disabilities, it is important to understand ways to support children and their families at various stages of a case to be able to provide early, appropriate, and consistent services. (See Chap. 3 for an in-depth discussion of child development; it identified indicators of developmental delays and disabilities and described how to ensure proper assessment and service provision.) Services designed for children with disabilities and their families often involve a number of individuals, stages, and a series of approvals as well as insurance coverage. Services should always be culturally grounded, trauma-informed, and family-centered. That means that support should be offered within the context of the family and the community in which they live.

Families (biological and substitute parents) are often a key part in supports and services designed for children with disabilities.

It is important to consider the impact of a child's disability on a family throughout a case. For example, during the investigation stage, parents and families may experience difficulty in balancing the demands of caring for a child with disabilities. There are often financial, social, emotional, and physical barriers to optimal care for a child with disabilities. This may lead to increased stress on the parent and family, which increases the risk for child maltreatment. Families often report feeling socially isolated, overburdened, and overwhelmed by the demands associated with the care and coordination of a child with disabilities. It is also important to note that disability and its cases are perceived differently among different socioeconomic, ethnic, racial, and organizational cultures and these groups and systems respond differently to acceptance and provision of support and services for families caring for children with disabilities. When a child with disabilities enters foster care, there may be different plans and provisions for ensuring their safety, permanency, and well-being. Further, children with disabilities may require specialized placement, care, and supervision.

Child welfare professionals can help to support biological families and substitute caregivers by understanding the child's disability and needs, help to identify strengths, set realistic expectations for the case plan, support a healthy environment for the child, and act as a liaison between the foster family and biological family to ensure both are aware of the care provided and to promote family reunification and permanency.

It is essential that the child welfare professional integrate multiple service providers and representatives from various systems to participate in child and family team meetings and communicate regularly with those parties to ensure the child's needs are being met. Child welfare professionals should be in touch regularly with any speech, occupational, or physical therapists, mental health professionals, physical health-care providers, and in-home supports. In addition, it is likely the child requires an individual educational plan (IEP) and supports at school, which child welfare professionals will be required to be a part. As child welfare profes-

---

Practice Highlight

The Role of the Child Welfare Professional when Working with Children with Disabilities and their Family

- Conduct a comprehensive assessment of the child and family
- Identify, coordinate, and monitor services for the child and family
- Identify the child and family's strengths and resources
- Advocate for the child and family
- Assist families to identify services and supports in their community

---

sionals learn more about the child's disabilities and needs, they are able to respond in a way that facilitates communication, comfort, and understanding. When interacting with the child, it is important to understand how they communicate, what they are and are not able to physically do, and what their daily living looks like. Communicating and interacting with the child directly shows care, respect, and concern for their well-being.

When children with disabilities who are involved with the child welfare system are in the home with biological parents or are ready to be reunified with their family, it is important to promote continuity of care and supports to ensure stability and permanency for the child. In order to do this, professionals working with the family should involve the family in treatment, promote family interaction, provide education about the child's needs, increase involvement of extended family and the family network as appropriate, and help the family in accessing supports in the community.

Achieving Permanency for Children with Disabilities

Achieving permanency for children with disabilities can be challenging. Children with disabilities often have greater needs and require additional time and services, which may include additional costs or investments on behalf of the caregiver. Caregivers may need to have additional training, resources, or equipment. However, many foster and adoptive parents are willing and able to provide a long-term placement for children with disabilities. States and child welfare agencies have been working towards providing additional training, support, and resources to ensure permanency for children with disabilities.

Not all children and cases are alike. Cases involving children with disabilities require additional practice competencies among child welfare professionals. When working with children with disabilities in foster care, child welfare professionals should be prepared to identify and coordinate specialized care as recommended by professionals. Children may need specialized medical care, developmental assessments, special education and supports, psychological or psychiatric services, financial assistance, and recreational programming. These may be services the child welfare agency is already contracted with to provide services; however, it may be that the child's caseworker must find an appropriate service provider to meet the needs of the child and/or their caregiver. These services should be assessed for and monitored throughout the case, including at the time of adoption.

Disabilities include mental, emotional, intellectual, and behavioral health challenges as well. Child welfare professionals should be prepared to identify and assess for such conditions and refer and monitor services to address those challenges. Interactions, such as interviewing, visiting, and meeting with children with disabilities, may also differ, and caseworkers should be adaptable and flexible to such accommodations.

LGBTQ Youth

Lesbian, gay, bisexual, transgender, queer, or questioning (LGBTQ) youth are overrepresented in the child welfare system. An estimated 15.5% of all child welfare system involved youth ages 11 or older identified as lesbian, gay, or bisexual

(Dettlaff et al., 2018). Lesbian and bisexual females as well as LGB youth of color are overrepresented in the child welfare system. An analysis of a nationally representative sample of children and youth found LGBTQ youth are almost 2.5 times likely as their heterosexual peers to be in foster care and are overrepresented in receiving child welfare services (Fish et al., 2019). One study of children and youth in foster care in Los Angeles found almost one-fifth (10%) identify as LGBTQ (Wilson et al., 2014).

The reasons that LGBTQ youth enter the child welfare system are varied, yet most of the reasons are similar to the reasons their heterosexual and cisgender peers become involved in the child welfare system. The sexual orientation, gender identity, or gender expression of LGBTQ youth may be one of the reasons they entered care. One study found more than two in five LGBTQ youth (44%) attributed their sexual orientation or gender identity as being related to the reason they were placed in out-of-home care (Ryan et al., 2009). These youth could have been maltreated by family due to the youth's identity or orientation by either being rejected or physically abused. The youth may have run away from their homes due to safety concerns.

Within the child welfare system, LGBTQ youth may experience problems with permanency and continued violence. LGBTQ youth have been found to have lower rates of permanency. LGBTQ youth experience have been found to have more movement among placements (Wilson et al., 2014). LGBTQ youth are more likely than their heterosexual peers to age out of the child welfare system (Courtney et al., 2010). There are higher rates of LGBTQ youth running away from placements. Many LGBTQ experience verbal harassment or physical violence when they are in foster care.

In many regards working with LGBTQ youth is like working with any other youth involved with the child welfare system. Their needs for safety, permanency, and well-being are the same as other youths' needs. However, their experiences as an LGBTQ youth may also have created circumstances different than their heterosexual peers in foster care (e.g., reasons for entering care, trauma due to abuse related to being LGBTQ). They may be facing homophobia and heterosexism and dealing with issues related to coming out. LGBTQ youth should be accepted for who they are, and they should be supported in their self-expression. There have been innovated initiatives such as the RISE Care Coordination Team that specifically integrate LGBTQ-specific education and support strategies to assist youth in care (Lorthridge et al., 2018). The Child Welfare League of America has practice recommendations for serving LGBT youth in out-of-home care which encourages child welfare agencies to adopt nondiscrimination policies and make sure to have protocols that address the needs of LGBT youth (Wilber et al., 2006).

Child welfare professionals have the obligation to understand how best to serve LGBTQ youth. This begins by adopting a stance where discrimination of any type, including homophobia and heterosexism, is not tolerated. LGBTQ youth notice when adults in their lives either use or do not address homophobic statements or name-calling. It is important for child welfare professionals to create a safe space for LGBTQ youth and communicate that they are affirming of people of all sexual orientations, gender identities, and gender expressions. To communicate this, child welfare professionals may display "hate-free zones" or signs that denote a safe space such as rainbow flags in their workspace. More importantly, child welfare professionals can signal that they are accepting by using inclusive language and not making assumptions. For example, when asking about romantic relationships, use gender-neutral language and do not assume that the relationship is heterosexual. Child welfare professionals can ask "are you dating someone?" rather than "do you have a boyfriend/girlfriend?" It is important that child welfare professionals use the youth's requested name and pronouns, even when these may be different than what parents or others have used.   When working with LGBTQ youth, child welfare professionals should refer to services that serving people from diverse sexual orientations and gender identities. Some LGBTQ youth may wish for services where they can explore their sexual orientation, gender identify, and gender expression. This could be in school with a gay-straight alliance group, a community center for LGBTQ people, or a therapist. It is important for child welfare professionals to be able to identify these appropriate resources. Above all, conversation therapy or any other intervention that seeks to change someone's sexual orientation or gender identity should never be used, as these interventions have been found to be extremely harmful (SAMHSA, 2015).

Research Brief

Pregnant and Parenting Foster Youth
Justin S. Harty, MSW, LCSW

Youth in foster care often have life experiences that increase the likelihood of them becoming pregnant (or for males getting a female pregnant). Furthermore, young parenthood among youth in foster care is difficult and may lead to adverse outcomes and conditions that make their transition to adulthood difficult.

Research has found several factors associated with early pregnancy among foster youth. Risk factors increasing the likelihood of early pregnancy among foster youth include being maltreated, experiencing trauma, early sexual intercourse, running away from placement, and low social supports. Sexual health education, family planning education, access to contraception, and having social connections with adults are some protective factors associated with lower probabilities of early pregnancy among this population.

The stress and struggles of parenting while in foster care are compounded by difficulties that foster youth in general experience such as victimization, behavioral problems, mental health issues, low educational attainment, employment difficulties, and housing instability. These added stressors may explain risks associated with early parenthood among youth in care such as lower educational attainment, decreased employment, homelessness, increased reliance on public assistance, and increased risk for maltreatment and child welfare involvement of their children.

Early pregnancy and parenthood among foster care youth are further complicated by three concurrent transitions they must face as they reach the age of majority. First, these youth are approaching an age where they must exit the foster care system and lose related care and support. Second, these youth must prepare for a transition to adulthood at an early age and without the preparedness and supports their non-foster care peers often have. Third, they have the added stressor of being a young parent, often without the support, preparation, and resources to be the kind of parent they desire to be.

There are strategies that child welfare practitioners can use to help prepare and support pregnant and parenting foster youth for young parenthood, including the following:

- Understanding the risk and protective factors associated with early pregnancy and parenthood and target prevention and services accordingly
- Knowing that not all pregnancies are unintentional and talking to youth about their desire to become pregnant as well as their reproductive rights
- For pregnancies that do not lead to childbirth, talking to parents about child loss and monitoring how the loss of a child may affect youth
- Talking to young parents about pre-/postnatal health, pediatric child health, and safe and appropriate childcare
- Discussing services and supports for youth designed to increase parenting skills, knowledge, and resources (including extended foster care if available)
- Understanding how young parenthood may affect youths' ability to meet requirements of extended foster care (if available)
- Connecting youth with financial, emotional, mental health, social, and parenting support that will help improve parent- and child-related outcomes
- Allowing youth to participate in normative activities that will help them develop as young parents
- Considering that the needs of fathers in care differ from mothers in care and tailor services for fathers appropriately

Youth Aging Out/Transition-Age Youth

Nationally, there are an estimated 400,000 children in the foster care system as a result of child maltreatment, with 28% between the ages of 12 and 18 (US DHHS, 2020). In the United States each year, it is estimated that about 20,000 youth "age out" of the foster care system when they are no longer eligible for services because of their age or reach the age of majority and decide to leave care. Youth transitioning into adulthood from the foster care system experience significant difficulties in adjusting to independent living. They also have overall poorer outcomes related to psychosocial adjustment, physical and mental health, financial stability, and early childbearing and pregnancy in addition to low educational attainment, homelessness, and poverty than children who have never been in foster care (e.g., Courtney et al., 2010). The heterogeneity among youth aging out means that there is a need for individualized transition planning and services offered (Miller et al., 2017).

The transition to adulthood is a period in life of particular heightened stress and uncertainty that includes critical decision-making related to relationships and career. This time is generally more difficult for youth in care because of their experiences involving traumatic events, emotional and social instability, and the lack of preparation for the transition. In addition, youth in care are expected to make this transition sooner, more quickly, and without parental support (Antle, et al., 2009; Sullivan, et al., 2010). Youth in care may not be engaged in school and experience educational difficulties (Mihalec-Adkins & Cooley, 2020). They graduate from high school at a lower rate and often lack the life skills, work experience, and the emotional and financial support other youth have (Dworsky & Perez, 2010; Greeson & Bowen, 2008). Youth in care often lose their housing, health insurance, and financial assistance upon reaching the age of eighteen (Antle et al., 2009). During this time, many youth in care are embracing the freedom they did not have while in state care and struggle with the responsibilities associated with this newfound independence. Youth in care are often ill-prepared to live on their own and to financially support themselves and are less likely to pursue postsecondary education (Courtney et al., 2010). Many are unemployed, become homeless within months of "aging out" of the foster care system, and experience mental health and substance abuse issues. Youth in care may have difficulty achieving financial stability as a result of low educational attainment, lack of employment, and overall independent living skill preparation. Despite research indicating postsecondary aspirations of youth in care, it is estimated that 7–13% of youth enroll in higher education, with approximately 3–5% of young adults with foster care histories going on to earn a bachelor's degree compared with a third of the general population (Courtney et al., 2010). The known financial and social benefits of postsecondary education are well documented; however there are few programs promoting education among youth in care in the United States (Dworsky & Perez, 2010; Geiger et al., 2018). Without education and adequate preparation to live independently, foster youth are at risk of living in poverty.

Youth in foster care have similar and very distinct needs from their same-aged peers who are not in foster care. They share many of the same developmental processes and want to be part of a family and have friends and romantic relationships. They want to experience normal adolescent experiences that their peers who are not in care have, such as dating, having a job, going to camp, and obtaining a driver's license. Being in care, however, can also create barriers to having these experiences. For example, some child welfare policies do not allow for youth to have sleepovers with friends, have a job, or drive a car. Child welfare professionals can play a key role in easing the transition to adulthood through early, consistent, and intentional development and implementation of case planning, setting goals, and service provision. They can also consider ways they can promote "normal" adolescent experiences for youth in care. Service provision during adolescence for youth in care can help them be ready for adulthood responsibilities; however, ensuring youth have long-term, supportive relationships is even more critical to ensure that youth have people in their lives they can count on to support them and serve as a safety net of sorts when they need them.

Federal law requires that the child welfare agency assist the youth in developing a personalized transition plan during the 90-day period before a youth turns 18 or is scheduled to leave foster care; however it is recommended that this planning occurs as early as possible to ensure referrals and services are in place when a youth turns 18. The plan must address specific options related to housing, education, employment, health insurance, mentoring, and support services. To develop the plan, the youth's caseworker will typically meet with the youth as well as other trusted adults of the youth's choosing,

Practice Tip

Ways to Help Youth with Transition to Adulthood

- Help to build supportive relationships and connections.
- Help youth to manage money.
- Encourage and support youth in pursuing educational and vocational opportunities.
- Provide opportunities for youth to find and maintain employment.
- Help youth secure safe and affordable housing.
- Support youth in maintaining physical and mental health wellness.
- Help youth in exploring identity and culture.

which may include a foster parent or another supportive adult. While the law refers to a 90-day period, most youth will benefit from more time to prepare.

Research Brief

The Risk of Suicidal Behavior for Transition-Age Youth in Foster Care

Colleen Cary Katz, PhD, LCSW

Youth who are preparing to emancipate from foster care are more likely than their peers in the general population to report suicidal ideation and attempt (Courtney et al., 2014). In a recent study of youth emancipating from care in California, over 40% of the participating youth reported having contemplated suicide and 24% reported having attempted suicide when they were asked at age 17 (Courtney et al., 2014). Rates appear to be even higher for female-identified participants, with 51% reporting past ideation and 30% reporting at least one past suicide attempt. These rates are alarming, especially in light of the fact that mental health service utilization tends to drop as youth formally emancipate from the system (Brown et al., 2015; Butterworth et al., 2017).

High rates of suicidal behavior are likely a result of interacting risk factors present in the lives of these youth. First, nearly all youth in the foster care system have a history of child maltreatment (U.S. DHHS, 2020), with many reporting more than one form (Havlicek, 2014; Katz et al., 2017). Youth who have a history of child maltreatment are known to be at enhanced risk for suicidal behavior, especially those youth with experiences of sexual maltreatment

(Norman et al., 2012; Ullman & Najdowski, 2009). This finding may relate to the high rates of ideation and attempt in girls, as they are more likely than boys to report past sexual maltreatment (Courtney et al., 2014). Second, relatedly, studies have shown that one third to one half of all youth preparing to emancipate from care have a mental health or behavioral health disorder, with major depression and substance abuse being two of the most common (McMillen et al., 2005; Courtney et al., 2016). Mental illness is the most robust predictor of suicidal behavior in the general population, with both depressive disorders and substance abuse disorders placing youth at particularly heightened risk (Cash & Bridge, 2009). Third, the transition from foster care is known to be extremely stressful, particularly if youth have inadequate social support to call upon when challenges arise (Iglehart & Becerra, 2002; Cunningham & Diversi, 2013; Samuels, 2008). Both stress and lack of social support are known risk factors for suicidal behavior (Zhang et al., 2012; Kleinman & Liu, 2013).

Despite these known risks, most youth who are preparing to transition from foster care are not routinely or systematically assessed for mental illness and suicidal behavior. While some youth may be known to child welfare staff as high risk, suicidal behavior in others may go undetected (especially when youth are high-functioning in other areas of their lives). Frontline child welfare caseworkers and independent living program staff members can access evidence-supported assessment tools that could enable the timely detection of suicidal behavior in the youth they are serving. Tools such as the Columbia Suicide Severity Rating Scale (Posner et al., 2011), the Suicide Behaviors Questionnaire-Revised (Osman et al., 2001), and the Adolescent Suicide Questionnaire (Horowitz et al., 2012) are some of the most appropriate assessment tools for use with youth preparing to emancipate from care. Child welfare professionals can save lives by referring these youth to appropriate mental health treatment once risk for suicidal behavior has been detected.

Transition planning is a process and requires thought, support, and guidance. A transition plan should include long- and short-term goals and objectives that the youth, caseworker, and provider can work toward. Transition plans should also include important documents (e.g., birth certificate, social security card, state ID or driver's license, health insurance information, and medical records). As with all matters concerning the youth, they should be engaged in the planning and execution of the transition plan. This can often be challenging, as with all youth, in considering options, making decisions about the future, and following through with plans.

Supporting Youth During the Transition

There are a number of ways that child welfare professionals can assist young people with the transition into adulthood. First, it is critical that they help youth to establish and build supportive relationships and connections with caring adults, family, and friends. When youth experience the grief and loss of being separated from their family, friends, and community, many have not had the opportunity to develop the social skills necessary that comes with safety and stability. A child welfare professional can ask youth to identify one reliable, caring adult in their life such as a teacher, coach, foster parent, or another person and help them make that connection through support and opportunities for connection. Many youth will benefit from a mentor, extra time with a family member, joining a group or team, or being involved with CASA or Big Brothers, Big Sisters. Many youth will return to their biological families upon their 18th birthday, so it is important to explore ways that youth can improve family relationships with the support of therapy or extended visitation while they are still in care. Case managers can have conversations about romantic relationships and have discussions about healthy relationships, sex, and plans for the future. Some youth transitioning out of foster care may be parenting, and the needs of the young family should be taken into consideration (Eastman et al., 2017).

Many young people struggle with managing money as they transition into adulthood and face challenges related to making ends meet, paying bills, and accessing financial support. Child welfare professionals can refer youth to programming that offers firsthand experience along with instruction on how to save, balance a checking account, invest, and make good choices with money. They can also use moments in conversations to talk about smart shopping, paying bills, and what credit is, establishing credit, and using credit. Additionally, child welfare professionals can help youth open bank accounts before they age out and help them to develop a budget in real time and when planning for the future.

Postsecondary education and training promote social mobility, especially for many marginalized populations and vulnerable groups. There are a number of financial, academic, and social supports available for youth to attend postsecondary educational programs; however, many youth face barriers while in high school related to being adequately prepared and meeting the institutional criteria (e.g., testing, grade point averages, application fees, etc.) as well as submitting materials on time.

In the past two decades, several federal laws have focused on supporting older foster youth in their transition to adulthood and creating opportunities to access postsecondary education, training, and employment. The most comprehensive legislation, first passed in 1999 and amended several times since, is the Foster Care Independence Act (FCIA). The FCIA allocates $140 million per year to states to offer independent living skills to youth in care. FCIA was amended in 2001 to create a separate program that funds up to $5000 per year in the form of education and training vouchers (ETV) for postsecondary education and training. Although states have discretion with age limits, youth who were in care on or after their 16th birthday can receive an ETV up to the age of 23 (and now up to age 26 under a 2018 federal law). Additionally, almost half of US states offer some form of a tuition and fee waiver program for postsecondary education and training for youth formerly in foster care (Hernandez et al., 2017); however, very little is known about waiver utilization among students across states or the impact of tuition and fee waivers on postsecondary education and employment outcomes. The Fostering Connections to Success and Increasing Adoptions Act (2008) was a monumental law that provides federal reimbursements for states to extend the foster care age limit beyond age 18 and up to the age of 21.

Child welfare professionals can connect youth with educational and vocational opportunities by ensuring they are adequately prepared, aware of their options, and provide the space for them to make decisions before and after high school. Specifically, child welfare professionals can talk with youth about their goals, interests, and talents and present them with options that might be a good fit. They can work with youth to organize documents and other materials they might need for applications and interviews (e.g., identification, school records and transcripts, application fees, etc.) and connect youth with a wide array of individuals who can give information or mentor them while also showing them their options through campus visits, talking to counselors, admissions, and financial aid offices. Further, child welfare professionals can provide youth with information about financial aid options. Many youth do not pursue postsecondary education and training because they think they cannot afford it; however, if done responsibly they can access a wide variety of financial aid through scholarships, waivers, student loans, and other programs. Finally, child welfare professionals must begin the discussion about the importance of education and employment early and create a norm of attending college or obtaining a certificate. In addition, when youth make the decision that is right for them, support them, check in on them, and provide guidance in accessing supports and community while they are enrolled.

Related, youth should be aware of what employment opportunities are available to them during and after high school. Research shows that youth who have early employment and internship opportunities have better economic and social outcomes (Dworsky, 2005; Goerge et al., 2002; Stewart et al., 2014). After high school, many youth struggle to find part-time and full-time employment and often earn lower wages than young people who haven't experienced foster care. Child welfare professionals can play a role in promoting employment by helping them to explore different job options, career paths, and what the requirements might be (degrees, licensures, experience, etc.) and accompanying them to job fairs. Child welfare professionals can sit down and help them develop a resume and cover letter and help them identify outlets to find jobs. They can give youth opportunities to gain experience through internships, volunteering, and job shadowing. Finally, child welfare professionals can find ways to include youth in networking events or opportunities to meet potential employers.

Obtaining safe and stable housing during the transition to adulthood is particularly challenging for many youth in care. While many young people who have not experienced foster care stay in their parents' home well after the age of 18, many youth in care do not have that option. They struggle with the costs of education, employment, and housing expenses, without experiencing short- and long-term homelessness after leaving care. Funding for housing is sometimes available through federal and state funds (e.g., Section 8, public housing, etc.) and child welfare funds (i.e., Chafee, ETV); however, there are often restrictions, regulations, and other issues that create barriers for youth formerly in care to access these benefits and supports. As a child welfare professional, we can ensure that housing is a critical part of the transition plan developed with youth and ensure all applications and outlets for housing supports are in place early and the youth is aware of what these options are for them. Child welfare professionals can spend time identifying safe and affordable housing with youth and discussing their responsibilities as a renter (e.g., rent, repairs, rules, etc.). Also, workers can help youth to identify a plan should they need assistance or need alternate housing arrangements in case of an emergency. They can serve as a safety net and help youth address barriers in obtaining stable and safe housing.

Youth aging out of foster care are at a greater risk for health and mental health issues (Courtney et al., 2011). Some receive regular treatment and care for chronic illnesses prior to leaving care, and their coverage and services may change when they turn 18. Child welfare professionals can support youth in ensuring a smooth transition with physical and mental health coverage, services, and supports prior to leaving care. This includes ensuring appointments, providers, and prescriptions are in order. While in care, youth should be educated and supported in engaging in a healthy diet and exercise, and child welfare professionals and caregivers can have discussions about mental and physical health and well-being. Further, child welfare professionals can help with gathering medical records, lists of providers, and insurance options and discuss managing health and well-being as an adult.

Youth in care are at a developmental phase where they are exploring their own identity and establishing a sense of self. With their experiences of foster care, it is common for them to have questions about their family, their identity, and their desire to understand the meaning of family and their background. There are ways to support healthy identity development for youth, such as helping them create a life-book or account of their family, personal history, key events, and photos; supporting them in their efforts to seek out culture and spirituality through activities, discussions, and experiences; and helping them to collect and safely organize their belongings and important documents.

Adolescents in foster care may have a different experience as they transition into adulthood than young people who have not been in care. As child welfare professionals, we are in a position to be a support, provide guidance, ensure a healthy transition through programs, provide information, and be available to youth during this process. It is also our responsibility to assist youth with developing a transition plan that will fit their needs and help them achieve independence and stability.

Note from the Field

The Importance of Unconditional Support

Kizzy Lopez, EdD

My life as a child and young adult was challenging and full of trauma. When I was 11 years old, my sisters and I were placed into foster care. At 18, I was homeless for the first 3 months of being enrolled in community college. Today, I have a beautiful family of my own, I have earned advanced degrees,

(continued)

and I have a successful career in education. Based on the statistics, though, my life should have looked very different. I am often asked how was I able to succeed given all of the challenges I faced.

There are many factors that contributed to my successful outcomes, but, in my opinion, the most important factor was my relationship with my sisters. My sisters provided me with my first experience of unconditional love and a trusting relationship. The connection with my sisters was critical in my ability to cope and survive the trauma. Fortunately, we were together during most of our time in foster care, which was a tremendous protective factor. Knowing the value of a healthy, permanent connection would give me a deep understanding of its importance in my relationships while shaping the way I served youth in the future.

Twenty-five years later, I went on to coordinate a program for students who experienced foster care or homelessness at the university. These lessons of unconditional love and support stayed with me. One example is Trey,[1] a student who transferred from a local community college, who had been living in his car with his partner and was primarily surviving off of financial aid. Trey had to travel almost an hour, one way, just to get to school.

I informed Trey that he could live on campus and the program would cover the cost for the first semester until we were able to develop a plan for him to move into an apartment. Trey asked if his partner could live on campus with him. Unfortunately, due to the campus restrictions, his partner was unable to stay on campus with him. Trey's relationship with his partner was critical to his emotional well-being and he was not willing to be without her. He explained that they had been living in a car for about a year and they found a way to make it work. I told Trey that I completely understood how important this person was to him. Instead of trying to convince him to stay on campus, I asked, "What support would be helpful to you?" He said gas cards to cover his travel costs and gift cards for food would give them some immediate relief. He also mentioned that assisting him with finding a job and an apartment would be helpful. This was something I could help with.

The practical thing for this student was to live on campus. It may seem strange to some that I did not push a little harder to encourage him to live on campus so that he could have free room and board and not commute. However, I understood that having a permanent connection is often one of the most critical factors to a person's ability to survive and thrive. Sometimes meeting young people where they are is more important than trying to do and get everything for someone. Showing you understand what and who is important to them can go a long way in helping them achieve stability and success.

---

[1]All names and other personal identifiers in cases and examples throughout this book have been changed to protect privacy and confidentiality.

Immigrant and Refugee Children and Families

Immigrants are a diverse group that includes foreign-born children and adults, as well as second-generation children and adults. All individuals and families have different stories related to their immigration journey. A relatively small proportion of immigrant and refugee families come into contact with the child welfare system. An analysis of the National Survey of Children and Adolescent Well-Being data found 8.6% of children reported to child protective services lived with a foreign-born parent and 82.5% of these children were born in the United States (Dettlaff & Earner, 2012). Approximately two-thirds (67.2%) of these children were Hispanic. Children of immigrants may enter the child welfare system when their parents are detained or deported. Immigrants with undocumented legal status may face significant challenges in accessing services to care for their children (Finno-Valasquez, 2014).

When immigrant and refugee families become involved in the child welfare system, it is important to recognize how their status and experiences as immigrants and refugees in the United States play a role in their case and service provision. Immigrant and refugee families may share similar and very different experiences than other families involved with the child welfare system based on their experiences of trauma, interaction with various law enforcement agencies and systems, potential language and cultural differences, and unfamiliarity with the structure of systems in the United States. It may also be influenced by racism and discrimination due to their race/ethnicity and/or immigration status in the United States.

There is a need to better understand the different experiences among immigrant and refugee families. Currently, research seeks to deepen the knowledge about risk and protective factors in different immigrant families. For example, recent research examining mothers born in Mexico who were raising their children in the United States found that mothers' depressive symptoms and economic hardship uniquely predicted increased parenting stress and their romantic relationship quality decreased parenting stress and that these influenced their engagement in harsh parenting practices (Mortensen & Barnett, 2015).

Given the growing number of immigrant children and families in the United States, it is important for child welfare professionals to be prepared to apply existing elements of family-centered, strengths-based, and trauma-informed practice in child welfare to working with immigrant families. This includes conducting sound and

> **Practice Tip**
>
> **Potential Questions to Ask Immigrant Parents About Their Family**
>
> - Tell me about your life as a child – what positive things do you remember? What was difficult?
> - How was your journey to this country?
> - What do hope for your children? What dreams do you have for them?
> - What is your relationship with your children? Your parents? Extended family?
> - What makes your children happy?
> - What can I do to help you and your family?

appropriate investigations, assessments, making necessary referrals for services, and monitoring progress on each case that are grounded in the culture and language that the family prefers. Although for some languages it may be challenging to find a translator, children should not be used as translators within cases. As with all families, child welfare professionals must assess strengths and resources, cultivate resilience, and focus on solutions in developing a case plan and supports for the child and family. With immigrant and refugee families, we must also learn and respect cultural norms and practices through our everyday interactions and through culturally grounded services and interventions.

While immigrant families have many strengths, they may be at an increased risk for poor outcomes with the child welfare system due to the effects of the traumatic experiences related to the immigration process (Dettlaff & Earner, 2012). These experiences may be exacerbated due to cumulative effects of other highly stressful conditions such as poverty, housing and employment instability, and anti-immigrant attitudes, policies, and behaviors that lead to fear, uncertainty, and social isolation.

A child welfare professional can effectively engage immigrant families by presenting with a warm, empathic, and supportive approach with families, avoiding stereotypes and assumptions, recognizing the importance of the family, respecting cultural and family traditions and preferences, and providing as much information and guidance as necessary for the family.

There are a number of ways the child welfare system can foster best practices to support immigrant families involved with the child welfare system. Many child welfare systems and states have begun to implement sound policies to support immigrant and refugee families; however many have work to be done. Child welfare agencies should promote cross-systems collaboration by establishing partnerships with local immigration legal clinics, developing relationships with foreign consulates, ensuring workforce, and training for child welfare professionals that includes information about legal relief options and how to prepare families for possible detention and/or deportation (e.g., safety planning, attorney information, custody/guardianship/power of attorney documentations).

Child welfare agencies can review and update policies and procedures to reflect a more immigrant family-friendly approach, which would include provisions about eligibility for noncitizen/undocumented caregivers and the development of clear policies on confidentiality and information sharing about families with authorities and ensure documents and forms are in languages needed by clients. Child welfare systems should continue to recruit and retain culturally and linguistically diverse groups of foster parents to care for children in care. The child welfare system should continue to develop and nurture community partnerships with agencies that advocate for immigrant families and provide culturally grounded services to immigrant and refugee families.

Practice Highlight

Interviewing Immigrant Families in Child Welfare Investigations

Elizabet Bonilla Escobar, MSW

The child welfare field is filled with a number of challenges. Anytime a new investigation comes in, families become uncomfortable and at times resistant to cooperate due to fear, frustration, anger, and many other reasons. When it comes to immigrant families in the United States, the feeling of fear, in particular, is often prevalent. A lack of knowledge and a perceived lack of power are the biggest contributors to such fear. Being faced with a child abuse or neglect investigation is preoccupying in any case, but for immigrant families, that feeling intensifies. Immigrant families often share stories about their upbringings and the way in which they were disciplined as children. Those stories may include details of actions that are deemed as "normal" in the family's culture, but that are considered abuse in the United States.

There was one occasion when a new investigation came in due to allegations that an 8-year-old child had gotten hit with a belt on the thighs and had received bruises as result. When first meeting with the family, who was originally from Mexico, the father indicated the following: "In Mexico, we used to get pulled by the hair, dragged around, and get hit with everything from shoes, chords, irons, and other things when we misbehaved." He added, "I have never done those things to my child... I have hit him with a belt when he talks back, but that's just discipline." This father's explanation was honest and direct. It's important as a child welfare worker to listen and validate the experiences of those who we interview. Once that's been done, the challenge lies in explaining that what may be within the "norm" in other cultures is considered abuse in the United States. The best way to do that, in my experience, is by avoiding being "preachy" and taking an educational approach. I let the parent know that I understand his/her perspective. However, I also add that there are rules and regulations that must be followed when residing in the United States and the state we live in and state that the regulations are there for the protection of all children. Parents often respond well when I explain that the goal of my work is to ensure that their children are safe.

At times, depending on the allegation (s) and the facts of the case, the allegations still need to be indicated. When this is the case, parents are often upset. While I cannot change the way they feel, I do find that when I work to build a relationship in which I take the time to listen and to answer any questions the parents may have, they appreciate it. Even when I have indicated reports before, families have thanked me at the conclusion of an investigation. I think that they come to understand that there is a protocol that I must adhere to, and they appreciate that I inform them as much as possible of why each step and decision must take place.

Overall, I think one of the most valuable lessons I've learned as a child protection specialist is that it's of utmost importance to be willing to listen and educate the families we work with while holding a nonjudgmental attitude.

Siblings in Foster Care

There is no doubt that sibling relationships are important in one's development and well-being throughout the lifespan. Sibling relationships can provide support, stability, and joy. Research shows that siblings placed together can increase the chance of reunification and other types of permanency (Jones, 2016, Akin, 2011) and experience more placement stability. Siblings placed together also experience fewer externalizing behaviors (Wojciak et al., 2013) and improved mental health (Jones, 2016) and school performance (Hegar & Rosenthal, 2011). Despite the known benefits of sibling relationships, it is not always possible for them to be placed together in out-of-home care. There are a number of barriers that can exist, such as siblings having different needs, difficulty in accommodating a large sibling group, difference in age, and entering care at different times. It is estimated at least one-third of children placed in care will be separated from at least one of their siblings while in foster care (Shlonsky et al., 2003).

Child welfare systems should make every effort to enact policies that support siblings staying together in placement. Systems can ensure that child welfare staff have adequate training about sibling placement and relationship promotion, recruit foster caregivers willing to foster sibling groups, and have events that promote sibling contact. Child welfare professionals should make every effort to place children together in the same setting when they are initially placed and when permanency options are explored later in the case. Assessment throughout the case is important as information may come at different times. Child welfare professionals should ask questions about who is considered a sibling and possible caregivers (e.g., relatives, teaches, other kin). In these cases, it is extremely important and often mandated that child welfare professionals go above and beyond to ensure siblings have regular in-person visits and regular contact via phone or video chat. Child welfare professionals should discuss the siblings' preferences for maintaining contact and visits. If children are placed apart, child welfare professionals can ensure that their respective placements have contact information to allow for phone calls and video chats and encourage visits, as appropriate. Child welfare professionals can arrange for sibling therapy, clinical support during visitation, and offer extracurricular activities, joint outings, or camp that both can participate in together. If siblings cannot be placed together, they could be placed in close proximity or in the same school district or school. Sibling relationships should be prioritized in child welfare, and those professionals and caregivers working with youth should ensure that they have optimal and appropriate contact and support.

Human and Sex Trafficking

Human trafficking has been referred to as "modern-day slavery." Through the use coercion, deception, fraud, threat, and force, traffickers exploit people and deprive them of their rights and freedoms. It is "involuntary servitude" that includes both forced labor and sexual exploitation. Labor trafficking includes having a person work against their will in any number of settings and types of work (e.g., service industry, manufacturing, housekeeping, agriculture, domestic servitude). It includes debt bondage where a person pledges their personal services to another person and the value of those services are not applied towards the debt or the length and nature of the services are not limited and defined. Sexual exploration includes forcing a person into sexual acts where there is financial gain for someone, such as prostitution or pornography. Sex trafficking includes the acts of recruiting, harboring, transporting, obtaining, patronizing, and soliciting a person for the purposes of any commercial sex act. Human trafficking is a multi-billion-dollar "industry" that exploits children and adults from the United States and other countries. While people who have been trafficked should not be punished for having been trafficking, it is an ongoing concern that survivors of trafficking are involved with the justice system because of events they did due to their circumstances of being trafficked (Marsh, 2019).

Annual estimates are that over 100,000 children are sex trafficked domestically in the United States and up to 325,000 more children are at risk of being trafficked (Estes & Weiner, 2001). Sex trafficking of children is also often referred to as the commercial sexual exploitation of children. Research has identified multiple risk factors for commercial sexual exploitation of children, although there is more work that needs to be done, especially to understand how to predict risk for sex trafficking (Panlilio et al., 2019). Risk factors include having experienced child maltreatment, having been involved in the child welfare or juvenile justice system, previously run away from home, homelessness, and identifying as LGBTQ (National Resource Council, 2013). Being in out-of-home care is a known risk factors for human trafficking. It is estimated between 50% and 90% of children who were involved in sex trafficking had a history of being involved in the child welfare system (ACF, 2013).

Traffickers are known to target youth in care because of their trauma history and their weaker social connections. They may lure youth away from their placements. Or they prey upon those who run away from placements (Gibbs et al., 2018). Traffickers do not just violently kidnap youth; they use a range of behaviors to build trust and convince youth to come with them. They may shower them with affection initially and promise to provide for their basic needs. Youth may see the trafficker as a romantic partner and not realize they are being manipulated into trafficking. Traffickers also use drugs and violence to continue to control youth they are trafficking.

The child welfare system is involved in the response to human trafficking and the commercial sexual exploitation of children (CSEC; Gibbs, et al., 2018). In several states commercial exploitation is a specific reportable child abuse offense (Bounds et al., 2015). Much of the child welfare system involvement with trafficking is in dealing with the aftermath. Many states have included trafficking of children as a form of child maltreatment regardless if the perpetrator is a parent or caregiver. Child welfare agencies have collaborated with systems to provide services to children and youth who were trafficked. Children and youth who were sex trafficked and engaged in pornography are recognized as victims and not arrested or prosecuted. There are "safe harbor" laws in many states that ensure that children who were trafficked are served by the child welfare system and not the juvenile justice system. Special services including specific housing are often required due to the nature of trafficking. Youth may run away from placement to return to those who were trafficking them. In providing housing for youth who have been trafficked, it is important to consider their wishes and needs (Dierkhising et al., 2020). It is imperative to understand that youth may not wish to disclose that they were involved in commercial sexual exploitation (Lavoie et al., 2019). They may not perceive themselves as victims and may not wish to be removed from those who were trafficking them.

Those working with children and youth who were trafficked must understand the nature of trafficking. Specialized training on understanding trafficking and working with youth who have been trafficked is available, and child welfare workers should participate in the trainings. Identification of trafficking is important as youth may not necessarily conceptualize the nature of what they experienced as trafficking. There are multiple screening tools available that can be used by agencies. Likewise, child welfare workers can be trained to recognized signs of trafficking. For example, the presence of an older boyfriend who is controlling, youth's loyalty to the trafficker, a youth working long hours, or a youth living with their employer or many other people (Center for the Human Rights for Children & International Organization for Adolescents, 2011). Awareness about trafficking is necessary as is knowing how to work with those who have experienced trafficking.

While in many regards working with children and youth who have been trafficked is like working with children and youth who have experienced other traumas, there is a uniqueness to trafficking (Bounds et al., 2015). (See Chap. 5 for information on trauma-informed care). Those who have been trafficked have experienced trauma and may react in a wide variety of ways. The range of reactions may be from rage and aggression to withdrawn and dissociated. Children and youth who have been trafficked may strongly seek their independence and find programs and services as restrictive. While they were being trafficked, youth may have felt more freedoms to engage in behaviors that are restricted in care (e.g., drink alcohol, do drugs, have sex). To address youth feeling the lack of control, engaging the youth in the case plan and empowering them to make decisions impacting their life can be helpful. Additionally, having more flexibility in how services are provided may be helpful. Building trust and rapport with youth who had been trafficked is important and can take time. Youth who have been trafficked may have a difficult time trusting someone and may not feel safe (Hurst, 2019). They may have had negative experiences with systems and authorities that contribute to their distrust. Their focus on safety and survival may result in behaviors and attitudes perceived as challenging. They may engage in risky behaviors or self-harm. Youth who have been trafficked may have health problems and experience delays in their development. Many youth who have been trafficked have had disruptions in their education.

Prevention of commercial exploitation of children is also relevant to child welfare because children and youth in foster care are at greater risk than their peers to being trafficked. Risk factors for being trafficked include not having a stable living environment, being isolated from family and friends, and emotional vulnerability, all of which are frequent characteristics of those in out-of-home care. Child welfare agencies have the responsibility to ensure that children in their care are not targeted by trafficking. This cannot be done alone though; collaboration across systems is necessary to prevent and address human trafficking.

Case Study: Commercial Sexual Exploitation
Carly B. Dierkhising, PhD

Brielle was born with drugs in her system and entered foster care the day after she was born. She was taken from her mother at the hospital. At this time, there were already substantiated allegations of emotional abuse and severe physical abuse of her siblings, which led to bruises and marks on their bodies. For the next several years, her mother worked to address her substance use issues so she could reunify with Brielle. Brielle lived in two foster homes during her first 3 years until she was able to return home to her mother. When Brielle was 13 years old, her brother was born with drug exposure which triggered a removal for Brielle who went to live with her aunt. Two years later, her mother passed away.

While grieving for her mother, Brielle began to leave her aunt's house without permission and would be gone for days at a time. Her aunt connected with the social worker who referred Brielle for a mental health assessment which indicated that she had been diagnosed with major depressive disorder and cocaine and methamphetamine abuse. Brielle reported using drugs to numb her grief and trauma reactions. The report also stated that she would trade sex for drugs or steal when needed. Brielle and her aunt were referred to trauma-focused cognitive behavioral therapy, but before services began, Brielle disappeared and her social worker reported her to the National Center for Missing and Exploited Children.

One month later, she was recovered by law enforcement in a sting operation focused on recovering commercially sexually exploited children and youth. At the station her social worker and a community-based survivor advocate were called. Brielle was able to go home to her aunt that night, but a few weeks later, her aunt called her social worker and said that Brielle had been in an altercation with her "boyfriend" and law enforcement had been involved. Brielle had bruises and cuts on her body. Her aunt told the social worker that she was no longer willing or able to take care of Brielle and asked that she find her another place to live. She was placed in short-term shelter care as her social worker looked to find a new place for her to live.

Conclusion

Child welfare practice is enhanced significantly through an understanding of the needs of those with unique experiences. Child welfare professionals can improve their practice by being flexible and understanding in meeting the needs of the children and families they serve. Best practice in child welfare also includes acknowledging varied approaches with special populations such as youth aging out of foster care, children with disabilities, and immigrant and refugee populations and in specific contexts such as sibling groups or human and sex trafficking.

Acknowledgments The authors thank Justin S. Harty, MSW, LCSW; Colleen Cary Katz, PhD, LCSW; Kizzy Lopez, EdD; Elizabet Bonilla Escobar, MSW; and Carly B. Dierkhising, PhD, for their contributions to in this chapter.

Discussion Questions

1. What are two ways to improve permanency among children with disabilities who are involved in the child welfare system?
2. How can child welfare professionals support pregnant and parenting youth in foster care?
3. What are strategies that child welfare professionals can use to support youth in their transition into adulthood and independence?
4. What are some ways that the child welfare system can foster best practices in supporting immigrant families?
5. How do human and sex trafficking intersect with the child welfare system?

Suggested Activities

1. Listen to the stories of youth transitioning out of foster care. Visit the Digital Stories of youth involved with Florida Youth SHINE: https://www.floridayouth-shine.org/digital-stories. Discuss with others these youths' experiences. Reflect about the importance of child welfare professionals and other adults in their lives in shaping the experiences of youth.
2. Visit The Center on Immigration and Child Welfare's website (https://cimmcw.org/), and review current events in the news. Write a brief paper on one of the events. Reflect on to what extent the child welfare system (or other systems) addressed the safety, permanency, and well-being of immigrant children and families.
3. Watch the Video: "Youth Voices: Life after Foster Care" https://www.davetho-masfoundation.org/library/video-youth-voices-life-after-foster-care-full-length/. Reflect on some of the similarities and differences between your experiences and those of the youth during the transition to adulthood. Consider what types of supports are necessary during this process.
4. Read Eastman et al. (2019), and discuss with others the similarities and differences between pregnant and parenting youth in foster care and (1) youth in care who do not have children, (2) youth without foster care experience who may be parenting, and (3) youth without foster care experience who are not parenting.

Eastman, A. L., Palmer, L., & Ahn, E. (2019). Pregnant and parenting youth in care and their children: A literature review. *Child and Adolescent Social Work Journal*, 36(6), 571–581. (Available: https://rdcu.be/cb8US).

Additional Resources

Child Welfare League of America Best Practice Guidelines, Serving LGBT Youth in Out-of-Home Care: https://www.nclrights.org/get-help/resource/child-welfare-league-of-america-cwla-best-practice-guidelines-serving-lgbt-youth-in-out-of-home-care/

The Center on Immigration and Child Welfare: https://cimmcw.org/

The Center on Immigration and Child Welfare, A Social Workers Tool Kit for Working with Immigrant Families: https://cimmcw.org/wp-content/uploads/Trauma-Immigrant-Families.pdf

Lambda Legal, Getting down to basics: Tools to support LGBTQ Youth in Care: https://www.lambdalegal.org/publications/getting-down-to-basics

Foster Care Alumni of America: https://fostercarealumni.org/

U.S. Department of Education, Foster Care Transition Toolkit: https://www2.ed.gov/about/inits/ed/foster-care/youth-transition-toolkit.pdf

Human Rights Campaign, LGBTQ Resources for Child Welfare Professionals: https://www.thehrcfoundation.org/professional-resources/all-children-all-families-lgbtq-resources-for-child-welfare-professionals

Child Welfare Information Gateway, Human Trafficking and Child Welfare: A Guide for Caseworkers: https://www.childwelfare.gov/pubs/trafficking-caseworkers/

The National Child Traumatic Stress Network, The 12 Core Concepts of Understanding Traumatic Stress Responses in Children and Families Adapted for Youth who are Trafficked: https://www.nctsn.org/resources/12-core-concepts-understanding-traumatic-stress-responses-children-and-families-adapted

ReSHAPING (Research on Sexual Health and Adolescent Parenting in Out-of-Home Environments Group): https://www.reshapingnetwork.org/reshaping

Child Welfare Information Gateway, Supporting your LGBTQ Youth: A Guide for Foster Parents: https://www.childwelfare.gov/pubs/LGBTQyouth/

Youth.Gov, LGBTQ youth in child welfare: https://youth.gov/youth-topics/lgbtq-youth/child-welfare

References

Administration on Children and Families. (2013) *Report to Congress: The child welfare system response to sex trafficking of children*. Retrieved from: https://www.acf.hhs.gov/sites/default/files/cb/report_congress_child_trafficking.pdf

Akin, B. A. (2011). Predictors of foster care exits to permanency: A competing risks analysis of reunification, guardianship, and adoption. *Children and Youth Services Review, 33*(6), 999–1011. https://doi.org/10.1016/j.childyouth.2011.01.008

Antle, B. F., Johnson, L., Barbee, A., & Sullivan, D. (2009). Fostering interdependent versus independent living in youth aging out of care through healthy relationships. *Families in Society, 90*(3), 309–315. https://doi.org/10.1606/1044-3894.3890

Bounds, D., Julion, W. A., & Delaney, K. R. (2015). Commercial sexual exploitation of children and state child welfare systems. *Policy, Politics, & Nursing Practice, 16*(1–2), 17–26. https://doi.org/10.1177/1527154415583124

Brown, A., Courtney, M. E., & McMillen, J. C. (2015). Behavioral health needs and service use among those who've aged-out of foster care. *Children and Youth Services Review, 58*, 163–169.

Butterworth, S., Singh, S. P., Birchwood, M., Islam, Z., Munro, E. R., Vostanis, P., et al. (2017). Transitioning care-leavers with mental health needs: 'They set you up to fail!'. *Child and Adolescent Mental Health, 22*(3), 138–147.

Cash, S. J., & Bridge, J. A. (2009). Epidemiology of youth suicide and suicidal behavior. *Current Opinion in Pediatrics, 21*(5), 613–619. https://doi.org/10.1097/MOP.0b013e32833063e1

Center for the Human Rights for Children & International Organization for Adolescents. (2011). *Building child welfare response to human trafficking.* https://www.luc.edu/media/lucedu/chrc/pdfs/BCWRHandbook2011.pdf

Courtney, M. E., Dworsky, A. L., Lee, J. S., & Raap, M. (2010). *Midwest evaluation of the adult functioning of former foster youth: Outcomes at ages 23 and 24.* Chapin Hall at the University of Chicago.

Courtney, M. E., Charles, P., Okpych, N. J., Napolitano, L., & Halsted, K. (2014). *Findings from the California youth transitions to adulthood study (CalYOUTH): Conditions of foster youth at age 17.* Chapin Hall at the University of Chicago.

Courtney, M. E., Okpych, N. J., Charles, P., Mikell, D., Stevenson, B., Park, K., Kindle, B., Harty, J., & Feng, H. (2016). *Findings from the California Youth Transitions to Adulthood Study (CalYOUTH): Conditions of foster youth at age 19.* Chicago, IL: Chapin Hall at the University of Chicago.

Cunningham, M. J., & Diversi, M. (2013). Aging out: Youths' perspectives on foster care and the transition to independence. *Qualitative Social Work, 12*(5), 587–602.

Dettlaff, A. J., & Earner, I. (2012). Children of immigrants in the child welfare system: Characteristics, risk, and maltreatment. *Families in Society, 93*(4), 295–303. https://doi.org/10.1606/1044-3894.4240

Dettlaff, A. J., & Washburn, M. (2018). Lesbian, gay, and bisexual (LGB) youth within in welfare: Prevalence, risk and outcomes. *Child Abuse & Neglect, 80*, 183–193. https://doi.org/10.1016/j.chiabu.2018.03.009

Dierkhising, C. B., Brown, K. W., Ackerman-Brimberg, M., & Newcombe, A. (2020). Recommendations to improve out of home care from youth who have experienced commercial sexual exploitation. *Children and Youth Services Review, 116*, 105263. https://doi.org/10.1016/j.childyouth.2020.105263

Dworsky, A. (2005). The economic self-sufficiency of Wisconsin's former foster youth. *Children and Youth Services Review, 27*(10), 1085–1118. https://doi.org/10.1016/j.childyouth.2004.12.032

Dworsky, A., & Pérez, A. (2010). Helping former foster youth graduate from college through campus support programs. *Children and Youth Services Review, 32*(2), 255–263. https://doi.org/10.1016/j.childyouth.2009.09.004

Eastman, A. L., Putnam-Hornstein, E., Magruder, J., Mitchell, M. N., & Courtney, M. E. (2017). Characteristics of youth remaining in foster care through age 19: A pre-and post-policy cohort analysis of California data. *Journal of public child welfare, 11*(1), 40–57.

Estes, R. J., & Weiner, N. A. (2001). *The commercial sexual exploitation of children in the US, Canada and Mexico.* University of Pennsylvania, School of Social Work, Center for the Study of Youth Policy.

Finno-Velasquez, M. (2014). *Barriers to support service use for Latino immigrant families reported to child welfare: Implications for policy and practice.* Available: http://childwelfaresparc.org/wp-content/uploads/2014/07/Barriers-to-Support-Service-Use-for-Latino-Immigrant-Families-Reported-to-Child-Welfare.pdf

Fish, J. N., Baams, L., Wojciak, A. S., & Russell, S. T. (2019). Are sexual minority youth over-represented in foster care, child welfare, and out-of-home placement? Findings from nationally representative data. *Child Abuse & Neglect, 89*, 203–211. https://doi.org/10.1016/j.chiabu.2019.01.005

Geiger, J. M., Piel, M. H., Day, A., & Schelbe, L. (2018). A descriptive analysis of programs serving foster care alumni in higher education: Challenges and opportunities. *Children and Youth Services Review, 85*, 287–294. https://doi.org/10.1016/j.childyouth.2018.01.001

Goerge, R.M., Bilaver, L., Lee, B.J., Needell, B., Brookhart, A., & Jackman, W. (2002). *Employment outcomes for youth aging out of foster care*. US Department of Health and Human Services, Office of the Assistant Secretary for Planning and Evaluation.

Gibbs, D. A., Feinberg, R. K., Dolan, M., Latzman, N. E., Misra, S., & Domanico, R. (2018). *Report to congress: The child welfare system response to sex trafficking of children*. U.S. Department of Health and Human Services, Administration for Children and Families.

Glidden, L. M. (2000). Adopting children with developmental disabilities: A long-term perspective. *Family Relations, 49*(4), 397–405. https://doi.org/10.1111/j.1741-3729.2000.00397.x

Greeson, J. K., & Bowen, N. K. (2008). "She holds my hand" the experiences of foster youth with their natural mentors. *Children and Youth Services Review, 30*(10), 1178–1188. https://doi.org/10.1016/j.childyouth.2008.03.003

Havlicek, J. (2014). Maltreatment histories of foster youth exiting out-of-home care through emancipation: A latent class analysis. *Child Maltreatment, 19*(3–4), 199–208. https://doi.org/10.1177/1077559514539754

Hegar, R. L., & Rosenthal, J. A. (2011). Foster children placed with or separated from siblings: Outcomes based on a national sample. *Children and Youth Services Review, 33*(7), 1245–1253. https://doi.org/10.1016/j.childyouth.2011.02.020

Hernandez, L., Day, A., & Henson, M. (2017). Increasing college access and retention rates of youth in foster care: An analysis of the impact of 22 state tuition waiver programs. *Journal of Policy Practice, 16*(4), 397–414. https://doi.org/10.1080/15588742.2017.1311819

Horowitz, L. M., Bridge, J. A., Teach, S. J., Ballard, E., Klima, J., Rosenstein, D. L., et al. (2012). Ask suicide-screening questions (ASQ): A brief instrument for the pediatric emergency department. *Archives of Pediatrics & Adolescent Medicine, 166*(12), 1170–1176.

Hurst, T. E. (2019). Prevention of child sexual exploitation: Insights from adult survivors. *Journal of Interpersonal Violence*. https://doi.org/10.1177/0886260519825881

Iglehart, A. P., & Becerra, R. M. (2002). Hispanic and African American youth: Life after foster care emancipation. *Journal of Ethnic and Cultural Diversity in Social Work, 11*(1–2), 79–107.

Jones, C. (2016). Sibling relationships in adoptive and fostering families: A review of the international research literature. *Children & Society, 30*(4), 324–334. https://doi.org/10.1111/chso.12146

Jonson-Reid, M., Drake, B., Kim, J., Porterfield, S., & Han, L. (2004). A prospective analysis of the relationship between reported child maltreatment and special education eligibility among poor children. *Child Maltreatment, 9*(4), 382–394. https://doi.org/10.1177/1077559504269192

Katz, C. C., Courtney, M. E., & Novotny, E. (2017). Pre-foster care maltreatment class as a predictor of maltreatment in foster care. *Child and Adolescent Social Work Journal, 34*(1), 35–49.

Kleiman, E. M., & Liu, R. T. (2013). Social support as a protective factor in suicide: Findings from two nationally representative samples. *Journal of Affective Disorders, 150*(2), 540–545. https://doi.org/10.1037/e556952013-003

Lavoie, J., Dickerson, K. L., Redlich, A. D., & Quas, J. A. (2019). Overcoming disclosure reluctance in youth victims of sex trafficking: New directions for research, policy, and practice. *Psychology, Public Policy, and Law, 25*(4), 225. https://doi.org/10.1037/law0000205

Lightfoot, E., Hill, K., & LaLiberte, T. (2011). Prevalence of children with disabilities in the child welfare system and out of home placement: An examination of administrative records. *Children and Youth Services Review, 33*(11), 2069–2075. https://doi.org/10.1016/j.childyouth.2011.02.019

Lorthridge, J., Evans, M., Heaton, L., Stevens, A., & Phillips, L. (2018). Strengthening family connections and support for youth in foster care who identify as LGBTQ: Findings from the PII-RISE evaluation. *Child Welfare, 96*(1), 53–78.

Marsh, E. (2019). *Relief not arrests: Strengthening laws for survivors of human trafficking.* Available: https://www.legalexecutiveinstitute.com/polaris-arrests-human-trafficking/

McMillen, J. C., Zima, B. T., Scott, L. D., Jr., Auslander, W. F., Munson, M. R., Ollie, M. T., & Spitznagel, E. L. (2005). Prevalence of psychiatric disorders among older youths in the foster care system. *Journal of the American Academy of Child & Adolescent Psychiatry, 44*(1), 88–95.

Mihalec-Adkins, B. P., & Cooley, M. E. (2020). Examining individual-level academic risk and protective factors for foster youth: School engagement, behaviors, self-esteem, and social skills. *Child & Family Social Work, 25*(2), 256–266. https://doi.org/10.1111/cfs.12681

Miller, E. A., Paschall, K. W., & Azar, S. T. (2017). Latent classes of older foster youth: Prospective associations with outcomes and exits from the foster care system during the transition to adulthood. *Children and Youth Services Review, 79*, 495–505. https://doi.org/10.1016/j.childyouth.2017.06.047

Mortensen, J. A., & Barnett, M. A. (2015). Risk and protective factors, parenting stress, and harsh parenting in Mexican origin mothers with toddlers. *Marriage & Family Review, 51*(1), 1–21. https://doi.org/10.1080/01494929.2014.955937

National Research Council. (2013). *Confronting commercial sexual exploitation and sex trafficking of minors in the United States.* National Academies Press.

Norman, R. E., Byambaa, M., De, R., Butchart, A., Scott, J., & Vos, T. (2012). The long-term health consequences of child physical abuse, emotional abuse, and neglect: A systematic review and meta-analysis. *PLoS Medicine, 9*(11), e1001349.

Osman, A., Bagge, C. L., Gutierrez, P. M., Konick, L. C., Kopper, B. A., & Barrios, F. X. (2001). The suicidal behaviors questionnaire-revised (SBQ-R): Validation with clinical and nonclinical samples. *Assessment, 8*(4), 443–454. https://doi.org/10.1177/107319110100800409

Panlilio, C. C., Miyamoto, S., Font, S. A., & Schreier, H. M. (2019). Assessing risk of commercial sexual exploitation among children involved in the child welfare system. *Child Abuse & Neglect, 87*, 88–99. https://doi.org/10.1016/j.chiabu.2018.07.021

Posner, K., Brown, G. K., Stanley, B., Brent, D. A., Yershova, K. V., Oquendo, M. A., et al. (2011). The Columbia-suicide severity rating scale: Initial validity and internal consistency findings from three multisite studies with adolescents and adults. *American of Psychiatry, 168*(12), 1266–1277. https://doi.org/10.1176/appi.ajp.2011.10111704

Ryan, C., Huebner, D., Diaz, R. M., & Sanchez, J. (2009). Family rejection as a predictor of negative health outcomes in white and Latino lesbian, gay, and bisexual young adults. *Pediatrics, 123*(1), 346–352. https://doi.org/10.1542/peds.2007-3524

Samuels, G. M. (2008). *A reason, a season, or a lifetime: Relational permanence among young adults with Foster Care backgrounds.* Chapin Hall Center for Children at the University of Chicago.

Shlonsky, A., Webster, D., & Needell, B. (2003). The ties that bind: A cross-sectional analysis of siblings in foster care. *Journal of Social Service Research, 29*(3), 27–52.

Stewart, C. J., Kum, H. C., Barth, R. P., & Duncan, D. F. (2014). Former foster youth: Employment outcomes up to age 30. *Children and Youth Services Review, 36*, 220–229. https://doi.org/10.1016/j.childyouth.2013.11.024

Substance Abuse and Mental Health Services Administration. (2015). *Ending conversion therapy: Supporting and affirming LGBTQ youth* (HHS Publication No. (SMA) 15-4928). Substance Abuse and Mental Health Services Administration.

Sullivan, M. J., Jones, L., & Mathiesen, S. (2010). School change, academic progress, and behavior problems in a sample of foster youth. *Children and Youth Services Review, 32*(2), 164–170. https://doi.org/10.1016/j.childyouth.2009.08.009

U.S. Department of Health & Human Services. (2020). *The AFSCARS report.* https://www.acf.hhs.gov/sites/default/files/cb/afcarsreport27.pdf

Ullman, S. E., & Najdowski, C. J. (2009). Correlates of serious suicidal ideation and attempts in female adult sexual assault survivors. *Suicide and Life-threatening Behavior, 39*(1), 47–57. https://doi.org/10.1521/suli.2009.39.1.47

Van Scoyoc, A., Marquardt, M. B., & Phelps, R. A. (2018). The challenge and importance of differentiating trauma and stress-related disorders from autism Spectrum disorders. In J. Fogler & R. Phelps (Eds.), *Trauma, autism, and neurodevelopmental disorders*. Springer. https://doi.org/10.1007/978-3-030-00503-0_5

Wilber, S., Ryan, C., & Marksamer, J. (2006). *CWLA best practice guidelines: Serving LGBT youth in out-of-home care*. Child Welfare League of America.

Wilson, B. D., Cooper, K., Kastanis, A., & Nezhad, S. (2014). *Sexual and gender minority youth in foster care: Assessing disproportionality and disparities in Los Angeles*. The Williams Institute.

Wojciak, A. S., McWey, L. M., & Helfrich, C. M. (2013). Sibling relationships and internalizing symptoms of youth in foster care. *Children and Youth Services Review, 35*(7), 1071–1077. https://doi.org/10.1016/j.childyouth.2013.04.021

Zhang, X., Wang, H., Xia, Y., Liu, X., & Jung, E. (2012). Stress, coping and suicide ideation in Chinese college students. *Journal of Adolescence, 35*(3), 683–690. https://doi.org/10.1016/j.adolescence.2011.10.003

Chapter 12
Supervision and Professional Development in Child Welfare

Introduction

To best serve children and families, child welfare professionals must be committed to accepting feedback and assistance as well as learning throughout their career. Child welfare agencies are structured to ensure that feedback, assistance, and learning opportunities are available for child welfare professionals. A large way in which this occurs is having child welfare professionals report to supervisors who oversee the cases and assist the child welfare professionals on their team. Child welfare professionals should take an active role in their supervision. Supervision is not something that is given to them; rather, it is a process in which they are engaged. Child welfare professionals should be committed to using supervision as a tool to improve how they work with children and families.

Learning occurs within supervision, but it extends beyond to professional development which broadly encompasses various learning opportunities that improve the skills and abilities to perform within their positions. While some professional development trainings may be required of child welfare professionals by a child welfare agency or certification, it also includes activities that child welfare professionals undertake to improve their ability to perform in the position. Taking classes, attending webinars, and reading books and articles are all forms of professional development. The topics of professional development are quite varied; they can be technical about a new protocol or broader and focus on something like self-care or safety. Child welfare professionals should actively participate in their professional development to ensure that they are effective in their work as well as the work brings meaning to their lives.

© Springer Nature Switzerland AG 2021

J. M. Geiger, L. Schelbe, *The Handbook on Child Welfare Practice*,
https://doi.org/10.1007/978-3-030-73912-6_12

Supervision in Child Welfare Practice

Supervision in child welfare practice involves the everyday practice that supervisors engage in that involve assigning, monitoring, and closing cases that they or their unit are responsible for. Supervision also includes the regular communication, support, and feedback that supervisors provide for their supervisees or caseworkers. Supervisors also serve as the liaison between the child welfare agency and the systems they work for and alongside (e.g., judicial, educational, mental health and behavioral, healthcare) and ensure the implementation of policies in the field. These policies and practices must be communicated effectively and timely with child welfare professionals working in the field. Supervisors hold an important role in decision-making and are ultimately responsible for the decisions and actions of the staff they supervise. Therefore, in addition to the case management and administrative role that supervisors have, they are also responsible for ensuring that departmental and permanency goals are reached and their staff are adhering to proper conduct in the field, following policies and protocols, and providing the best service to the children and families they interact with. Other administrative supervision includes a focus on job performance and how it relates to the agency's mission. For example, supervisors in child welfare establish performance objectives, measure and monitor work performance, track required client contacts and other mandates, and enforce discipline.

Supervisors act as supporters, case consultants, teachers, advocates, and experienced colleagues. They provide emotional support to reduce barriers in practice while helping the staff they supervise explore their role in child welfare practice. They often assist in resolving conflict and help to foster self-awareness and empathy. As case consultants, they offer advice and leadership in difficult and routine situations and how to implement practice effectively and intervene appropriately in cases as needed. Supervisors are typically more experienced than the individuals they supervise and can offer their expertise, knowledge, and wisdom from their time working in the field. They can share resources and advice about professional development, models of practice, and intervention techniques. Supervisors are charged with ongoing training regarding policies, assessing staff knowledge and skills, providing an orientation in practice to the agency's policies and procedures, and helping to develop a plan for ongoing professional development. Supervisors are often in positions to advocate for the needs of their staff so they can better serve their communities. Supervisors can support child welfare professionals by initiating policy changes and sharing feedback about policies and procedures to improve systems. They listen and act on staff concerns and issues and create a positive environment for staff. In addition to supervising, they serve their staff in a variety of ways that can improve practice, morale, and well-being.

Importance of Supervision in Child Welfare

Research has shown that the quality and capacity of child welfare supervision in child welfare practice is critical to service delivery that ensures child safety and well-being (Kadushin & Harkness, 2002). Supervisors have an impact on the quality and effectiveness of staff and can influence child welfare professional retention and the culture and climate at the agency (Collins-Camargo & Royce, 2010; Landsman, 2007). Supervisors and their staff can be effective in ensuring child safety and family well-being when working in settings that support high, yet reasonable expectations (e.g., caseloads), supportive, timely, and high-quality supervision. The impact of quality supervision goes beyond retention in that it can reduce stress, improve critical thinking and decision-making (Lietz, 2009; Rezepnicki & Johnston, 2005), improve job satisfaction (Faller et al., 2010), and offer important guidance as frontline workers negotiate challenging situations associated with child welfare practice (Mor Barak et al., 2001; Kadushin & Harkness, 2002). Supervision can also improve perceived worker empowerment (Cearley, 2004), help with retention of frontline staff (DePanfilis & Zlotnik, 2008), and support the implementation of child welfare practice models (Frey et al., 2012). Accessing supervisory support often requires workers to take initiative (Radey & Schelbe, 2020).

As child welfare professionals, supervision can improve our practice. It helps to ensure that we are acting in the best interest of the children, gives us the opportunity to learn from our supervisor and colleagues, affords needed emotional support from our supervisor, and provides accountability in our work. Having a good relationship with our supervisor as they are the one who completes our annual performance evaluations teaches us how to do our job effectively and can improve our satisfaction with our work. There are several times of supervision in child welfare practice, including clinical supervision and administrative supervision.

Clinical Supervision

Clinical supervision focuses on the work that caseworkers do with children and families. Good clinical supervision is critical to building worker competencies, including reinforcing positive social work ethics and values, encouraging self-reflection and critical thinking skills, building upon training to enhance performance, and supporting

---

Practice Tip

Common Components of Clinical Supervision

Collins-Camargo and Millar (2010) outlined common components of clinical supervision, which include the following:

- Scheduling regular or group supervision meetings
- Enhancing caseworker critical thinking skills
- Encouraging and providing caseworkers with time to engage in self-reflection so as to examine and consider ways to improve their own practice
- Facilitating the identification of crucial casework questions that are meant to critically evaluate issues related to family maltreatment and applying knowledge gained from the critical thinking sessions to assessment and treatment activities
- Developing workers' skills and focusing on evidence-based practice by looking to the professional literature for guidance in casework and implementing successful programs that promote positive outcomes for children and families
- Using case review and observation to assess workers' skills and evaluate progress

the worker through casework decision-making and crises. Clinical supervision can also help promote a trauma-informed approach to casework. In clinical supervision, supervisors discuss safety and risk factors in specific cases with their staff, review service plans and family progress towards permanency goals, help to determine possible service needs, and help in making critical decisions. Clinical supervision focuses more on providing knowledge and support to caseworkers to apply in practice with children and families. These interactions build competence in practice, self-reflection, critical thinking, and making connections between training and performance.

Supervisors are often required by policy to support staff and/or approve staff's critical case decisions, as well as provide clinical guidance related to case work. In many states, supervisors often have to approve decisions related to placement changes, change of case plan, change of parental visitation schedule, and a child's placement in congregate care and/or with siblings. Supervisors can help to identify underlying conditions they observe or suspect in cases (e.g., intimate partner violence, substance abuse), identify parallel processes (e.g., transference and counter-transference), identify the impact of personal beliefs and values on practice, and help to recognize knowledge and skills as well as area for growth.

Several models of supervision in child welfare have been developed and adopted in various child welfare agency settings, including strengths-based supervision, trauma-informed supervision in group supervision, solution-focused supervision, and family-centered supervision. Child welfare agencies and supervisors may use one of these specific models of supervision. It is helpful for child welfare professionals to understand the model they are functioning within.

Strengths-Based Supervision

Strengths-based supervision is based in a family-centered framework of practice in child welfare (Lietz, 2013) that focuses on six organizing principles: (1) prioritizing the family as the unit of attention, (2) creating and maintaining supportive partnerships with families to create change, (3) being grounded in empowerment, (4) allowing for individualized practice to meet the needs of the family, (5) using a holistic view of the family, and (6) using a strengths-based perspective. A core principle of family-centered practice is to keep families together when possible and draw on family strengths and resources to meet the needs of families and children. Strengths-based supervision is a model of supervision that "enhances the intentionality and quality of supervision provided in public and private child welfare organizations. The purpose is to support implementation of family-centered practice by using supervisor activities that are theoretically consistent with this model" (Lietz & Julien-Chinn, 2017, p. 146). Strengths-based supervision involves four components: (1) parallel processes, (2) integration of crisis-oriented and in-depth supervisory processes, (3) individual and group clinical supervision, and (4) administrative, educational, and support functions to supervisees (Lietz et al., 2014). Strengths-based supervision is associated with higher levels of satisfaction with supervision among child welfare specialists (Lietz & Julien-Chinn, 2017) and self-reported positive changes in supervision provided (Lietz et al., 2014).

Research Note

Strengths-Based Supervision

Cynthia A. Lietz, PhD, LCSW

Providing quality supervision is essential to supporting the child welfare workforce. An extensive body of literature demonstrates the connection between supportive supervision and the ability of agencies to ensure the retention and job satisfaction of their workers. As a young child welfare professional, I remember experiencing this reality firsthand. I was just 21 years old when I first started working as an ongoing caseworker for a nonprofit organization that contracted with the Department of Children and Family Services in Illinois. I was young, enthusiastic, and completely unprepared for the important yet complex work of ensuring the safety, permanency, and well-being of the children and youth in my care. My first child welfare supervisor took her role as my supervisor quite seriously. She understood the duality of both monitoring and mentoring her workers. She paid close attention to my work and held me accountable to ensure my practice was consistent with federal, state, and agency policies and procedures. At the same time, she offered me quick feedback and ongoing coaching such that I was able to learn quickly how best to engage, assess, and intervene with the clients we served. She also taught me about documentation, court procedures and testimony, and how best to manage my workload. Not only was my career positively influenced by her, but more importantly, the children, youth, and families I served also were better off as a result of her commitment to providing quality and consistent supervision.

Because of this and other ongoing experiences as a supervisee and supervisor in social work, I have become committed to advancing the practice of child welfare supervision. I developed Strengths-Based Supervision (SBS; Lietz, 2013), a model of supervision that was created to support effective implementation of family-centered practice. SBS has four components that can be helpful as supervisors consider how best to support investigators and ongoing workers in ensuring the quality of child welfare practice. First, child welfare supervisors should think about parallel process and consider how their modeling influences the ways in which their workers develop professional relationships with their clients. Supervisors simultaneously provide support and feedback to their workers. They set goals and hold their workers accountable. They have to effectively lean on their supervisory authority when necessary. In the same ways, workers much also build professional relationships with clients that involve goal-setting, support, and effective use of authority. These similarities create an opportunity for supervisors to not just tell but actually show their workers how to conduct these professional activities.

(continued)

Child welfare supervisors should also consider ways to integrate the use of scheduled supervisory conference while also meeting urgent decision-making through crisis supervision. Too often, child welfare settings rely heavily on crisis supervision. It is true that being available in a crisis is fundamental to successful child welfare supervision. However, to only provide supervision in an emergency means that important yet nonurgent questions and concerns are overlooked. Child welfare workers need the ability to develop critical and analytical thinking skills. Having some scheduled, in-depth supervisory conferences is equally as important to mentoring the child welfare workforce.

Third, supervisors should consider utilizing both one-on-one and group supervisory modalities. Individual supervision is important for coming to know the strengths, needs, and competency of each worker. Individual supervisory sessions also allow for supervisory support. On the other hand, group supervision is important for developing a team approach and for cultivating peer-driven mutual aid. The diversity of perspectives that emerge in group supervisory conferences also allows for enhancing critical thinking.

Finally, child welfare supervisors should be sure to fulfill all three functions of supervision; the administrative, educational, and support roles are all essential. Monitoring the quality of practice, mentoring workers to grow in their knowledge and skills and doing all of this in the context of a supportive professional relationship allow supervisors to oversee child welfare practice effectively.

Let me close by saying how grateful I am that several wonderful supervisors were so influential for me and my work in my early years as a social worker.

Trauma-Informed Supervision

Trauma-informed supervisory practice involves using a trauma-informed approach to supervising child welfare professionals or caseworkers in their practice (e.g., working with clients, decision-making), as well as using this approach to better understand supervisees as individuals and attempt to minimize secondary trauma responses, burnout, and compassion fatigue. According to the National Child Traumatic Stress Network (NCTSN, 2020), "a trauma-informed child and family service system is one in which all parties involved recognize and respond to the impact of traumatic stress on those who have contact with the system including children, caregivers, and service providers. Programs and agencies within such a system infuse and sustain trauma awareness, knowledge, and skills into their organizational cultures, practices, and policies. They act in collaboration with all those who are involved with the child, using the best available science, to maximize physical and psychological safety, facilitate the recovery of the child and family, and support their ability to thrive." Trauma-informed care in child welfare refers to a systems approach to all aspects of administration and service delivery, including supervision.

When using a trauma-informed approach to supervision, a trauma-informed lens is used when assessing clients and their families, making decisions, and mitigating the effects of trauma and secondary trauma on direct service workers such as child welfare professionals. This approach, therefore, ensures regular screenings and check-ins regarding trauma exposure and symptoms, whether that be a particularly difficult interaction with a client, reviewing a difficult case, or managing possible transference with a client or case. A trauma-informed system and supervisor uses evidence-based, culturally responsive assessments and treatments, highlights strengths and resilience among clients and workers, and recognizes parent and child experiences of trauma and their impact on the family and/or circumstances. Trauma-informed supervision also ensures the continuity of care and collaboration among various systems to minimize re-traumatization. Strategies within this approach include building meaningful relationships and partnerships within and outside of the child welfare agency and addressing the intersection of trauma with history, race, gender, and culture (NCTSN, 2020).

Solution-Focused Supervision

The solution-focused supervision approach is rooted in principles of solution-focused brief therapy (SFBT) based on the work of Steve de Shazer and Insoo Kim Berg and their team at the Milwaukee Brief Family Therapy in the early 1980s. The overall philosophy to therapeutic intervention is to focus on solutions rather than the problems clients are facing. Main assumptions of the approach are that (1) all clients have strengths and resources; (2) the relationship between the client and therapist has significant therapeutic value; (3) change happens all the time; (4) the focus remains on the present and future, rather than the past; (5) small change leads to bigger change, (6) clear goals are essential, and (7) it is not essential to know the cause of a problem in order to find a solution.

By using a solution-focused approach in supervision, supervisors guide child welfare professionals to support families in identifying and building strengths while developing clear goals and strategies to address the problem the family is currently facing. Solution-focused supervision also involves a reciprocal and supportive process where supervisors identify and promote solutions to professional behavior (e.g., work with clients, professional development and training). Child welfare professionals on the frontline may feel more empowered, supported, and motivated in their work with clients. They also can use similar strategies used in the supervision relationship with their own clients.

Group Supervision

In addition to individual consultation and supervision, child welfare professionals often have the opportunity for group supervision with caseworkers organized in units or groups assigned to one supervisor. This type of organization is efficient and allows teams to work together, communicate, share accountability, and peer support (Hanna & Potter, 2012). Within child welfare, having the ability to be safe psychologically can reduce worker turnover (Kruzich et al., 2014). Group supervision sessions should be structured, have an agenda that is created by all members, and include discussion and sharing opportunities and themes for learning. Supervisors can provide education and feedback, offer opportunities for practice or role-playing, and learn from supervisees about their experiences to gauge their needs personally and professionally. This type of supervision allows for brainstorming and critical thinking by bringing multiple perspectives, idea sharing, and developing solutions. With caseworkers often sharing similar experiences, it is advantageous to learning to hold group supervision sessions regularly and consistently.

Note from the Field

It Takes Time to Learn the Ropes!

Lisa Garcia, MSW

I discovered my passion for social work and the child welfare field during my undergraduate program where I learned about abuse and neglect and the effects of these adverse childhood experiences, especially on adults. As a new worker coming into the field of child welfare, I had this mentality that I want to help and save these children. Case managers are the people who are first on the scene and the ones who build the rapport with these families. This can be very scary, especially as a new worker.

When you become a child welfare worker, you go through a long, tedious training and are required to take several exams to make sure you know the material. These exams are supposed to train you to know the policy and procedure. However, the real exam is when you get "thrown to the sharks" and you are expected to know what you're doing, straight out of training.

For the first 6 months on the job, I was just going through the motions and really had no idea what I was doing. How horrible is that? As a social worker, I hold the power to make decisions that affect the lives of these families, and I get to go in front of the judge and tell the court whether these parents can have their children back in their care. Throughout my experience as a worker in the field, I have discovered a possible solution to bridge the gap of sending workers straight out of training to the field. The child welfare field *requires* hands-on experience and training to really know what you are doing. After the first 6 months of trial and error and guessing my way through, I finally felt confident enough to say I knew what my job consisted of.

To be in the child welfare field, you must advocate for yourself in order to be able to advocate for your families. Here is my best advice: ask questions, ask for supervision, and ask for a timeline for your expectations. Luckily, my agency was able to see my strength to train, and I was able to create a handbook with the most used procedures with step-by-step instruction on how to complete the task. Ask for this! Ask for more training when you need it, and ask to shadow another worker. As a new worker coming to the field, you will experience other workers who have been in the field for decades and workers who are burned out; be that breath of fresh air for your agency, and be confident enough to find a gap and try to bridge it. The child welfare system is broken, and it needs workers who truly care to help these children and families. It took me a couple years to get to this point, and I'm still learning, but I want to be the worker who the children remember 20 years from now.

Maximizing Supervision

As a child welfare professional receiving supervision, there are several things child welfare professionals can do to maximize the time and interaction with their supervisors. First, they should ask to schedule a regular time to meet with their supervisor. With a regular time to meet, child welfare professionals can be better prepared and have a set aside time to talk to their supervisor every week or every other week. It also means that they can discuss cases outside of a crisis. Along with the supervisor, child welfare professionals should make some "guidelines" about their supervision time. For example, what will be talked about and for how long? Will the meeting be structured or not? Where will the meet take place? Will the meeting be one-on-one or in a group or both? Child welfare professionals should acknowledge that it will take some time to feel comfortable talking about things that are beyond cases (e.g., feelings, burnout, conflict, etc.). Most importantly, it is necessary for the child welfare professional and the supervisor to find a system that works for both of them.

Child welfare professionals should be prepared and proactive when going to supervision. They should think about a case or cases that they would like to discuss and obtain feedback about or ideas going forward. It is important that child welfare professionals pay attention and listen to their

> **Practice Highlight**
>
> **Reflective Supervision**
>
> Weatherston et al. (2010) outline 3 key components of reflective supervision:
>
> 1. **Reflection:** use active listening and thoughtful questions by both parties.
> 2. **Collaboration:** share ideas and responsibilities to inform decision-making.
> 3. **Regularity:** meeting regularly to reflect and collaborate.

supervisors. Supervisors have been doing this work for a longer period of time and have experience with the system, community partners, and children and families. When an issue presents itself, child welfare professionals should be honest and tell the whole story. Supervisors are looking out for child welfare professionals' well-being and want to have all the information when supporting them in difficult situations. Child welfare professionals should know agency protocol and be sure to follow the chain of command. If they do not like the supervisor's answer, they should not "shop around" for other answers. However, if they believe the supervisor is asking them to do something inappropriate or unethical, they should contact an administrator. Child welfare professionals should ask for help when they need it. This is sound social work practice and will help child welfare professionals get what they need. These are good guidelines when approaching supervision as a student intern as well as a child welfare professional employed at an agency.

Agency Responsibility for Supervision

It is the child welfare agency's responsibility to support and create a pipeline of supervisory leadership. Child welfare agencies should prioritize the recruitment of skilled supervisors and provide them with appropriate support and training in this role. This type of recruitment should include cultivating internal child welfare professionals who have the experience and knowledge of the system and whose skills align with that of the organization. In addition to selecting qualified candidates as supervisors, who possess skills

> **Practice Tip**
>
> **Child Welfare Professionals' Responsibilities in Supervision**
>
> - Tell the whole story as it is known.
> - Follow the chain of command.
> - Be prepared when going to supervision.
> - Be proactive.
> - Pay attention.
> - Listen to the supervisor's advice.

such as empathy, motivation, mentoring, and leadership, supervisors should be provided with ongoing training regarding new and effective models of supervisory practice and field work. Practice standards should also include investing in a diverse group of supervisors that reflect the community and workforce. Child welfare administration should clearly define what is expected of supervisors and train them appropriately to fulfill this role. Training should also include best practices for using data, provide tools and resources to provide clinical and administrative supervision (e.g., education, professional development, space, and time), and provide guidance and supervision to supervisors themselves. There are a number of toolkits and resources available to supervisors as well as models to guide and structure their supervisory practice. It is also important to note that not all practice models fit each community and group of people and may often need to be modified to meet the needs of families and children in a specific community.

Supervision Practices and Strategies

The supervisory interaction may present itself like many helping relationships. For example, good supervisory skills include listening skills, reflecting, good questions, appropriate feedback, and follow-up. An important component of supervision is being present and available to those being supervised – psychologically and physically. When child welfare workers need support, guidance, and assistance with making a decision, it is important that their supervisor is available and willing to provide that support. Supervisors should create an environment where supervisees feel safe and able to be honest about their feelings and thoughts. Mostly, they must feel supported. Supervisors should have strong active listening skills while making eye contact, providing verbal cues to indicate understanding. In supervision, supervisors should reflect and ask questions to show understanding of what is being said. Supervisors should ask follow-up or clarifying questions that lead to exploring options and problem-solving. When appropriate, supervisors shod provide feedback, give advice, and share experiences to help caseworkers in formulating their own plans and decisions. Supervisors should be keen on following up and providing accountability for such interactions. This shows the supervisor's attention to matters and helps caseworkers ensure follow-through.

Practice Conversation

Example of Supervision Discussion

Supervisor: Hi there! I wanted to check in with you to see how the Hernandez family[1] is doing. How have you been able to engage the family in services?

Child welfare professional (CWP): I'm feeling okay. Mom has been difficult to get on board with services, but I have been checking in with her every week to ask her how I can help.

Supervisor: Has she been receptive? In what ways has it been difficult to engage her in services?

CWP: She is really fixated on getting her kids back, but struggles with understanding what services she needs to complete in order for reunification to occur.

Supervisor: That does sound challenging, but it also sounds like you have done a great job with staying in touch and supporting mom through this. Have you offered services like transportation and counseling for her?

CWP: Yes. I have started using some of the motivational interviewing techniques with her, too, and I think that is working.

Supervisor: That's great! What techniques have you used, and how have they been helpful?

(continued)

CWP: I think she really wants someone to listen to her concerns about the case. So, I am using active listening and summarizing her statements. I also work with her resistance and challenge her when she pushes back about completing tasks.

Supervisor: This is great! I think if you continue to use these skills and show empathy, compassion, and genuineness, she will feel comfortable with you and be more open and motivated to work through her case plan.

CWP: I agree. I will continue to check in with her, and I'll be sure to support her in these ways.

_____

[1]All names and other personal identifiers in cases and examples throughout this book have been changed to protect privacy and confidentiality.

Practice Conversation

Supervision When Child Welfare Professional Is Beginning to Feel Burnout

Supervisor: Hi Alison, how are you doing? I've noticed you seem a bit down lately. Is there anything going on that I can support you with?

CWP: Actually, yeah. I am really starting to question my ability to do this work. I feel like no matter what I do, I can't help these kids or their parents.

Supervisor: I can understand where you're coming from and why you might be feeling this way. This is really hard work. We often work with families that we are not able to reunify and families who come to us with a lot of needs. I also know that the work you do has helped a lot of families. For example, the Brown family – remember when you started working with them, it seemed like everyone was having a hard time. You worked with them for a long time and were able to get the services that the kids needed to work through some of their challenges. You also worked really hard so that the siblings could stay together in the foster home and stay at their school together. I also remember how you sat down with their parents and encouraged them to get treatment for their substance use. You show families compassion, support, and work closely with them to empower them to understand the system and how they can complete their case plan so their kids can come home safely.

CWP: Yeah, that was a tough case. But I really saw in them the ability to get better and strengthen their family. I don't know why I am feeling this way all of a sudden.

Supervisor: I think it's OK for us to feel this way some time. It's important for us to reflect on our cases and our work and see the things we've done well and recognize where we could improve. I know we've talked about burnout and compassion fatigue that comes with this kind of work. What things have you been doing to keep yourself well outside of work?

CWP: Well, maybe that is the problem. I have been working later on most days to make sure I get all of my paperwork done and complete all of my case visits. Then, when I get home, my partner is unhappy that I can't spend more time with them. I used to work out in the evenings, but I haven't had the time lately. So, I am feeling more tired and deflated a lot. I also feel like I have been worrying more about the families on my caseload and questioning my decisions.

Supervisor: Hmmm. OK. It sounds like you are overextended with your cases. Maybe we can take a look at your caseload numbers and the demands they have had on you. I think it's important for you to stay healthy and happy, so let's review your cases and go from there. Maybe we can also map out your time to see if we can reduce the amount of time you're spending on cases after-hours so you can get back to working out and spending time with your family. Is there anything else I can do to support you right now?

CWP: No, I think this is a good start. Maybe we can talk again in a week to see where I am. Maybe I am just in a funk right now and needed someone to listen. Thank you.

Practice Conversation

Supervision at Key Decision Points: Investigation

Supervisor: So, how did the initial visit go? What did you determine about the safety of the child?

CWP: Based on my assessment, if the child stayed in the home, she would be at risk for moderate to severe abuse in the near future. The parents did not acknowledge what happened to the child, were verbally aggressive with me and the child during the interview. She was physically injured and we are concerned for her safety and well-being. We are recommending that the child be removed and placed with her aunt.

Supervisor: Ok, let's make sure everything is documented in your notes. What family strengths did you note?

(continued)

CWP: There are a lot of family members who want to help. The child is attentive, kind, and clearly loved her mom. Mom said that she did well in school and was helpful. Mom obviously cares for the child, but was and is unable to protect her from her boyfriend.

Supervisor: Great! Do you think there were any family strengths that would mitigate the safety concerns that you have?

CWP: No, unfortunately not. Mom's boyfriend was abusive with the child and he will not leave the home. I think protective custody is needed.

Supervisor: OK. Let's talk about what services you think are appropriate for this family.

CWP: To start, I think the family should be referred for counseling, parenting classes, and a drug and alcohol screening. The mother should have regular visits with the child, without mother's boyfriend present. Information about housing and financial resources should be offered and provided to help with mom to take care of the family independently from the boyfriend. Further, I would recommend counseling with someone who is familiar with intimate partner violence to help mom advocate for her needs and that of the child.

Supervisor: Ok, that sounds like a good plan. What services need to be in place for the child and her caregiver, her aunt?

CWP: I will make a referral for counseling for the child as well as a forensic interview regarding the incident. I will ensure that the caregiver has the resources to schedule an appointment with a medical provider and counselor. I will also make sure they are enrolled to receive financial support from the agency and know where to find support groups and education. I will also spend time with her to talk about the system, parameters for visitation, and so forth.

Supervisor: This is a great starting point. Keep me posted on how things are going. Great job with this case!

Practice Conversation

Supervision at Key Decision Points: Case Closure

Supervisor: Let's talk about the Miller family. I believe they might be at a point where we can close the case. Is that your sense, too?

CWP: Yes, as I refer to the case plan, I believe that the father has completed all of the requirements related to the reason the child came into care. He has been able to access stable and safe housing, is working full time and has set up childcare while he works. He also successfully completed counseling and parenting education and participated in all visitation with the child.

Supervisor: Great. Have you received reports from all of the providers regarding his services and talked to them about their recommendations?

CWP: Yes, I have all of the reports and I have shared them with all the parties in the case.

Supervisor: Have you been to the home to do a home safety assessment and talked to the father and child?

CWP: Yes, the home is appropriate and has been deemed safe for the child. I talked to both the father and child and believe that they are ready to move forward. They have supports in place and family to rely on should they need assistance.

Supervisor: OK. Do you think there are any services they could benefit from going forward? Are there any court mandates we need to address?

CWP: There are no mandates. There was a recommendation that the father obtain custody of the child and he has been able to do that. I told the father that I thought he should continue the family therapy after the case closes and he agreed with this.

Supervisor: Great work. You've really done an excellent job with this case. It was challenging to get the father on board, but you were able to really empower him to take on the role of sole provider and take advantage of all the services provided to have the child be placed with him. Next, I would put a call in to the attorney to make a motion to dismiss and close the case.

Professional Development for Child Welfare Professionals

The goal of professional development is to support child welfare professionals in their work and help them hone their skills and learn policy and procedures. Professional development must remain ongoing throughout a child welfare worker's career. Child welfare professionals must engage in professional development to ensure they have the most up-to-date skills and knowledge about policies, programs, and procedures. The children and families whom child welfare workers serve benefit from the professional development.

The field of child welfare is ever-changing as the knowledge base grows and society changes and new trends emerge. Professional development of child welfare professionals is important. Child welfare professionals must be thoroughly educated about the etiology and aspects of child maltreatment and the child welfare system and profession as they enter their positions; however, their knowledge will not stop there. Throughout their careers, child welfare professionals must participate in trainings and continue to network to ensure they are up to date on information in child welfare as well as policies and procedures. As new evidence-based practices are developed, child welfare professionals need to be trained in how to implement the practices with high fidelity (Akin et al., 2016).

Professional development gives workers opportunities to learn about best practices while refining their skills. Opportunities for professional development can be facilitated by experts in person at agencies or conferences, or they may be live or previously recorded webinar. There are multiple opportunities for training virtually through podcasts, videos, and webinars that are self-directed or hosted by the child welfare agency. The National Child Welfare Workforce Institute is an example of a resource for professional development. Universities may have training and research centers that also provide trainings such as the Center for Advanced Studies in Child Welfare at the University of Minnesota or the Pennsylvania Child Welfare Resource Center at the University of Pittsburgh. Workers should prioritize professional development and advocate for themselves to get professional development.

Professional Goals

Child welfare workers are the backbone of the child welfare system. They are responsible for ensuring the safety, permanency, and well-being of children. While the goals for the system are clearly defined, it is necessary that child welfare professionals set professional goals for themselves. Often these goals can be around professional growth and development. These goals can be connected to promotions that offer more responsibilities and compensation. Perhaps a worker wants to become a mentor, supervisor, or a trainer within the unit where they work. Perhaps the promotion is moving into administration at the local or state level. Many of these goals may involve completing additional training or education.

Professional goals could also include developing expertise in a specific area of child welfare, for example, becoming specialized in handling cases involving a specific issue or population such as child sexual abuse, older foster youth, or human trafficking. Along with the expertise, a professional goal could be to help improve the system and how children and families are served. As the child welfare system is forever evolving, a professional goal could be part of shaping the future of the system.

There are a whole range of goals about job satisfaction that are professional goals. One goal could be finding fulfillment within the work. Another goal could be helping create a supportive work environment through connecting with colleagues. Maybe the goal is to informally mentor recently hired workers to work as a field supervisor for student interns. Perhaps the goal is to find work-life balance and to have a vibrant, fulfilling life outside of working in child welfare.

Everyone's professional goals are going to be slightly different. Regardless of what the goals are, workers should determine what they value and create a plan to achieve the goal. To set a professional goal, workers can ask themselves broad questions such as what they want their legacy to be and where they want to be in 5 or 10 years. These questions can help identify a professional goal. In working towards a goal, it will be helpful to create objectives that are specific, measurable, achievable, relevant, and timed (SMART). This will ultimately assist in evaluating progress towards the professional goal. Additional strategies to achieving professional goals is revisiting plans and finding a way to be accountable. This could be telling a colleague or supervisor about the goal or keeping a journal about specific professional goals and progress.

Ethics and Legal Issues

Ethics are central to the child protection in behaviors and making decisions. Child welfare workers must perform their work with integrity while they prioritize the best interests of the child. Some of the key ethical issues within child welfare work include confidentiality, conflicts of interest, client self-determination, and informed consent. Child welfare professionals will encounter ethical dilemmas throughout their careers and must be able to work with their supervisors and teams to make decisions.

While there is not a single set of ethics that guide all child welfare professionals follow, various states have codes of ethics. For example, Illinois and Florida are two states that have a code of ethics. In Florida, employees of the Department of Children and Families are obligated to follow the Florida Code of Ethics, CF Operating Procedure, NO. 60-05, Chapter 05, and there are additional requirements after becoming a certified child welfare professional that are outlined by the Florida Certification Board. The code of ethics covers a wider range of topics outlining professionals' responsibilities and behaviors. Additionally, the National Association of Social Workers (2013) has standards for social work practice in child welfare. These standards outline expectations for child welfare practices and provide guidance for child welfare social workers. Informed by the National Association of Social Workers (NASW) Code of Ethics, the standards present expectations on topics including professional development, advocacy, collaboration, confidentiality, cultural competence, assessment, engagement, supervision, and administration.

Child welfare professionals must remain current in their knowledge about legal statutes and policy and procedures. Each state has specific statutes regarding child maltreatment and child welfare. These statutes align with federal regulations, although implementation may vary across states and jurisdictions. Child welfare professionals must maintain current knowledge about the statues as they pertain to working with children and families. Legislation is ever-changing, which results in changes in policies and procedures. Therefore, there is an ongoing need for training and information. While child welfare agencies are responsible for training workers on the legal issues and implementation of the legislation, child welfare workers must prioritize attending trainings and mastering the materials.

Racial Equity and Cultural Humility

With the well-documented racial disparities and disproportionalities within child welfare, professional development in the areas of ensuring racial equity and using a cultural humility approach is paramount. Racial equity is when there is fairness and justice due in regard to race. This means that the color of a person's skin does not limit their opportunities or predict their outcomes. Racial equity increasingly is prioritized as a goal in child welfare. To achieve equity, it requires a commitment at the organizational level where an examination of institutional policies and systematic racism is addressed.

Child welfare professionals and other professionals who work with children and families need to be committed to addressing racism within their work with children and families (e.g., Madison, 2016). There are various training programs that seek to improve the ways that child welfare professionals serve children and families from different cultures and reduce racism. The trainings are one way to ensure that child welfare workers have the most up-to-date information about practice skills and policies related to reducing racial and ethnic disparities and disproportionalities. While workshops on specific topics such as working with families of various racial and ethnic backgrounds are helpful, it is important also that child welfare professionals have opportunities to explore their personal beliefs and biases.

Professional development regarding racial equity and cultural humility often begins with a reflection of our own beliefs and biases as well as our behaviors. We are a product of our environment. How we were raised has shaped our outlook in the world, which we often tend to feel is the "normal" or "right" worldview. Being open-minded and acknowledging that we all hold different views is central to being able to learn about how we can work towards racial equity. It is important that we also critically examine our behaviors in addition to our beliefs. This may be challenging and uncomfortable to do, but it is central to our challenging racism and promoting racial equity.

One way that child welfare professionals are being trained is in cultural humility. Cultural humility can be understood as a commitment to self-awareness about cultural differences where someone accepts and connects with a person from a different culture while valuing their culture and seeking to minimize power imbalances. Rather than trying to learn how best to work with people from different cultures and learn the beliefs, values, and norms of specific cultures, which is sometimes referred to as cultural competence (e.g., "In Mexican cultures, people often believe…."), a cultural humility approach posits there is a need to reflect upon personal biases and beliefs and seeing how these may perpetuate power structures, especially in the helping relationship (Tervalon & Murray-Garcia, 1998). The cultural humility approach, as the name suggests, is based in professionals adopting a humility mindset, whereas they suspend beliefs of superiority and they honor others' cultures. There is an openness to differences without the judgment that another culture is flawed.

Much of cultural humility in child welfare is parallel to general social work practice. For example, it includes meeting the client where they are, having empathy, identifying the family strengths, and acknowledging historical injustices, systematic barriers, and power imbalances (Ortega & Coulborn, 2011). Using cultural humility in child welfare practice can help child welfare professionals engage children and families. Skills relevant to cultural humility in child welfare practice include active listening, reflecting, reserving judgment, and entering the client's world (Ortega & Coulborn, 2011). Cultural humility in child welfare can be seen to compliment the cultural competence practices where child welfare professionals are provided information about different cultures (Ortega & Coulborn, 2011).

There are also trainings for child welfare professionals focused on implicit bias and how this impacts decision-making in child welfare. Implicit bias is our unconscious beliefs about groups of people that are shaped by our life experiences including what we see in the media. These internalized messages may influence our behaviors. The implicit biases of child welfare professionals are seen as important as if they can negatively impact children and families of racial and ethnic groups that have historically been discriminated against as well as other groups of people. For example, a child protective investigator who holds an implicit bias against Black single mothers may be more likely to remove a child from a Black single mother than removing a child from a married White couple even when there are identical assessments of risk and safety. Being aware of implicit bias can assist child welfare professionals in understanding how their own decision-making and actions can be impacted by their beliefs. An assessment tool, the Implicit Association Test, can measure someone's positive or negative attitudes towards different groups of people (Greenwald et al., 1998). Additionally, self-examination about our thoughts and behaviors can be useful in determining the extent to which implicit biases are present and may impact our work in child welfare.

Licensing and Certification

The purpose of licensure and certification is to ensure the worker has a set of standards of skills and training to demonstrate competence in child welfare practice. States have different licensing standards and certification processes. In general, states that have licensing for child welfare workers require that the workers complete specific training, pass an exam, and/or complete a required number of supervision hours. The supervision may include both direct individual one-on-one supervision and supervisor's observations of the worker interacting with children and families. There are typically other conditions including passing a criminal background check and agreeing to follow professional guidelines. Once someone is licensed or certified, ongoing continuing education credits are required. Additionally, there may be a renewal process every few years to ensure that the workers are current on their knowledge and skills. With certification and licensure, there is often a state board that is made up of individuals who review applications and complaints for professional misconduct and works with the Office of the Inspector General to conduct hearings, write reports, and determine punitive measures and license/certification suspensions and revocations.

Practice Highlight

Child Welfare Licensing in Illinois

In most states and jurisdictions, a degree, experience, and training are required to assume the role of child welfare practitioners. As described in earlier chapters, there are a number of roles in child welfare work; however, practitioners working directly with children and families often require more experience and training. In some states, like Illinois these practitioners are required to obtain Child Welfare Employee Licensure (CWEL) to assume direct practice roles. In order to qualify, individuals must have a degree (bachelor's, preferably a master's); complete classroom and/or virtual training related to special populations, policies and practices, and basic social work skills (e.g., engagement); and complete and pass a series of exams (risk and safety assessment, placement specialty, and CWEL). Applicants must not be in default of an educational loan and not be subject of a child abuse/neglect investigation or conviction, and they must have a valid driver's license and fingerprint clearance. CWEL licenses are monitored by an office within the Illinois Department of Children and Family Services and work closely with the Illinois Office of the Inspector General (OIG) to monitor any complaints, infractions, and oversight. Many schools of social work in Illinois offer training and exams to students enrolled in their programs to prepare them for licensure upon graduation.

Child Welfare Professional Safety

Safety rightfully is a concern for child welfare workers. A national study reported that approximately 70% of child welfare workers in the United States have been victims of violence or threat of violence in the workplace (American Federation of State, County, and Municipal Employees, 2011). A statewide study of child protective services workers found within the first 6 months of employment 75% experienced nonphysical violence, 37% experienced threats, and 2.3% experienced physical violence (Radey & Wilke, 2018). According to Occupational Safety and Health Administration (OSHA) standards, child welfare workers are at risk to experience violence in the workplace. The OSHA standards highlight 10 different risk factors for workplace violence. Eight can be considered elements of child welfare workers' job responsibilities: contact with the public; delivery of passengers, goods, or services; having a mobile workplace such as a taxicab or police cruiser; working with unstable or volatile persons in healthcare, social service, or criminal justice settings; working alone or in small numbers; working late at night or during early morning hours; working in high-crime areas; and working in community-based settings (NIOSH, 2016). Child welfare workers often work alone during various hours of the day in the homes of families where there is a perceived adversary and conflict related to allegations of child maltreatment and in neighborhoods that are disproportionately of lower socioeconomic levels and may have high levels of crime.

Training for child welfare professionals should include information on safety. The goal of the trainings should be to increase worker safety through familiarizing workers with risk factors for violence and agency policies and resources related to safety. Workers must master techniques to handle potential violence such as de-escalation. It is important to recognize that empathy and engagement skills proactively contribute to keeping workers safe. (See Chap. 6 for information about engagement.)

Worker safety begins with the commitment to safety and open communication. Agency leaders and workers alike must prioritize creating an environment where child welfare professionals can work free from violence and threats of violence. Safety concerns must be taken seriously. Efforts should be proactive; rather than waiting to respond to violence, violence can be avoided. Awareness of the situation as well as environment is key. Workers should have the available information about the families they are serving. They should know if there is a history of violence and any concerning issues that could escalate violence. Many agencies have the ability to conduct background checks which can provide relevant information. Within the work environment, there should be easy access to exiting a workspace and a system to alert others to immediate safety concerns. This could be predetermined code words or a silent panic button. There can be policies of workers meeting with potentially volatile or violent people with a colleague present. Within office spaces, objects that could be used to hurt someone (e.g., scissors, staplers) should not be in the space where meeting with clients. If possible, child welfare workers should avoid meeting in spaces where objects could easily become weapons (e.g., knives, tools). While most home visits are conducted individually, workers typically can request a colleague to accompany them, and in some instances law enforcement can be present.

In addition to training workers, child welfare agencies are responsible for creating a culture of safety to assist with prevention of client-perpetrated violence. The NASW (2013) Guidelines for Social Work Safety in the workplace emphasizes that agencies must "establish and maintain an organizational culture that promotes safety and security for their staff" and "create a culture of safety that adopts a proactive preventative approach to violence management and risk." (p. 9). While having policies and procedures that focus on safety are important, it is also crucial that agencies respond appropriately when an incident of violence occurs. A response begins with supporting the worker who experienced the violence. Also important in the response includes proper documentation and a debriefing where agencies can process how to learn from the incident to hopefully minimize the likelihood of future incidents. The Capacity Building Center for States' Child Welfare Worker Safety Guide (2017) comprehensively explores the key issues about worker safety and provides direction for how agencies can increase safety in the workplace.

Retention and Job Satisfaction

The average length of child welfare employment is less than 2 years (US GAO, 2003). Studies have reported the worker turnover in child welfare workers within the first few years of hire ranging from 20% to 50%, with highest rates during the first 3 years of starting the position (Chenot et al., 2009; Smith, 2005). Worker turnover is a concern for multiple reasons. Changes in child welfare professionals assigned to a case are related to poorer outcomes for children and families (US GAO, 2003). Reducing turnover increases timely investigations and more client contact, both key elements of quality service delivery and can contribute to increasing child safety, permanency, and well-being. In addition to worker retention being important due to its connection with outcomes for children and families, worker turnover costs a lot. Training new workers is both time-consuming and expensive. When workers do not stay long, the investment of training them is not recuperated. Worker turnover also has a negative impact within the work environment and colleagues. When people leave, especially those who leave with little notice, colleagues must take over their cases and their work burden increases.

The importance of child welfare workers' satisfaction with their job extends beyond avoiding burnout and secondary trauma. Helping families and seeing positive changes are important aspects contributing to job satisfaction (McGowan et al., 2010; Johnco et al., 2014). A study of recently hired frontline child welfare professionals reported their satisfaction with the work largely was due to helping and making a difference (Schelbe et al., 2017). Additionally, the autonomy of the position and variety in the work was cited as contributing to their job satisfaction.

There are multiple stressors that workers experience that can erode their satisfaction with the job. Excessive workload and large caseloads are especially concerning in contributing to dissatisfaction (US GAO, 2003). Aspects of the work that create tension and dissatisfaction have been found to include administrative requirements, workload, unsupportive colleagues, and working with challenging parents and hurt children (Schelbe et al., 2017). Additionally, working in a trauma-filled environment can be stressful. (See Chap. 5 for information about trauma-informed practice.)

Burnout and Secondary Traumatic Stress

Child welfare workers are at risk for burnout, secondary traumatic stress, and vicarious traumatization. One study found almost a third of child welfare workers in their sample experienced high levels of burnout (30%) and secondary trauma (29%; Salloum et al., 2015). This finding has been replicated elsewhere where approximately a third of child welfare workers experience vicarious traumatization (Middleton & Potter, 2015). Burnout, caused by administrative stress or burden, is one of the main reasons that child welfare professionals cite for leaving their positions. Burnout develops over time. Factors that contribute to burnout include high caseloads, immense amount paperwork and documentation, demanding work environment, rigid procedures, communication problems, and inadequate training (Barak et al., 2006). An unsupportive environment where supervisor and peer support are limited or the unit does not function as a team can contribute to burnout. When workers perceive unfairness or have few opportunities to influence their work and policies, they may experience burnout. Symptoms of burnout include a wide range of negative reactions such as physical and emotional exhaustion; chronic fatigue; feeling hopeless and helpless; feeling disillusioned; feeling negative about self and holding a negative outlook towards others and life; high absenteeism and tardiness; inability to cope; experiencing depersonalization; not performing work to meet the needs of clients; and not completing assigned work responsibilities (Barak et al., 2006).

Related to burnout are secondary traumatic stress and vicarious traumatization. Secondary traumatic stress is when someone experiences trauma indirection through hearing about another person's firsthand experience of trauma. Unlike burnout, secondary trauma can occur from one event, although it can also be the accumulation of the impact of the work. The symptoms mirror those of posttraumatic stress disorder. Vicarious trauma occurs when someone works with people who have experienced trauma and through their repeated exposure to other people's trauma their worldview is impacted and behaviors change.

Secondary traumatic stress and vicarious trauma have a range of outcomes for workers including impaired judgment, low motivation, decreased productivity, poorer quality of work, decreased compliance with agency requirements, absenteeism, and quitting (Barak et al., 2006). These outcomes result in problems for agencies in terms of issues with quality of services provided, staff friction, and higher staff turnover (Barak et al., 2006). All of which can have negative impacts on children and families served by child welfare professionals.

Prevention of burnout, secondary trauma stress, and vicarious trauma may seem to rest on the shoulders of child welfare professionals and their need to better manage stress and trauma. However, in actuality, child welfare agencies have the responsibility and ability to reduce the likelihood of burnout and secondary traumatic stress in child welfare workers. There are multiple strategies to do so including effective recruitment, training, increasing knowledge, developing coping skills, quality supervision, social support, addressing workplace culture and climate, and recognizing diversity of workforce.

Self-care

Self-care is the activities and practices that someone regularly engages in to maintain and enhance their current and future health and well-being. Child welfare professionals have been found to engage only in modest amounts of self-care although it is promising to maintain well-being and retention within child welfare (Miller et al., 2019). Self-care is multidimensional and consists of various components:

body, mind, and spirit. The caring for the body is attending to physical health at a basic level including ensuring proper nutrition and hydration as well as adequate sleep. Self-care includes seeing healthcare providers for routine checkups and timely appointments should health concerns arise. It includes getting exercise and staying active. Some people get massages or acupuncture as part of their physical healthcare. Taking a bath or soaking in a hot tub could also be self-care.

The mind aspect of self-care focuses on attending to someone's mental and emotional state. In many regards, it starts with the noticing of feelings. Self-care involving the mind is ensuring that negative feelings and thoughts do not become all consuming. It includes addressing and decreasing stressors. Maintaining a positive outlook is one of the goals of self-care. To do so, some people talk to others or journal. They spend time proactively looking for the positive aspects of life and focusing on being aware of their feelings. To address negative feelings, self-care can include spending time relaxing and doing activities that are fun or restorative. This could include reading a book, putting together a puzzle, knitting, crafting, or other hobbies. It can also include spending time with friends and family.

The spirit component of self-care can be understood as taking care of the soul and connecting to something larger than oneself. For some, this could be in the form of religion and being active in a church, synagogue, or mosque. Others may embrace spirituality outside of an organized religion. Spending time in nature and admiring the beauty of the world can be components of self-care related to the spirit. Likewise, reading poems or books that inspire can also be considered self-care. Some consider their creative outlets, including art, music, and dance to be elements of spiritual self-care.

Self-care includes practices in and outside the workplace. Within the workplace, self-care practices include setting healthy boundaries with clients and colleagues, creating a strategy to address the different work tasks, and finding time to eat lunch and take breaks during the day. A support system within the workplace with colleagues and supervisors can be central to self-care and can be fostered through regularly scheduled supervision or routine check-ins with colleagues. As the paperwork demands can be great and require extensive time at a computer, workers should explore ways to be active at work. For example, standing up during a phone call or having a "walking meeting" with a colleague instead of sitting at their desks.

Outside the workplace, self-care mirrors the workplace. Ensuring that work does not "splash over" outside working hours. While arguably child welfare workers working hours may be different from a 9-to-5 job, setting boundaries and not engaging in work activities (i.e., phone calls, paperwork, consultations) during nonwork hours is an important part of self-preservation and self-care. While it may be difficult, trying not to think about work responsibilities and cases when "off the clock" is important. To establish a delineation between professional and personal lives, some workers practice a ritual to establish the transition between the two. This could be as simple as listening to a playlist on the drive home or coming home, changing clothes, feeding a pet, and opening the mail.

Developing a Self-care Plan

The adage "if you fail to plan, you plan to fail" is apropos in regards to child welfare professionals developing a self-care plan. Self-care does not happen accidentally; it must be intentionally planned and tailored to the need of individual workers. Child welfare professionals need to develop a plan for their self-care. A good plan goes beyond identifying activities that can help relax and unwind after a stressful incident. It should include details about being proactive in securing support and managing the ongoing demands of the work. The development of a plan for self-care should be intentional. It should be specific for the person, based on individual preferences and life circumstances. For some people, the physical aspects of a self-care plan mean running multiple times a week, whereas for others it may be yoga classes or playing in an adult kickball league. People need to determine what will work best for themselves, although they may wish to try something that they have not tried before.

There are many resources that can also be used to develop a plan for self-care. The State University of New York at Buffalo (2019) has online materials to guide the creation of plans starting with an assessment of current "negative" and "positive" coping strategies. In addition to creating a plan to use to address typical daily stressors, it also includes a plan for self-care in a crisis. Another resource for self-care is *The A-to-Z Self-Care Handbook for Social Workers and Other Helping Professionals* (Grise-Owens et al., 2016). The book highlights 26 different aspects of self-care, encouraging readers to find balance in their professional lives. Other websites and books seek to assist with the similar message: self-care cannot be optional or accidental. To be an effective child welfare professional, it is necessary to plan self-care. The importance of child welfare professionals practicing self-care cannot be overstated.

Developing a plan for self-care early is helpful when done thoughtfully and early in one's career. The self-care plan is meant to evolve depending on work responsibilities, family responsibilities, and interests. The plan should be individualized to meet all of those areas and should address psychological, emotional, physical, spiritual, and professional needs. Trying to find a balance in work and personal life is often challenging, but not impossible. As a child welfare

---

Reflection

Assessing Boundaries: Personal Boundary Vulnerabilities

1. What are influences of your past and current experiences?
2. Think about influencing factors and how they impacted your boundaries (e.g., family, gender, culture, religion, and generation.)
3. What are your personal tendencies as a result?
4. What types of clients and scenarios might cause you to be entangled or to become rigid?
5. Think about professional experiences, what are two to three most influential events that mark developmental boundaries development?

professional, it can be easy to work extra hours and begin to give up areas of personal development (e.g., exercise, healthy diet, relationships); however, recognizing when these behaviors begin is important in order to intervene and correct. Establishing boundaries with co-workers, clients, and in personal relationships is important in self-care. As individuals, we all have levels of comfort around the physical, emotional, professional, and personal boundaries. We choose who we spend time with, when we answer the phone, and the number of hours we work. As professionals who may hold a significant amount of trust and power with our clients and their families, it is important to be aware of this and ensure balance.

Boundaries

Professional relationship boundaries can be understood within a continuum as it ranges from entangled boundaries to rigid boundaries. Entangled boundaries refer to a consistent over-involvement, where a worker may be investing more of their time, emotional energy, or favor in his relationship than in others, in a manner that is unhelpful for the client. A worker with entangled boundaries meets their own emotional, social, or physical needs through the relationship with their client, at the expense of the client. Rigid professional boundaries refer to those who go forward with their own agenda, inflexibly, condescendingly, and without attending to the unique and multifaceted needs of the client. Their lack of authenticity and sensitivity while attending to the client's needs contravenes their ethical responsibility to honor the dignity and worth of the individual. Responding rigidly exploits the client's vulnerabilities and is an abuse of the professional's position of power as it accentuates and even exaggerates the power differential between them. Equally between rigid and entangled boundaries is a balance. Professionals with balanced boundaries are authentic and caring while maintaining clear boundaries. They use their authority appropriately; remaining aware of their position of power, they take care to neither exploit their client's vulnerabilities nor infringe on their rights. Those functioning in a balanced manner use professional judgment and self-reflection skills in their assessments and make decisions that are professionally despoiled and accountable to other professionals.

Conclusion

In child welfare, clinical and administrative supervision are critical to ensure client, worker, and agency standards, as well as personal well-being and safety. There are many ways one can engage in supervision, whether it be individual, group, clinical, and/or administrative. In general, a strengths-based, solution-focused, and trauma-informed approach to supervision is optimal for the supervisor and child welfare professional and for ideal case outcomes. Both supervisor and child welfare professional must be invested and committed to consistent, organized supervision to ensure best outcomes and satisfaction. To continue to develop professional skills and practices, child welfare professionals should engage in continuing education and training and continue to set and work towards goals of improving knowledge and skills. Supervision and professional development include developing a plan for self-care and setting boundaries that can help with reducing the incidence of burnout and secondary traumatic stress, which, in turn, could improve longevity in child welfare practice and improve individual well-being.

Acknowledgments The authors thank Cynthia A. Lietz, PhD, LCSW, and Lisa Garcia, MSW, for their contributions to Chap. 12.

Discussion Questions

1. What are two reasons that supervision in so critical in child welfare practice?
2. What are the child welfare professional's responsibilities and role in supervision?
3. What are two ways that child welfare professionals can engage in professional development?
4. How can child welfare systems promote child welfare professional retention and job satisfaction?
5. What are two ways child welfare professionals can engage in self-care and avoid burnout?

Suggested Activities

1. Complete the self-care assessment at https://socialwork.buffalo.edu/content/dam/socialwork/home/self-care-kit/self-care-assessment.pdf, and come up with two strategies for each domain to improve your personal and professional self-care.
2. Join a professional group (e.g., NASW, CSWE, APSAC, etc.), and find local and national opportunities for professional development.
3. Interview a child welfare professional, and ask about how they engage in professional development and self-care.
4. Find an article or a podcast about self-care in child welfare, and consider new ways to engage in your own self-care.
5. Research the licensure and certification requirements for the state you live in or a state you might want to live in. What steps would you have to take to become licensed or certified to be a child welfare professional?
6. Participate in an online training designed to reduce racism and implicit bias (e.g., https://kirwaninstitute.osu.edu/implicit-bias-101).
7. Complete the Implicit Association Test (IAT), which measures if there are positive or negative attitudes towards a concept or social group. (Available: https://implicit.harvard.edu/).

   Reflect on your results. How has your life experience shaped your results? How could your results impact the way that you serve children and families involved in the child welfare system?

8. Read Akin et al. (2016), and write a reflection paper about ideas to improve training for frontline child welfare professionals.

   Akin, B. A., Brook, J., Byers, K. D., & Lloyd, M. H. (2016). Worker perspectives from the front line: Implementation of evidence-based interventions in
   child welfare settings. *Journal of Child and Family Studies*, *25*(3), 870–882.
   (Available https://rdcu.be/ccaNs).

Additional Resources

American Professional Society on the Abuse of Children: Forensic Interviewing
   training clinics and institutes: https://www.apsac.org/forensicinterviewing
Child Welfare Information Gateway, Ethics: https://www.childwelfare.gov/topics/
   management/ethical/
Child Welfare Information Gateway, Worker safety: https://www.childwelfare.gov/
   topics/management/workforce/workforcewellbeing/safety/
Kirwan Institute, Exploring Implicit Bias in Child Protection training: https://kirwa-
   ninstitute.osu.edu/implicit-bias-101
State University of New York at Buffalo School of Social Work Self Care
   Information: http://socialwork.buffalo.edu/resources/self-care-starter-kit/
   introduction-to-self-care.html
National Child Welfare Workforce Institute: https://www.ncwwi.org/
National Child Welfare Workforce Institute, Racial Equity Resources:
   https://ncwwi.org/index.php/resourcemenu/racial-equity

References

Akin, B. A., Brook, J., Byers, K. D., & Lloyd, M. H. (2016). Worker perspectives from the front
   line: Implementation of evidence-based interventions in child welfare settings. *Journal of
   Child and Family Studies, 25*(3), 870–882. https://doi.org/10.1007/s10826-015-0283-7
American Federation of State, County and Municipal Employees. (2011).
   Double jeopardy: Caseworkers at risk helping at-risk kids. Retrieved from
   http://www.afscme.org/news/publications/workplace-health-and-safety/
   double-jeopardy-caseworkers-at-risk-helping-at-risk-kids
Barak, M. E. M., Levin, A., Nissly, J. A., & Lane, C. J. (2006). Why do they leave? Modeling child
   welfare workers' turnover intentions. *Children and Youth Services Review, 28*(5), 548–577.
   https://doi.org/10.1016/j.childyouth.2005.06.003
Capacity Building Center for States. (2017). *The child welfare work safety guide*. Retrieved from
   https://library.childwelfare.gov/cwig/ws/library/docs/capacity/Blob/115592.pdf?r=1&rpp=10
   &upp=0&w=+NATIVE(%27recno=115592%27)&m=1
Cearley, S. (2004, October). The power of supervision in child welfare services. In Child and Youth
   Care Forum (Vol. 33, No. 5, pp. 313–327). Kluwer Academic Publishers-Plenum Publishers.
Chenot, D., Benton, A. D., & Kim, H. (2009). The influence of supervisor support, peer support,
   and Organizational culture among early career social workers in Child Welfare Services. *Child
   Welfare, 88*(5), 29–148.
Collins-Camargo, C., & Millar, K. (2010). The potential for a more clinical approach to child wel-
   fare supervision to promote practice and case outcomes: A qualitative study in four states. *The
   Clinical Supervisor, 29*(2), 164–187. https://doi.org/10.1080/07325223.2010.517491

Collins-Camargo, C., & Royse, D. (2010). A study of the relationships among effective supervision, organizational culture promoting evidence-based practice, and worker self-efficacy in public child welfare. *Journal of Public Child Welfare, 4*(1), 1–24. https://doi.org/10.1080/15548730903563053

DePanfilis, D., & Zlotnik, J. L. (2008). Retention of front-line staff in child welfare: A systematic review of research. *Children and Youth Services Review, 30*(9), 995–1008. https://doi.org/10.1016/j.childyouth.2007.12.017

Faller, K. C., Grabarek, M., & Ortega, R. M. (2010). Commitment to child welfare work: What predicts leaving and staying? *Children and Youth Services Review, 32*(6), 840–846. https://doi.org/10.1016/j.childyouth.2010.02.003

Frey, L., LeBeau, M., Kindler, D., Behan, C., Morales, I. M., & Freundlich, M. (2012). The pivotal role of child welfare supervisors in implementing an agency's practice model. *Children and Youth Services Review, 34*(7), 1273–1282. https://doi.org/10.1016/j.childyouth.2012.02.019

Greenwald, A. G., McGhee, D. E., & Schwartz, J. L. (1998). Measuring individual differences in implicit cognition: The implicit association test. *Journal of Personality and Social Psychology, 74*(6), 1464. https://doi.org/10.1037/0022-3514.74.6.1464

Grise-Owens, E., Miller, J., & Eaves, M. (2016). *Self-care handbook.* White Hat Communications.

Hanna, M. D., & Potter, C. C. (2012). The effective child welfare unit supervisor. *Administration in Social Work, 36*(4), 409–425. https://doi.org/10.1080/03643107.2011.604403

Johnco, C., Salloum, A., Olson, K. R., & Edwards, L. M. (2014). Child welfare workers' perspectives on contributing factors to retention and turnover: Recommendations for improvement. *Children and Youth Services Review, 47*, 397–407. https://doi.org/10.1016/j.childyouth.2014.10.016

Kadushin, A., & Harkness, D. (2002). *Supervision in social work.* Columbia University Press.

Kruzich, J. M., Mienko, J. A., & Courtney, M. E. (2014). Individual and work group influences on turnover intention among public child welfare workers: The effects of work group psychological safety. *Children and Youth Services Review, 42*, 20–27. https://doi.org/10.1016/j.childyouth.2014.03.005

Landsman, M. (2007). Supporting child welfare supervisors to improve worker retention. *Child Welfare, 86*(2), 105. https://doi.org/10.1037/e522532014-205

Lietz, C. A. (2009). Critical thinking in child welfare supervision. *Administration in Social Work, 34*(1), 68–78. https://doi.org/10.1080/03643100903432966

Lietz, C. A. (2013). Strengths-based supervision: Supporting implementation of family-centered practice through supervisory processes. *Journal of Family Strengths, 13*(1), 6.

Lietz, C. A., Hayes, M. J., Cronin, T. W., & Julien-Chinn, F. (2014). Supporting family-centered practice through supervision: An evaluation of strengths-based supervision. Families in Society, 95(4), 227–235. https://doi.org/10.1606/1044-3894.2014.95.29

Lietz, C. A., & Julien-Chinn, F. J. (2017). Do the components of strengths-based supervision enhance child welfare workers' satisfaction with supervision? *Families in Society, 98*(2), 146–155. https://doi.org/10.1606/1044-3894.2017.98.20

Madison, M. (2016). *Dear ECE, we need to talk about racism.* Available https://ecepolicyworks.com/dear-ece-we-need-to-talk-about-racism/

McGowan, B. G., Auerbach, C., Conroy, K., Augsberger, A., & Schudrich, W. (2010). Workforce retention issues in voluntary child welfare. *Child Welfare, 89*(6), 83.

Middleton, J. S., & Potter, C. C. (2015). Relationship between vicarious traumatization and turnover among child welfare professionals. *Journal of Public Child Welfare, 9*(2), 195–216. https://doi.org/10.1080/15548732.2015.1021987

Miller, J. J., Donohue-Dioh, J., Niu, C., Grise-Owens, E., & Poklembova, Z. (2019). Examining the self-care practices of child welfare workers: A national perspective. *Children and Youth Services Review, 99*, 240–245. https://doi.org/10.1016/j.childyouth.2019.02.009

Mor Barak, M. E., Nissly, J. A., & Levin, A. (2001). Antecedents to retention and turnover among child welfare, social work, and other human service employees: What can we learn from past research? A review and metanalysis. *Social Service Review, 75*(4), 625–661. https://doi.org/10.1086/323166

National Association of Social Workers. (2013). *NASW standards for social work practice in child welfare*. NASW Press.

National Child Traumatic Stress Network. (2020). *Creating trauma-informed systems*. Retrieved from: https://www.nctsn.org/trauma-informed-care/creating-trauma-informed-systems

NIOSH. (2016). https://www.cdc.gov/niosh/docs/96-100/risk.html

Ortega, R. M., & Coulborn, K. (2011). Training child welfare workers from an intersectional cultural humility perspective: A paradigm shift. *Child Welfare, 90*(5), 27–49.

Radey, M., & Schelbe, L. (2020). Gender support disparities in a majority-female profession. *Social Work Research, 44*(2), 123–135. https://doi.org/10.1093/swr/svaa004

Radey, M., & Wilke, D. J. (2018). Client-perpetrated violence among frontline child welfare workers. *Journal of Interpersonal Violence*. https://doi.org/10.1177/0886260518812792

Rzepnicki, T., & Johnston, P. (2005). Examining decision errors in child protection: A new application of root cause analysis. *Children and Youth Services Review, 27*, 393–407. https://doi.org/10.1016/j.childyouth.2004.11.015

Salloum, A., Kondrat, D. C., Johnco, C., & Olson, K. R. (2015). The role of self-care on compassion satisfaction, burnout and secondary trauma among child welfare workers. *Children and Youth Services Review, 49*, 54–61. https://doi.org/10.1016/j.childyouth.2014.12.023

Schelbe, L., Radey, M., & Panish, L. (2017). Satisfactions and stressors experienced by recently-hired frontline child welfare workers. *Children and Youth Services Review, 78*, 56–63. https://doi.org/10.1016/j.childyouth.2017.05.007

Smith, B. D. (2005). Job retention in child welfare: Effects of perceived organizational support, supervisor support, and intrinsic job value. *Children and Youth Services Review, 27*(2), 153–169. https://doi.org/10.1016/j.childyouth.2004.08.013

State University of New York at Buffalo. (2019). http://socialwork.buffalo.edu/resources/self-care-starter-kit/developing-your-self-care-plan.html

Tervalon, M., & Murray-Garcia, J. (1998). Cultural humility versus cultural competence: A critical distinction in defining physician training outcomes in multicultural education. *Journal of Health Care for the Poor and Underserved, 9*, 117–125. https://doi.org/10.1353/hpu.2010.0233

United States. General Accounting Office. (2003). *Child welfare: HHS could play a greater role in helping child welfare agencies recruit and retain staff: Report to congressional requesters*. US General Accounting Office.

Weatherston, D., Weigand, R. F., & Weigand, B. (2010). Reflective supervision: Supporting reflection as a cornerstone for competency. *Zero to Three, 31*(2), 22–30.

Index

© Springer Nature Switzerland AG 2021
J. M. Geiger, L. Schelbe, *The Handbook on Child Welfare Practice*,
https://doi.org/10.1007/978-3-030-73912-6